MEDICAL DRUG
THERAPY

National Medical Series for Independent Study

NMS
CLINICAL MANUALS

MEDICAL DRUG
THERAPY

EDITOR

Josephine Pressacco, MD, PhD
PhD, Pharmacology
MD, University of Toronto
Resident, Department of Diagnostic Radiology
McGill University
Montreal, Canada

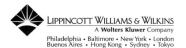

LIPPINCOTT WILLIAMS & WILKINS
A **Wolters Kluwer** Company
Philadelphia • Baltimore • New York • London
Buenos Aires • Hong Kong • Sydney • Tokyo

Executive Editor: Neil Marquardt
Managing Editor: Emilie Linkins
Marketing Manager: Scott Lavine
Development Editors: Emilie Linkins and Carol Koetke
Senior Production Editor: Karen Ruppert
Designer: Risa Clow
Compositor: Lippincott Williams & Wilkins
Printer: RR Donnelley

Copyright (c) 2003 Lippincott Williams & Wilkins

351 West Camden Street
Baltimore, MD 21201

530 Walnut St.
Philadelphia, PA 19106

All rights reserved. This book is protected by copyright. No part of this book may be reproduced in any form or by any means, including photocopying, or utilized by any information storage and retrieval system without written permission from the copyright owner.

The publisher is not responsible (as a matter of product liability, negligence, or otherwise) for any injury resulting from any material contained herein. This publication contains information relating to general principles of medical care that should not be construed as specific instructions for individual patients. Manufacturers' product information and package inserts should be reviewed for current information, including contraindications, dosages, and precautions.

Printed in the United States of America

Library of Congress Cataloging-in-Publication Data

Medical drug therapy / [edited by] Josie Pressacco.
    p. ; cm. - - (National medical series for independent study) (NMS clinical manuals)
  Includes bibliographical references and index.
  ISBN 0-7817-3711-7
    1. Chemotherapy--Handbooks, manuals, etc. I. Pressacco, Josie, 1968- II. Series. III. Series: NMS clinical manuals
    [DNLM: 1. Drug Therapy--methods--Handbooks. 2. Pharmaceutical Preparations--Handbooks. WB 39 M48752 2003]
    RM263 .M39 2003
    615.5′8--dc21

                                                                    2002035288

The publishers have made every effort to trace the copyright holders for borrowed material. If they have inadvertently overlooked any, they will be pleased to make the necessary arrangements at the first opportunity.

To purchase additional copies of this book, call our customer service department at **(800) 638-3030** or fax orders to **(301) 824-7390**. International customers should call **(301) 714-2324**.

Visit Lippincott Williams & Wilkins on the Internet: http://www.LWW.com. Lippincott Williams & Wilkins customer service representatives are available from 8:30 am to 6:00 pm, EST.

03 04 05 06 07
1 2 3 4 5 6 7 8 9 10

CONTRIBUTORS

Patrick Bellemare, MD, FRCPC
Assistant Professor of Medicine
University of Montreal
Division of Respirology and Intensive Care Medicine
Hôpital du Sacré-Coeur de Montréal
Montreal, Canada

Bernard F. Bissonnette, MD, FRCPC
Assistant Professor of Medicine
University of Montreal
Division of Rheumatology
Hôpital du Sacré-Coeur de Montréal
Montreal, Canada

Aline Boulanger, MD, MPH, FRCPC
Associate Professor
University of Montreal
Director, Pain Management Clinic
Department of Anesthesia
Centre Hospitalier de l'Université de Montréal-Hôpital Hotel-Dieu
Montreal, Canada

Christine M. Derzko, MD, FRCSC
Associate Professor of Obstetrics and Gynecology and Internal Medicine
(Endocrinology)
University of Toronto
Head, Division of Reproductive Endocrinology and Infertility
Department of Obstetrics and Gynecology
St. Michael's Hospital
Toronto, Canada

Jean G. Diodati, MD, FRCPC, FACC
Associate Professor of Medicine
University of Montreal
Chief, Coronary Care Unit
Division of Cardiology
Hôpital du Sacré-Coeur de Montréal
Montreal, Canada

Heather E. Edwards, MSc, MD, PhD
Resident, Department of Obstetrics and Gynecology
University of Calgary
Calgary, Canada

Ivy M. Fettes, PhD, MD, FRCPC
Associate Professor of Medicine
University of Toronto
Division of Endocrinology
Sunnybrook and Women's College Health Sciences Center
Toronto, Canada

Sergio B. Giancola, MD
Resident, Department of Surgery
Division of Urology
University of Toronto
Toronto, Canada

Wayne L. Gold, MD, FRCPC
Staff Physician
Division of General Internal Medicine and Infectious Diseases
University Health Network-Toronto General Hospital
Toronto, Canada

Karen Groneau, MD
Resident, Department of Obstetrics and Gynecology
University of Toronto
Toronto, Canada

Tomy Hadjis, MD, MS, FRCPC
Assistant Professor of Medicine
McGill University
Division of Cardiology
McGill University Health Center
Montreal, Canada

David W. Hedley, MD, MRCP
Associate Professor of Medicine
University of Toronto
Departments of Medicine, Pathology and Medical Biophysics
University Health Network–Princess Margaret Hospital
Toronto, Ontario

Shinya Ito, MD
Associate Professor
University of Toronto
Head, Division of Clinical Pharmacology and Toxicology
Hospital for Sick Children
Toronto, Ontario

Adrian L. James, MA, FRCS(ORL-HNS)
Clinical Fellow, Department of Surgery
University of Toronto
Division of Otolaryngology
Hospital for Sick Children
Toronto, Ontario

Gabor Kandel, MD, FRCPC
Associate Professor of Medicine
University of Toronto
Division of Gastroenterology
St. Michael's Hospital
Toronto, Canada

Arnon M. Katz, MD, FRCPC

Instructor
University of Toronto
Division of Dermatology
Toronto, Canada

Nathalie Labrecque, MD, FCRSC

Lecturer, Laval University
Staff Ophthalmologist
Director, Department of General Ophthalmology
Centre Hospitalier Universitaire de Quebec–Pavillon Saint-Francoise D'Asisse
Quebec City, Canada

Colin D. Lambert, BM, FRCPC, FRCP

Associate Professor of Medicine
University of Toronto
Division of Neurology
St. Michael's Hospital
Toronto, Canada

Roger S. McIntyre, MD, FRCPC

Assistant Professor of Psychiatry
University of Toronto
Head of the Mood Disorders and Psychopharmacology Division
Department of Psychiatry
University Health Network–Toronto Western Hospital
Toronto, Ontario

Rajin Mehta, MD, FRCPC

Assistant Professor
Division of Geriatric Medicine and General Internal Medicine
Sunnybrook and Women's College Health Sciences Center
Toronto, Ontario

Clifford A. Ottaway, MD, PhD, FRCPC

Associate Professor of Medicine
University of Toronto
Division of Gastroenterology
St. Michael's Hospital
Toronto, Canada

Amit M. Oza, MD, MRCP, FRCPC

Associate Professor of Medicine
University of Toronto
Division of Oncology
University Health Network–Princess Margaret Hospital
Toronto, Canada

Blake C. Papsin, MD, MSc, FRCSC

Assistant Professor of Surgery
University of Toronto
Division of Otolaryngology
Director, Cochlear Implant Program
Hospital for Sick Children
Toronto, Canada

Ian Paterson, MD, FRCPC
Fellow, Division in Cardiology
McGill University
McGill University Health Center
Montreal, Canada

M. Jane Poulson, MSc, MD, CM, FRCPC
Assistant Professor of Medicine
University of Toronto
Department of Medicine
Division of Palliative Care
University Health Network–Toronto General Hospital
Toronto, Canada

Ian C. Quirt, BSc, MD, FRCPC
Professor of Medicine
University of Toronto
Division of Oncology
University Health Network–Princess Margaret Hospital
Toronto, Canada

Sidney B. Radomski, MD, FRCSC
Associate Professor of Surgery
University of Toronto
Division of Urology
Department of Surgery
University Health Network–Toronto Western Hospital
Toronto, Canada

Martin Schreiber, MD, FRCPC, MMEd
Associate Professor of Medicine
University of Toronto
Division of Nephrology
St. Michael's Hospital
Toronto, Canada

Dat J. Tran, MD, FRCPC, FAAP
Formerly, Associate Staff
Division of Infectious Diseases
Department of Pediatrics
Hospital for Sick Children
Toronto, Canada

Adam Waese, MD
Resident, Department of Psychiatry
University of Toronto
Toronto, Ontario

Renaud Whittom, MD, FRCPC
Lecturer, University of Montreal
Nucleus Member, Specialty Committee in Medical Oncology
The Royal College of Physicians and Surgeons of Canada
Staff Hematologist-Oncologist
Division of Hematology and Oncology
Hôpital du Sacré-Coeur de Montréal
Montreal, Canada

Kerry A. Wilson, MD
Resident, Department of Obstetrics and Gynecology
University of Toronto
Toronto, Canada

Michelle R. Wise, MD
Resident, Department of Obstetrics and Gynecology
University of Toronto
Toronto, Canada

Samuel Wong, MD, FRCPC
Member
Canadian Association of Physical Medicine and Rehabilitation
Newmarket, Canada

DEDICATION

To my mentors in pharmacology from the University of Toronto—

Drs. L. Endrenyi, D. Kadar, W. Kalow, W.H.E. Roschlau, and A.K. Sen—

thank you for your kind encouragement and genuine support.

CONTENTS

PREFACE

Derived from the popular *National Medical Series (NMS)*, *NMS Clinical Manual of Medical Drug Therapy* is part of a series of books intended to present need-to-know information in an easily retrievable format, with emphasis on the pharmacologic treatment of commonly encountered disease entities.

A template has been developed to convey the salient points about each disease entity and its pharmacologic treatment quickly and consistently:

KY **Key information:** Pathophysiology and other crucial facts concerning the disease.

TX **General explanation of drug treatment:** Appropriate options available for management of the patient.

RX **Generic (brand) name for the drug used for treatment:** The generic drug names and their respective brand names are provided; however, the omission of any brand name does not imply that it is less effective than that listed. For certain disease entities, there may be more than one line of treatment options (e.g., first line, second line), and this is denoted as RX1, RX2, and so forth. Use-in-pregnancy ratings are also provided in brackets.

DS **Dose and route of administration for the treating agent described in RX:** Adult doses and, when applicable, pediatric doses are provided. The units of measurement for drug doses and levels are expressed in Conventional Units. See the Appendix for the conversion table between Conventional Units and Système International (SI) Units of commonly used measurements.

SE **Side effects or adverse drug reactions, contraindications, and drug-drug interactions:** Only the most common and most dangerous are listed in this section. The *American Society of Health-System Pharmacists (ASHSP) Drug Information* and the Canadian publication *Compendium of Pharmaceuticals and Specialties (CPS)* provide more detailed information. (When available, the lifesaving antidote or treatment for a side effect or drug overdose is provided.)

This manual serves as a convenient and comprehensive reference aid for medical students, interns, and residents. It is our hope that it will help you locate important information quickly and will guide you in decision making for more effective treatment for your patients.

Josie Pressacco, MD, PhD

ACKNOWLEDGMENTS

Thank you to all the contributing authors and to the staff at Lippincott Williams and Wilkins (LWW). Special appreciation to Emilie Linkins, Managing Editor at LWW, for her dedication and professionalism. A special thank you to my family and friends for supporting me through this project.

ABBREVIATION LIST

5'ASA	5'aminosalicylate
AA	aplastic anemia
ACE	angiotensin-converting enzyme
ACh	acetylcholine
ACTH	adrenocorticotropic hormone
ADH	antidiuretic hormone
AED	antiepileptic drug
AH	alcoholic hepatitis
ALA	δ-aminolevulinic acid
ALL	acute lymphoblastic leukemia
ALP	alkaline phosphatase
ALT	alanine transaminase
AML	acute myelogenous leukemia
Anti-Xa	anti factor Xa
AP	action potential
aPTT	activated partial thromboplastin time
ARF	acute renal failure
ASA	acetylsalicylic acid
AST	aspartate transaminase
AT III	antithrombin III
ATC	acute tubular necrosis
AV	atrioventricular
BAL	bronchoalveolar lavage
BL	bladder
BP	blood pressure
BPH	benign prostatic hyperplasia
CAD	coronary artery disease
CD	Crohn disease
cGMP	cyclic guanosine monophosphate
CHF	congestive heart failure
CK	creatine kinase
CLL	chronic lymphocytic leukemia
CML	chronic myelogenous leukemia
CMV	cytomegalovirus
CNS	central nervous system
COPD	chronic obstructive pulmonary disease
COPROgen	coproporphyrinogen
CPPD	calcium pyrophosphate dihydrate
CR	controlled release
CRF	chronic renal failure
CSF	cerebrospinal fluid
CSF	colony-stimulating factors
CT	computed tomography
CX	cervix
dBP	diastolic blood pressure
DHE	dihydroergotamine

DHT	dihydrotestosterone
DI	diabetes insipidus
DIC	disseminated intravascular coagulation
DKA	diabetic ketoacidosis
DM	diabetes mellitus
DMARDs	disease-modifying antirheumatic drugs
DS	double strength
DTaP	diphtheria, tetanus, and acellular pertussis vaccine
DVT	deep vein thrombosis
ECF	extracellular fluid
ECG	electrocardiogram
ED_{95}	effective dose corresponding to 95% twitch depression of the adductor pollicis [produced by a neurostimulator on the ulnar nerve]
EEG	electroencephalogram
EPC	emergency postcoital contraception
EPO	erythropoietin
EPS	extrapyramidal symptoms
ESR	erythrocyte sedimentation rate
FEV_1	forced expiratory volume in 1 second
FFP	fresh frozen plasma
FSH	follicle-stimulating hormone
FVC	forced vital capacity.
G-6-PD	glucose-6-phosphate dehydrogenase
GABA	gamma-aminobutyric acid
GABA-A	γ-aminobutyric acid-A
GBS	group B streptococcal
GC	germ cell
G-CSF	granulocyte colony-stimulating factor
GDM	gestational diabetes mellitus
GFR	glomerular filtration rate
GH	growth hormone
GI	gastrointestinal
GITS	gastrointestinal therapeutic system
GM-CSF	granulocyte-macrophage colony-stimulating factor
GN	glomerulonephritis
GnRH	gonadotropin-releasing hormone
HBIG	hepatitis B immune globulin
HBsAg	hepatitis B surface antigen
HBV	hepatitis B virus
HCV	hepatitis C virus
HDL	high-density lipoprotein
Hep A	hepatitis A vaccine
Hep B	hepatitis B vaccine
HHS	hyperosmolar hyperglycemic state
Hib	*Haemophilus influenzae* type b vaccine
HIT	heparin-induced thrombocytopenia
HIV	human immunodeficiency virus
HL	Hodgkin's lymphoma

HMG-CoA	hydroxymethyl glutaryl coenzyme A
HMWK	high-molecular-weight kininogen
HRT	hormone replacement therapy
HSV	herpes simplex virus
IA	intra-arterial
IBD	inflammatory bowel disease
ICU	intensive care unit
Ig	immunoglobulin
IGF-I	insulin-like growth factor I
IM	intramuscular
INH	isoniazid
INR	international normalized ratio
IPF	interstitial pulmonary fibrosis
IPV	inactivated polio vaccine
ITP	idiopathic thrombocytopenia
IV	intravenous
JRA	juvenile rheumatoid arthritis
LDH	lactate dehydrogenase
LDL	low-density lipoprotein
LFT	liver function test
LH	luteinizing hormone
LHRH	luteinizing hormone-releasing hormone
LMWH	low-molecular-weight heparin
LP	lumbar puncture
Lung NSC	non–small cell lung cancer
Lung SC	small cell lung cancer
MAC	minimum alveolar concentration
MAC	*Mycobacterium avium* complex
MAO	monoamine oxidase.
MAOIs	monoamine oxidase inhibitors
MCA	middle cerebral artery
MH	malignant hyperthermia
MI	myocardial infarction
MMR	measles, mumps, and rubella vaccine
MRSA	methicillin-resistant *Staphylococcus aureus*
MRSE	methicillin-resistant S*taphylococcus epidermidis*
NaCl	sodium chloride
NaHCO$_3$	sodium bicarbonate
NASCET	North American Symptomatic Endarterectomy Trial
NaSSA	noradrenergic/specific serotonergic antidepressant
NDRI	norepinephrine dopamine reuptake inhibitor
NG	nasogastric tube
NHL	non-Hodgkin's lymphoma
NMDA	*N*-methyl-D-aspartate
NNRTI	nonnucleoside reverse transcriptase inhibitor
NRTI	nucleoside reverse transcriptase inhibitor
NSAID	nonsteroidal anti-inflammatory drug
OA	osteoarthritis
OC	oral contraceptive

OCP	oral contraceptive pill
OE	otitis externa
OGTT	oral glucose tolerance test
PABA	para-aminobenzoic acid
PBG	porphobilinogen
PBP	penicillin-binding protein
PCH	paroxysmal cold hemoglobinuria
PCOS	polycystic ovarian syndrome
PCP	*Pneumocystis carinii* pneumonia
PCV7	heptavalent conjugate pneumococcal vaccine
PDE	phosphodiesterases
PE	phenytoin equivalent
PE	phenytoin sodium equivalent
PE	pulmonary embolism
PEF	peak expiratory flow
PID	pelvic inflammatory disease
PK	pyruvate kinase
PL	phospholipids
PNH	paroxysmal nocturnal hemoglobinuria
PPH	postpartum hemorrhage
PPI	proton pump inhibitor
PRCA	pure red cell aplasia
PROTOgen	protoporphyrinogen
PSA	prostate specific antigen
PT	prothrombin time
PTH	parathyroid hormone
PTT	partial thromboplastin time
RA	rheumatoid arthritis
RBC	red blood cell
Rh	rhesus
RIMA	reversible inhibitor of MAO-A
RS	regular strength
RSV	respiratory syncytial virus
RSV-IGIV	RSV immune globulin intravenous
SA	sinoatrial
SARI	serotonin-2 antagonists/reuptake inhibitor
SC	subcutaneous
SERM	serum estrogen receptor modulator
SIADH	syndrome of inappropriate secretion of ADH
SIADH	syndrome of inappropriate secretion of antidiuretic hormone
SLE	systemic lupus erythematosus
SNRI	serotonin norepinephrine reuptake inhibitor
SR	slow release
SSRI	specific serotonin reuptake inhibitor
T_3	triiodothyronine
T4	levothyroxine
T_4	tetraiodothyronine (thyroxine)
TB	tuberculosis

TCA	tricyclic antidepressants
Td	tetanus and diphtheria "adult-type" vaccine
TDM	therapeutic drug monitoring
TF	tissue factor
TI	Therapeutic index
TIA	transient ischemic attack
TIPS	transjugular intrahepatic portosystemic shunt
TMP-SMX	trimethoprim and sulfamethoxazole
TMTase	thiopurine methyltransferase
TOA	tubo-ovarian abscess
tPA	alteplase
t-PA	tissue plasminogen activator
TSH	thyroid-stimulating hormone
UC	ulcerative colitis
UFH	unfractionated heparin
UROgen	uroporphyrinogen
URTI	upper respiratory tract infection
UTI	urinary tract infection
Var	varicella vaccine
Vd	volume of distribution
VLDL	very low-density lipoprotein
VTE	venous thromboembolus
WPW	Wolff-Parkinson-White

USE-IN-PREGNANCY RATINGS FOR DRUGS

Category A: Controlled studies show no risk to fetus.

B: No evidence of risk in humans. Either animal data show risk but human findings do not or animal findings are negative.

C: Risk cannot be ruled out. Human studies are lacking and animal studies either show risk or are also lacking. Potential benefits may outweigh risk.

D: Positive evidence of risk. Data show possible risk to the fetus. Potential benefits may outweigh risk.

X: Contraindicated in pregnancy. Studies show fetal risk that clearly outweighs benefit to the patient.

CHAPTER 1

Fundamentals of Pharmacology

SHINYA ITO

NOMENCLATURE OF DRUGS

An understanding of the nomenclature of drugs can help eliminate confusion about drug names:

Chemical name—the scientific designation that describes the atomic or molecular structure of a drug. Example: N-(4-hydroxyphenyl) acetamide

Nonproprietary name ("generic" name)—an official name that is given to the drug after it is developed by the drug company. It is usually shorter and more convenient than the complex chemical name, although it may be a simple form of the chemical name (e.g., sodium bicarbonate). Example: acetaminophen

Proprietary name ("brand" or "trade" name)—the name established by the manufacturer to represent the drug; by law, only the manufacturer's drug may carry that name. Example: Tylenol

Common name—a name commonly given to a drug depending on the environment in which it is used (i.e., hospital versus street setting). Example: "AZT" for the drug azidothymidine

ROUTES OF DRUG ADMINISTRATION

It is essential that the route chosen for drug administration provides a favorable environment for that drug to be absorbed to reach the desired site of action and to interact with the target site or tissue. Hence, the choice of route depends on the therapeutic objectives of the physician and on the properties of the drug that allow for its absorption and metabolism in the body. Routes of administration include the following:

By mouth: Oral administration of drugs depends on many factors to achieve drug absorption and therapeutic effects: gastric pH, gastric emptying (some drugs exhibit delayed absorption when taken after a meal), intestinal motility, drug solubility and concentration, stability of the drug in the gastrointestinal milieu, and binding of the drug to gastrointestinal contents. The greatest variable in drug absorption is the amount of time the drug remains in the stomach.

Rectal: Administration of a drug to the rectal mucosa is often chosen when the oral route is unsuitable, for example, if the patient is unconscious, vomiting, nauseous, or restricted from eating (e.g., after surgery) or if the drug has a bad taste or odor. Drugs that are applied to the lower part of the rectum (not the upper part) bypass liver metabolism (and the first-pass effect). Therefore, if a drug is sensitive to breakdown by liver enzymes, rectal administration may be favorable.

Sublingual: The area under the tongue provides a site for absorption and is a common site for administration of nitroglycerin tablets or spray.

The advantage of this route is that drugs are rapidly absorbed without being exposed to gastric or intestinal juices and enter the circulation directly, bypassing liver metabolism (and the first-pass effect).

Topical: Drugs administered topically—usually in the form of ointments, creams, lotions, powders, and sprays—act at the site of application.

Transdermal: Drugs administered by this route are often given by the application of a patch to the skin (e.g., nitroglycerin, scopolamine, hormone replacement therapy). Absorption is proportional to the lipid solubility of the drug.

Parenteral: Parenteral administration includes intramuscular, intravenous, and subcutaneous injection of a drug. It is a more rapid and predictable route for drug absorption than the oral route. **Intramuscular** (IM) administration of a drug in an aqueous solution allows for rapid absorption and is therefore useful in emergencies. Absorption of drugs by this route can also be steady and slow if the drug is dissolved in oil, allowing for the formation of a depot in the muscle. **Intravenous** (IV) administration of a drug directly into a vein allows relatively rapid injection and relatively slow infusion. Rapid injection allows instantaneous appearance of the drug in the circulation and is suitable for emergency situations. Slow infusion (usually over a 20-minute interval or longer) allows the concentration of the drug in the blood to be titrated to the desired level and maintained over a long period. **Subcutaneous** (SC) administration is through a needle inserted under the skin. This route allows for even and slow absorption, but large volumes of drugs cannot be given because the ensuing tissue distension may be painful. Other routes for injection are used as well, including the following: **Intra-arterial** (IA) is used when the physician wants to direct a small volume of a highly concentrated drug solution to a specific target organ, such as the heart or brain, while minimizing the drug's effects on other parts of the body. **Intrathecal** injection administers drugs directly into the cerebrospinal fluid (CSF), bypassing the blood-brain barrier and the blood-CSF barrier. **Intraperitoneal** injection of a drug into the peritoneal cavity permits rapid entry of drugs into the circulation because of the large absorptive surface, but it is seldom used in clinical practice because it carries the risk of infection, intestinal injury, vascular injury, and adhesions.

PLASMA CONCENTRATION TIME PROFILES

Pharmacokinetics is the kinetic principle behind changes in plasma concentrations of drugs.

Distribution Phase

Typically, plasma drug concentrations rise rapidly after drug administration. Distribution into tissues begins immediately; however, the amount of drug entering the plasma is initially so abundant that plasma concentrations continue to rise. Once drug input (i.e., absorption or infusion) is almost complete, plasma concentrations decrease rapidly, reflecting the distribution process (i.e., distribution phase).

Elimination Phase

Although elimination of a drug starts the moment after the drug appears in plasma, the elimination process is not evident because the amount of drug distributing into tissues is much larger than that being eliminated. As the distribution approaches completion, the decline of plasma drug concentration starts slowing down because of the slower elimination phase. In contrast to the distribution phase, the elimination phase is characterized by parallel decrease of the plasma and tissue concentrations because the elimination is usually slower than the distribution-redistribution process. The mismatch between the plasma and tissue levels happens again whenever there is a rapid change in plasma concentrations (i.e., the next dosing).

PATIENT-DRUG INTERFACES

Adherence

Compliance is a goodness of conformity of the actual dosing pattern with the planned dosing schedule. Usually, it is expressed as a percentage of planned doses (e.g., 80% if 8 of 10 planned tablets were consumed). Reasons for noncompliance range from simple forgetfulness to intentional neglect. Risk factors for significant noncompliance include adolescence, chronic therapy, multiple medications (polypharmacy), and lack of a clear understanding of the treatment regimen.

Bioavailability

Bioavailability of a drug is the fraction of unchanged drug that has reached the systemic circulation, and it is defined as the proportion of the administered dose that appears in the bloodstream. An important note: even after complete intestinal absorption, a substantial portion of the drug may be eliminated because of metabolism by the intestinal epithelium and liver. This is called **first-pass effect.**

Volume of Distribution

Volume of distribution (Vd) relates the amount of drug in the body to the plasma concentration. This is an "apparent" volume because it is not necessarily equal to a physical water volume of the anatomical space; if drug is sequestered in a tissue, Vd becomes much greater than the actual tissue water volume (e.g., tricyclic antidepressants have a Vd greater than 10 L/kg). Using Vd, one can estimate the dose required to achieve a given peak plasma concentration:

$$C_{peak} = Dose/Vd$$

Protein Binding

Most drugs are bound to plasma proteins, mainly albumin or α_1-acid glycoprotein. Because unbound drugs are the major active components, changes in plasma protein binding alter drug effects. Plasma protein binding of drugs ranges from 0% (e.g., lithium) to 99% (e.g., warfarin). Changes in plasma protein binding have greater clinical implications when the drug is more than 90% protein bound because a "relative" change in the unbound fraction is large (a change from 99% to 98% protein binding results in a twofold increase in the unbound fraction). Indeed, many drugs enhance the effects of warfarin by displacing it from the protein binding site.

Elimination (Metabolism and Excretion)

Clearance refers to the **efficiency of drug elimination** and is expressed as a volume per unit of time (i.e., plasma volume from which drug is cleared per unit of time). **Half-life** ($t1/2$) is the duration of time that is required to decrease the plasma concentration of a drug by one-half. **Half-life is proportional to Vd and inversely proportional to clearance.** In **first-order kinetics,** a fixed fraction of the drug is eliminated per unit of time. Most drugs follow this mode of elimination. In **zero-order kinetics,** however, clearance progressively slows down as the plasma drug concentration increases, that is, only a fixed amount (i.e., not a fraction) of drug can be eliminated. An enzymatic reaction is a first-order process at a lower substrate concentration, shifting toward zero-order kinetics at a higher concentration. Therefore, zero-order kinetics is also called saturation kinetics, because the capacity of the enzymatic process is saturated at higher substrate concentrations. A clinical consequence of saturation kinetics is that **when the dose is increased, the mean plasma concentrations increase more than would be expected from the increase in drug dose,** for example, a twofold increase in the dose may cause a fourfold rise in mean plasma concentration at steady state.

    Steady state is achieved when drug input (i.e., dose) and output (i.e., eliminated amount) per unit of time are virtually identical. When plasma concentrations reach 90% of the theoretical steady-state level, a "steady state" can be declared. It takes about 4 half-lives to achieve the steady state when a fixed dose is given at a fixed interval. **Drug dosing schedules are designed so that steady-state concentrations are equal to therapeutic concentrations. Loading dose** is used when a therapeutic level of drug must be attained quickly.

THERAPEUTIC INDEX

Therapeutic index (TI) is a measure that compares the dose required to produce a desired effect with the dose that produces a toxic effect. The greater the TI, the greater the margin of safety of the treatment. The TI is defined as follows:

$$TI = \text{Median toxic dose} / \text{Median therapeutic dose}$$

THERAPEUTIC DRUG MONITORING

To guide, assess, and optimize therapy, **feedback information based on therapeutic and toxic effects** is needed. This strategy is not appropriate

Table 1–1. Drugs That Qualify for Therapeutic Drug Monitoring

Drug Category	Generic (Brand) Name
Antibiotics	Amikacin (Amikin) [C]
	Gentamicin (Gentacidin, Cidomycin) [C]
	Tobramycin (Tobrex) [C]
	Vancomycin (Vancocin) [C]
Anticonvulsants	Carbamazepine (Tegretol) [D]
	Phenytoin (Dilantin) [D]
	Phenobarbital (Luminal—*U.S.*; Barbilixir—*Can.*) [D]
	Valproic acid (Depakene) [D]
Antiarrhythmics	Amiodarone (Cordarone, Pacerone) [D]
	Digoxin (Lanoxin) [C]
Immunosuppressants	Cyclosporine (Neoral, Sandimmune) [C]
	Tacrolimus (Prograf) [C]
Other drugs	Caffeine (for neonatal apnea)
	Lithium (Lithonate, Carbolith) [D]
	Methotrexate (high-dose therapy) (Rheumatrex, Trexall) [D]
	Salicylic acid (high-dose therapy: >60 mg/kg/day)
	Theophylline [C]

when the effect and toxicity cannot be objectively assessed within a reasonable time. This may not be a problem if there is no toxicity, even with a high dose (i.e., a high TI). However, to fine-tune a regimen of drugs with low TIs, a surrogate end point is required. The most common surrogate end point is plasma drug concentration. The surrogate end point is valid only after a reliable correlation with effects has been proven. Otherwise, the data cannot be interpreted in terms of clinical significance. **Guiding the therapy based on plasma drug concentration is called therapeutic drug monitoring** (TDM). Table 1-1 lists drugs that fulfill the requirements outlined above and are justified for TDM. As described herein, the time required to monitor the drug concentration depends on the individual drug. For example, the distribution phase of digoxin continues until about 6 hours after dosing. Therefore, plasma sampling for TDM of digoxin should be carried out no sooner than 6 hours following the administration of the last dose.

CHAPTER 2

Anesthesiology

ALINE BOULANGER

During anesthesia, four conditions are needed: analgesia, amnesia, muscle relaxation, and loss of consciousness. To satisfy these four conditions simultaneously, drugs and agents have to be combined. This chapter presents a **review of medications used during anesthesia** and a brief discussion of **malignant hyperthermia**.

INHALATION ANESTHETICS

Volatile Anesthetics and Nitrous Oxide

Inhalation agents provide **unconsciousness, amnesia,** and **some muscular relaxation** by interrupting neuronal transmission in many areas of the central nervous system (CNS). Their principal site of action seems to be proteins present in the neuronal membranes. During anesthesia, inhaled anesthetics are rapidly transferred from the lung to the bloodstream, and then to the CNS. At the end of administration, a large part of the agent has been exhaled, and metabolism, excretion, and redistribution are minimal. The **minimum alveolar concentration (MAC)** is the percentage of inhaled agent that prevents movement in response to a surgery stimulus in 50% of patients. The MAC is different for each gas (Table 2–1). **During surgery, an end-tidal concentration of inhaled agent of 1.3 × MAC is needed. Factors that may increase the MAC:** hyperthermia and chronic ethanol abuse. **Factors that decrease the MAC:** increasing age, hypothermia, pregnancy, and coadministration of CNS depressant medications. All volatile agents decrease blood pressure, depress the ventilatory response to hypercarbia and hypoxemia, and relax airway smooth muscle. Table 2–2 lists the hemodynamic effects of volatile anesthetics. Halothane (Fluothane) and sevoflurane (Sevorane, Ultane) are well known to produce bronchodilation.

Table 2–1. Physiological Properties of Volatile Anesthetics and Nitrous Oxide

Generic (Brand) Name	MAC	% Metabolites
Desflurane (Suprane) [B]	6.6	0.02
Enflurane (Ethrane)	1.63	2.4
Halothane (Fluothane) [C]	0.75	20
Isoflurane (Forane) [C]	1.17	0.2
Nitrous oxide	104	0
Sevoflurane (Ultane—*U.S.*; Sevorane—*Can.*)	1.8	2–5

MAC = minimum alveolar concentration, which is the percentage of inhaled agent that prevents movement in response to a surgery stimulus in 50% of patients.

Table 2–2. Hemodynamic Effects of Volatile Anesthetics

Generic (Brand) Name	Heart Rate	Myocardial Contractility	Vascular Resistance
Desflurane (Suprane) [B]	↑ ↑	0	↓
Enflurane (Ethrane)	↑ ↑	↓	↓
Halothane (Fluothane) [C]	0	↓ ↓	0
Isoflurane (Forane) [C]	↑ ↑	0	↓
Sevoflurane (Ultrane—*U.S.*; Sevorane—*Can.*)	0	0	↓

0 = none or no effect; ↓ = decrease; ↑ = increase

Nitrous oxide is a low-potency gas (MAC = 104%). Except for an increase in the pulmonary vascular resistance, nitrous oxide has no side effects on cardiovascular and respiratory functions. It does not produce skeletal muscle relaxation, but analgesic effects have been reported. Because of its poor solubility, it has the tendency to diffuse across blood through to air-filled spaces (e.g., bowel, middle ear, pneumothorax, or air emboli). Nitrous oxide expands these spaces until its partial pressure in the space equals that of blood or until sufficient pressure inside the compliant spaces blocks its entrance. A pneumothorax may triple in size when exposed to 75% nitrous oxide. **Particular risks for volatile anesthetics and nitrous oxide are listed in Table 2–3.**

Contraindications: Volatile agents are contraindicated in patients with malignant hyperthermia. **Nitrous oxide** is contraindicated in cases of bowel obstruction, pneumothorax, and tympanoplasty.

Table 2–3. Side Effects of Particular Volatile Anesthetics and Nitrous Oxide

Generic (Brand) Name	Side Effects
Desflurane (Suprane) [B]	Transient tachycardia, hypertension, and laryngospasm
Enflurane (Ethrane)	Seizurelike activity on EEG Renal insufficiency due to its metabolite fluoride
Halothane (Fluothane) [C]	Arrhythmias caused by sensitization to epinephrine **Immune-mediated hepatitis**
Isoflurane (Forane) [C]	May produce cardiac steal* as a result of coronary vasodilation; can increase intracranial pressure, cause arrhythmias, and reduce blood flow to kidneys, spleen, and liver; is a trigger of malignant hyperthermia
Nitrous oxide [B]	Drug's ability to expand air-filled structures and bubbles
Sevoflurane (Ultrane—*U.S.*; Sevorane—*Can.*) [B]	Nephrotoxicity caused by vanyl halide (compound A)

*Cardiac, or coronary, steal syndrome—preferential dilation of small coronary resistance vessels—may cause blood redistribution from ischemic to relatively nonischemic areas.

INTRAVENOUS HYPNOTICS

Barbiturates, propofol, benzodiazepines, and etomidate give their hypnotic effect by decreasing the excitability of neurons through an interaction with different components of the inhibitory gamma-aminobutyric acid (GABA) receptor complex at the CNS level. Ketamine (Ketalar) acts through its capacity to inhibit the excitatory response to glutamate at the central N-methyl-D-aspartate (NMDA) receptors. The rapid onset of action of hypnotics is related to their high lipid solubility together with considerable blood flow in the brain. Redistribution from the CNS to larger compartments explains their fast recovery, and elimination takes place in the liver, followed by renal excretion. Except for ketamine, these drugs have no analgesic effect. **Dosage requirements for each agent described are listed in Table 2–4.**

Contraindication: Intravenous hypnotics are contraindicated if knowledge or equipment to manage an apneic patient is lacking.

Etomidate (Amidate) [C]

Etomidate is a carboxylated imidazole compound. Emergence is short even after repeated bolus or continuous infusion. Etomidate is indicated for patients with severe cardiovascular, and cerebrovascular disease because of its hemodynamic stability during induction (Table 2–5). Its use for maintenance of anesthesia as been questioned because of its capacity to inhibit adrenocortical function for 5–8 hours. Involuntary myoclonic movements, unrelated to seizure activity, are common during the induction period, but convulsion in the epileptic patient has been reported. Etomidate is associated with nausea and emesis in the postoperative period.

Ketamine (Ketalar) [D]

Ketamine is an arylcyclohexylamine related to phencyclidine. Ketamine produces a dissociative anesthetic state characterized by profound analgesia and amnesia, while maintaining consciousness and protective reflexes. The high incidence of psychomimetic reactions (hallucination and nightmare) can be reduced by benzodiazepines. **Analgesic effects at low-dose infusion of 4 µg/kg/min are reported to be equivalent to morphine 2 mg/hr IV. It is useful in the presence of hypovolemic shock, cardiac tamponade, and acute bronchospastic states.**

Contraindication: Ketamine is contraindicated in patients with intracranial hypertension.

Midazolam (Versed) [D]

Midazolam is a water-soluble **short-acting benzodiazepine.** It has anxiolytic, amnesic, sedative, hypnotic, anticonvulsant, and muscle relaxant properties. **Premedicant dose** of midazolam is 0.04–0.08 mg/kg IV/IM. The **usual induction dose** is 0.05–0.20 mg/kg IV, with a **maintenance**

Table 2–4. Dosage Requirements for Sedative-Hypnotic Drugs

Generic (Brand) Name	IV Induction Dose (mg/kg)	Onset (sec)	Duration (min)	IV Maintenance Dose
Etomidate (Amidate) [C]	0.2–0.3	15–45	3–12	10 μg/kg/min
Ketamine (Ketalar) [D]	1–2	45–60	10–20	15–90 μg/kg/min
Midazolam (Versed)* [D]	0.5–2	30–90	10–30	0.25–1.00 μg/kg/min
Propofol (Diprivan) [B]	0.5–0.2	15–45	5–10	25–75 μg/kg/min 50–200 μg/kg/min for hypnosis
Thiopental (Pentothal) [C]	Adults: 3–5 Children: 5–6 Infants: 6–8	<30	5–10	Adults: 25–100 mg as needed Children: 1 mg/kg as needed

*There is an antidote (specific antagonist) for benzodiazepines: flumazenil (Anexate), which is described in the text.

infusion rate of 0.25–1.00 μg/kg/min. When used for induction or maintenance of anesthesia, return of consciousness takes substantially longer than with other sedative-hypnotic drugs. **Its most significant problem is respiratory depression when it is given for conscious sedation.**

ANTIDOTE

There is a specific antagonist for benzodiazepines: flumazenil (Anexate). Flumazenil is a benzodiazepine with minimal intrinsic activity that acts as a competitive antagonist in the presence of other benzodiazepines. **Dosage should be titrated** by repeating 0.2 mg IV increment every 1–2 minutes until the desired level of reversal is reached. About 45–90 minutes of antagonism can be expected following 3.0 mg IV of flumazenil. If sustained antagonism is desired, repeated bolus or continuous infusion is necessary. Flumazenil may cause seizures if the dose is high or administered at too fast a rate.

Propofol (Diprivan) [B]

Propofol is an alkyl phenol compound emulsified in egg lecithin. The **induction dose in healthy adults** is 1.0–2.5 mg/kg IV. The **recommended maintenance infusion varies** from 25–75 μg/kg/min for sedation to 50–200 μg/kg/min for hypnosis. **Induction and maintenance doses**

Table 2–5. Characteristics of Sedative-Hypnotic Drugs

Generic (Brand) Name	Excitatory Activity	Pain on Injection	Heart Rate	Blood Pressure	Intracranial Pressure
Etomidate (Amidate)	+++	+++	0	0	↓
Ketamine (Ketalar)	+	0	↑↑	↑↑	↑
Midazolam (Versed)	0	0	0	0-↓	0-↓
Propofol (Diprivan)	+	++	0-↓	↓↓	↓
Thiopental (Pentothal)	+	0-+	↑	↓	↓

0 = none or no effect; + = minimal; ++ = moderate; +++ = severe; ↓ = decrease; ↑ = increase.

require adjustment for patient age, associated medications, and health status. Propofol is the drug of choice for ambulatory surgery because patients become rapidly alert when they emerge from anesthesia. Recovery from a prolonged perfusion of propofol is rapid because of its extensive hepatic metabolism and its rapid renal clearance rate (1.5–2.2 L/min). **Subanesthetic doses** of propofol (10–20 mg IV) seem to possess antiemetic properties and also decrease the pruritus associated with spinal opioids. Induction with propofol is occasionally accompanied by nonepileptic myoclonus. Because fat emulsions allow growth of microorganisms, contamination can occur with fractionated use and a vial that is open for hours.

Contraindication: Propofol is contraindicated in patients with known egg allergies.

Thiopental (Pentothal) [C]

Thiopental is **an ultra-short-acting barbiturate.** The **usual intravenous induction dose** is 3–5 mg/kg IV in adults (5–6 mg/kg in children and 6–8 mg/kg in infants). Geriatric patients, pregnant women, and premedicated patients may require lower dosages. **In the presence of hypovolemia or preexisting cardiovascular disease, thiopental may lead to acute cardiocirculatory depressant effects;** therefore, a much lower dose is necessary. Intracranial hypertension and intractable convulsions might be treated with an infusion of thiopental at 2–4 mg/kg/hr.

Contraindication: Thiopental is contraindicated in patients with acute intermittent porphyrias.

LOCAL ANESTHETICS

Local anesthetics block the neural generation and propagation of the impulses mainly at the sodium channel level. **Two types of local anesthetic agents are available: amides,** which are metabolized by the liver, and **esters,** which are metabolized by plasma cholinesterases. Central nervous system toxicity may happen and is related to the vascular absorption of local anesthetic agents. With increasing blood levels, patients may feel lightheadedness, tinnitus, numbness around the mouth and tongue, convulsion, or coma; **at high levels (resulting generally from an intravascular injection), cardiovascular depression may result.** Toxicity will depend on the total amount of medication injected, the site of injection (e.g., intercostal > epidural > brachial plexus), and the presence of epinephrine in the solution (see Table 2–6 for recommended maximal doses).

MUSCLE RELAXANTS

Muscle contraction involves the interaction of a receptor, located on a specialized portion of the muscle membrane (the endplate), and acetylcholine (ACh), produced and released at the terminal portion of the axon. When an impulse reaches the nerve ending, ACh is released in the synaptic cleft and combines with the receptor, resulting in depolarization of the muscle fiber and its contraction. To end the process, acetylcholinesterase, an enzyme located at the neuromuscular junction, rapidly hydrolyzes the ACh molecules. Curares block neuromuscular transmission by their interaction at the ACh receptor level. The effect of muscle relaxants is evaluated by observation of the contractions of the muscle in answer to nerve stimulation. **Two classes of curare are available: (1) depolarizing drugs, which exhibit depolarization of the receptor or produce inactivation of the sodium channel, and (2) nondepolarizing drugs, which bind to the receptor in a competitive way.**

Table 2–6.   Recommended Maximal Doses of Local Anesthetics

Generic (Brand) Name	Duration (hr)	Recommended Maximal Single Dose	
		Alone	With Epinephrine
Amides			
Bupivacaine (Marcaine, Sensorcaine) [C]	2–12	175	225
Etidocaine (Duranest) [B]	2–12	300	400
Lidocaine (Xylocaine) [B/C]	0.5–4	300	500
Mepivacaine (Carbocaine, Isocaine, Polocaine) [C]	1–4	400	500
Prilocaine (Citanest) [B]	0.5–6	600	*
Ropivacaine (Naropin) [B]	2–8	200	*
Esters			
Chloroprocaine (Nesacaine) [C]	0.5–1	800	1,000
Procaine (Novocain) [C]	0.5–1	1,000	*
Tetracaine (Pontocaine—*U.S.;* Supracaine—*Can.)* [C]	2–6	20	*

*Epinephrine formulations not available.

Depolarizing Drugs

Succinylcholine depolarizes the neuromuscular junction, producing curarization and muscle fasciculations. (A small dose of a nondepolarizing drug may prevent fasciculations.) The **dose required for intubation** is 1.0 mg/kg IV (and it must be increased to 1.5–2.0 mg/kg if nondepolarizing curare is used). For children and infants, precurarization is unnecessary, and the succinylcholine dose has to be increased to 2.0–3.0 mg/kg. **Succinylcholine onset of action is less than 1 minute, and its duration is less than 8 minutes.** It is rapidly hydrolyzed by pseudocholinesterase. This enzyme is decreased during pregnancy, liver disease, burns, and uremia, resulting in a slight increase in the curarization time. It has been reported that 1:1,500–1:2,000 patients have either an absence or an abnormal form of plasma cholinesterase. In these cases, paralysis will persist for hours, and patients will need to be sedated and ventilated. **Succinylcholine may induce bradycardia,** especially in children and after a second dose in adults. **Atropine will reverse this effect.** Intraocular and intracranial pressure may increase with succinylcholine. Serum potassium increases by 0.5–1.0 mEq/L after succinylcholine. Severe hyperkalemia was reported in patients with burns, trauma, nerve damage, neuromuscular disease, and renal failure.

Nondepolarizing Neuromuscular Blocking Drugs

Nondepolarizing drugs block the neuromuscular junction by competitive inhibition of ACh receptors. The choice of the nondepolarizing drug depends on the urgency to intubate and the duration of the procedure (Table 2–7). For tracheal intubation, two to three times the ED_{95} (effective dose corresponding to 95% twitch depression of the adductor pollicis [produced by a neurostimulator on the ulnar nerve]) is needed.

ANTIDOTE

The effect of nondepolarizing drugs can be reversed by anticholinesterase agents. Neostigmine (Prostigmin) and edrophonium (Tensilon), both anticholinesterase drugs, inhibit the hydrolysis of ACh, which increases the concentration of ACh at the neuromuscular junction and allows it to compete with nondepolarizing curare. Anticholinesterases also block ACh hydrolysis at the muscarinic receptors at the autonomic ganglia, the heart, and salivary glands. To prevent bradycardia that may result, an antimuscarinic agent, such as atropine or glycopyrrolate (Robinul), is given with anticholinesterase.

Hypotension may result from atracurium (Tracrium) and rocuronium (Zemuron) because of histamine release. Pancuronium (Pavulon) and doxacurium (Nuromax) have vagolytic action and may induce tachycardia.

Contraindications: Muscle relaxants are contraindicated if knowledge or equipment to manage an apneic patient is lacking. **Succinylcholine**

Table 2–7. Neuromuscular Blocking Drugs

Generic (Brand) Name	ED$_{95}$ (mg/kg)	Onset (min)	Recovery (min)
Succinylcholine (Anectine, Quelicin) [C]	0.5	0.34	8
d-tubocurarine chloride	0.5	6	70–90
Atracurium (Tracrium) [C]	0.2	5–6	20–25
Cisatracurium (Nimbex) [C]	0.05	5–6	20–25
Doxacurium (Nuromax) [C]	0.025	10–14	80–100
Mivacurium (Mivacron) [C]	0.08–0.15	2–3	20
Pancuronium (Pavulon) [C]	0.6	4–5	60
Rocuronium (Zenuron) [C]	0.3	2–3	20
Vecuronium (Norcuron) [C]	0.08	5–6	20

ED$_{95}$ = effective dose corresponding to 95% twitch depression of the adductor pollicis (produced by a neurostimulator on the ulnar nerve).

is contraindicated in patients with malignant hyperthermia and those at risk for hyperkalemia.

OPIOIDS

Opioid analgesia is produced by the interaction of the opioids with receptors at the brain, spinal cord, and peripheral tissues. They are used in premedication for anesthesia in combination with other medications (balanced anesthesia) or alone (high opioid anesthesia) and for the treatment of postoperative pain. Doses are titrated for anesthesia or analgesic purposes (Table 2–8). **Dosage needs may decrease with age, unstable hemodynamic status, and liver disease.** Opioids have a rapid onset of action, offer good cardiovascular stability, have no active metabolites, and do not induce histamine release. **They may create muscle rigidity, respiratory depression, bradycardia, pruritus, nausea, and vomiting.**

ANTIDOTE

For respiratory depression related to opioids, naloxone (Narcan) can be administered repetitively at increased doses: 0.025–0.100 mg IV q5min until a respiratory rate >10 beats/min is achieved. Onset of action of naloxone is 1–2 minutes, and its duration of effect is 30–60 minutes.

SERIOUS SIDE EFFECT

Malignant Hyperthermia

KV Malignant hyperthermia (MH) is a hypermetabolic disease of the muscles involving a disorder of intracellular calcium. This disorder has a

Table 2–8. Anesthetic Use of Opioids

Generic (Brand) Name	For Anesthesia		Combined With Nitrous Oxide 60%–70%		IV Analgesia for Painful Procedures (µg/kg/hr)
	IV Loading Dose (µg/kg)	Intermittent IV Bolus (µg)	Continuous IV Infusion (µg/kg/hr)		
Fentanyl (Actiq, Duragesic, Sublimaze) [B/D]	2–10	25–100	2–10		0.3–3
Sufentanil citrate (Sufenta) [C]	0.25–2.0	2.5–10	0.5–1.5		0.1–0.6
Alfentanil (Alfenta) [C]	25–100	250–500	30–120		15–45
Remifentanil (Ultiva) [C]	1–2	5–50	6–60		3–12

genetic component and is predominant in children. Generally, soon after the administration of **trigger agents, volatile anesthetic agents (not including nitrous oxide), and succinylcholine,** the manifestations appear. **Signs** are characterized by elevation of blood pressure, tachycardia, arrhythmias, muscular and mainly masseter rigidity, hyperthermia, hypercarbia, acidosis, hyperkalemia, and myoglobinuria.

TX The use of dantrolene has decreased the extremely high mortality rate associated with MH. If a patient or one of his relatives is known to carry the metabolic defect, premedication with 2.0 mg/kg IV of dantrolene, the use of an anesthetic agent that is not known to trigger MH, and close follow-up after surgery are recommended. In the situation of a hyperthermia crisis, recommendations are:

1. Discontinue inhalation agents and succinylcholine
2. Oxygen 100%
3. Dantrolene 2.5 mg/kg IV up to 10.0 mg/kg
   NB: Each ampule contains 20 mg of dantrolene to be diluted in 50 mL of sterile water.
4. Treat acidosis with hyperventilation and bicarbonate injections (see Ch 11 Nephrology)
5. Treat arrhythmias (lidocaine is safe) (see Ch 3 Cardiology)
6. Treat hyperthermia (ice pack, gastric irrigation)
7. Treat hyperkalemia (see Ch 11 Nephrology)
8. Follow-up for recurrence of the MH crisis, disseminated intravascular coagulation (see Ch 9 Hematology), and renal failure secondary to myoglobinuria

RX Dantrolene (Dantrium)[C]: Interferes with the release of calcium into the myoplasm from the sarcoplasmic reticulum.

DS 2.5 mg/kg IV up to 10.0 mg/kg IV

SE Generalized muscle weakness and drowsiness can occur.

3

Cardiology

IAN PATERSON, JEAN G. DIODATI, TOMY HADJIS

ACUTE CORONARY SYNDROME

KY An acute coronary syndrome occurs when an atherosclerotic plaque becomes unstable and ruptures or erodes, thus exposing a thrombogenic lipid core. Platelets aggregate and release inflammatory mediators, causing thrombus propagation and coronary vasoconstriction. When a thrombus occludes the lumen of the vessel, the subtended myocardium is deprived of oxygen and becomes ischemic. If no reperfusion occurs within 30 minutes of onset of ischemia, myocardial necrosis (infarction) occurs. Acute coronary syndromes can be classified into persistent ST-segment elevation acute coronary syndrome and non–ST-segment elevation acute coronary syndrome. The goal of therapy in ST-segment elevation acute coronary syndrome is to reestablish coronary blood flow with reperfusion therapy using either coronary angioplasty or thrombolytic therapy (clot dissolution). The goal of therapy in non–ST-segment elevation acute coronary syndrome is to prevent thrombotic coronary artery occlusion using antithrombotic therapy (clot prevention).

TX The pharmacotherapy of an acute coronary syndrome is designed to **reestablish coronary blood flow** and **prevent irreversible myocardial damage** (Fig. 3–1). Calcium channel blockers have **not** been shown to improve patient outcomes during an acute coronary syndrome. (Short-acting nifedipine has been associated with increased mortality rates when given to patients during a myocardial infarction [MI].)

RX1 **Thrombolytic therapy:** Drugs in this category lyse fibrin cross-links by directly or indirectly activating the endogenous fibrinolytic system (Table 3–1).

DS1 Table 3–1

SE1 Intracerebral hemorrhage is the most serious complication of thrombolysis. **Agents' specific side effects** are listed in Table 3–1. **Contraindications** to the administration of a thrombolytic agent are listed in Table 3–2.

with

RX2 **Acetylsalicylic acid (aspirin)** [C/D in third trimester]

DS2 ≥ 160 mg PO, crushed

SE2 Table 3–3

with or without

RX3 **Eptifibatide** (Integrilin) [B]: Glycoprotein IIB/IIIA receptor inhibitor that acts by blocking activated platelets from binding fibrin

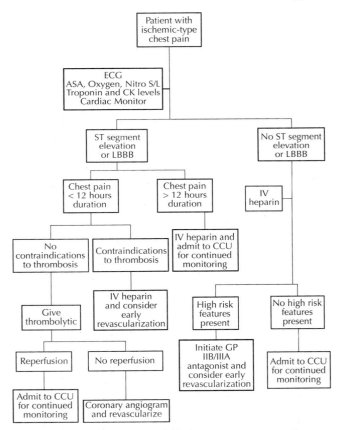

ASA: aspirin, LBBB: left bundle branch block, CCU: coronary care unit.

FIGURE 3–1 Management of acute coronary syndrome.

and, thus, neutralizes the final common pathway of platelet aggregation. Shown to provide modest benefit in reducing cardiovascular events in patients with non–ST-segment elevation acute coronary syndromes.

DS3 180 μg/kg/min IV bolus followed by 2 μg/kg/min IV infusion

SE3 Major bleeding and thrombocytopenia. **Contraindications** as in Table 3–2.

Table 3–1. Summary of Thrombolytic Agents

Generic (Brand) Name	Dose	Concomitant Heparin Administration	Fibrin Affinity	Side Effects and Cautions
Alteplase (tPA) (Activase) [C]	Weight-adjusted bolus*; then, 0.5 mg/kg (not to exceed 35 mg) over 60–90 minutes	Yes	High	Serious side effects: severe bleeding, hemorrhagic stroke Common side effect: minor bleeding **Contraindications:** See Table 3–2.
Reteplase (rPA) (Retavase) [C]	Two 10-U IV boluses No weight adjustment	Yes	Very high	Same as for tPA.
Streptokinase (STK) (Streptase) [C]	1.5 million U IV over 1 hour	No	Moderate	Serious side effects: anaphylaxis, serious bleeding, hemorrhagic stroke Common side effects: hypotension, minor bleeding, fever **Contraindications:** See Table 3–2. **Caution:** Streptokinase is antigenic and can cause immunologic sensitization and allergic reactions with repeated administration.
Tenecteplase (TNK-tPA) (TNKase) [C]	Single 30–40 mg IV bolus No weight adjustment	Yes	Very high	Same as for tPA.

*For patients > 67 kg, the total dose is 100 mg over 90 minutes. Infuse 15 mg IV over 1–2 minutes, followed by 50 mg IV over 30 minutes. For patients < 67 kg, the total dose is 1.25 mg.

**Table 3–2. Contraindications to the Administration of
Thrombolytic Agents**

Contraindications*
Active internal bleeding
Cerebral stroke within 1 year
Cerebrovascular events within 1 year
Previous cerebral hemorrhagic stroke
Suspected aortic dissection

Major Relative Contraindications
Acute pericarditis
Recent ($<$ 3 months) cerebrovascular accident or head trauma
Recent ($<$ 3 weeks) gastrointestinal or genitourinary bleeding
Recent (2–4 weeks) major surgery or serious trauma
Severe uncontrolled hypertension ($>$ 180/110 mm Hg)
Cardiopulmonary resuscitation
Streptokinase and anistreplase previously
Traumatic or prolonged ($>$ 15 minutes)

Minor Relative Contraindications
Current use of anticoagulants in therapeutic doses (international normalized ratio $>$ 2)
Endocarditis
Intracavitary cardiac thrombus
Known bleeding diathesis
Pregnancy
Proliferative diabetic retinopathy

*For streptokinase and anistreplase, avoid use if a previous exposure occurred 5 days to 2 years
earlier or if there is a history of previous allergic reaction.

or

RX4 **Tirofiban** (Aggrastat) [B]: Glycoprotein IIB/IIIA receptor inhibitor.

DS4 0.4 μg/kg/min IV bolus over 30 minutes followed by 0.1 μg/kg/min
IV infusion

SE4 Same as for eptifibatide.

with or without

RX5 **Unfractionated heparin** [C]: Exerts its anticoagulant activity by
reversibly binding to antithrombin III, thus accelerating the ability of
antithrombin III to neutralize thrombin and activated coagulation factor X
(Xa). The heparin–antithrombin III complex also inactivates activated coagulation factors IX, XI, and XII and plasmin (also see Ch 9 Hematology).
Heparin is not a thrombolytic agent, but it prevents progression of the existing clot by inhibiting any further clotting processes, allowing naturally
occurring thrombolytics to slowly affect clot lysis. Intravenous heparin therapy in ST-segment elevation MI is indicated when alteplase (tPA) or one of
its derivatives is used. Late patency rates of the involved coronary artery and
survival rates are higher in patients receiving dual therapy than in those
receiving tPA alone. Intravenous heparin does not offer a survival advantage
when given with streptokinase. In patients with non–ST-segment elevation
acute coronary syndromes, intravenous heparin has been shown to reduce
the mortality rate when given as a bolus and an infusion for at least 48 hours.

Table 3-3. Pharmacologic Treatment of Chronic Ischemic Heart Disease

Class	Generic (Brand) Name	Dose	Mechanism of Action	Side Effects and Contraindications
Angiotensin-converting enzyme inhibitors	Ramipril (Altace) [C/D in second and third trimesters]	2.5–10 mg PO qd	Inhibits formation of angiotensin II Improves endothelial function Inhibits degradation of bradykinin	Serious side effects: acute renal failure, hyperkalemia, angioedema (especially in African Americans) Common side effect: dry cough in 10%–15% of patients **Contraindicated** in patients with hyperkalemia, renal artery stenosis, and pregnancy; caution with chronic renal failure.
Antiplatelet agents	Acetylsalicylic acid (aspirin) [C/D in third trimester] Clopidogrel (Plavix) [B]	80–325 mg PO qd 75 mg PO qd	Inhibits platelet aggregation through either: Inhibition of platelet cyclooxygenase enzyme and subsequent prostaglandin formation or Inhibition of ADP release	Serious side effects: peptic ulcers with aspirin and clopidogrel; thrombocytopenia and leukopenia with clopidogrel Common side effects: bruising, minor bleeding, gastrointestinal complaints **Contraindicated** in patients with known hypersensitivity or in those with bleeding disorders.
Beta-blockers	Atenolol (Tenormin) [D] Metoprolol (Lopressor, Toprol—U.S.; Betaloc—Can.) [C/D in second and third trimesters] Nadolol (Corgard) [C] Propranolol (Inderal—U.S.; Detenso—Can.) [C/D in second and third trimester]	25–100 mg PO qd 25–100 mg PO bid 40–240 mg PO qd 20–200 mg PO bid	Predominantly inhibits β-1 receptors Improves symptoms by reducing myocardial oxygen demand	Serious side effects: heart failure, bronchospasm Common side effects: fatigue, impotence, decreased libido, nightmares, depression **Contraindicated** in patients with asthma, decompensated heart failure, significant heart block, bradycardia, and hypotension.

| Calcium channel blockers | Amlodipine (Norvasc) [C]
Diltiazem (Cardizem) [C]

Nicardipine (Cardene) [C]
Nifedipine (Adalat, Procardia) [C]
Verapamil (Isoptin) [C] | 5–10 mg qd PO
120–360 mg PO qd

20–40 mg PO tid
30–90 mg PO qd
80–120 mg PO tid–qid | Inhibits calcium entry into myocytes and causes smooth muscle relaxation
Improves symptoms by reducing myocardial oxygen demand, and may also increase oxygen supply | Serious side effects: (predominantly verapamil and diltiazem) heart failure, bradyarrhythmias
Common side effects: fatigue, gastrointestinal complaints, headache, dizziness, edema
Contraindications: hypotension for all and heart failure and significant bradycardia and heart block for verapamil and diltiazem. |
| Nitrates | Isosorbide mononitrate (Imdur, ISMO, Monoket) [C]
Nitroglycerin sublingual (Nitroglyard Buccal, Nitrolingual spray, Nitrostat Sublingual) [C]
Nitroglycerin sustained release (Deponit Patch, Minitran Patch, Nitrek Patch, Nitrodisc Patch, Nitro-Dur Patch, Transderm-Nitro Patch) [C] | 30–120 mg PO qd

0.4 mg sublingually prn for chest pain

0.2–0.8 mg topical application 12 hr/day | Relaxes smooth muscle of vessel media
Improves symptoms by reducing myocardial oxygen demand | Common side effects: headaches, dizziness, flushing
Contraindicated in patients with hypotension and hypertrophic obstructive cardiomyopathy. |

DS5 70 U/kg IV bolus followed by 15 U/kg/hr infusion. Aim for a partial thromboplastin time of 1.5–2 times control levels.

SE5 See Ch 9 Hematology.

or

RX6 **Enoxaparin** (Lovenox) [B]: See Ch 9 Hematology.

DS6 1 mg/kg SC bid (maximum, 100 mg)

SE6 See Ch 9 Hematology.

with or without

RX7 **Warfarin** (Coumadin) [D]: Inhibits vitamin K–dependent coagulation factors II, VII, IX, and X and prolongs the prothrombin time. Routine administration in all patients with acute coronary syndromes does not offer an advantage over conventional medical therapy. However, anticoagulation is recommended for all patients suffering an ST-segment elevation anterior wall MI or any extensive MI. Warfarin administration for 3–6 months improves patient outcomes by preventing cardioembolic events.

DS7 See Ch 9 Hematology.

SE7 See Ch 9 Hematology.

plus

RX8 **Beta-blockers:** Early beta-blocker administration during ST-segment elevation MI has been shown to reduce arrhythmic death and nonfatal reinfarction. Similar benefits have not been observed in non-Q wave MI and unstable angina. However, routine use of beta-blockers is still advocated as anti-ischemic therapy. In addition to oral beta-blockers, intravenous beta-blockers should be given at initial presentation to all patients with ST-segment elevation in addition to high-risk non–ST-segment elevation MI (Table 3–4).

DS8 Table 3–4

SE8 Table 3–3 and Table 3–4

with or without

RX9 **Angiotensin-converting enzyme (ACE) inhibitors:** The beneficial effect of ACE inhibitors likely stems from inhibition of postinfarction left ventricular remodeling and preservation of left ventricular function. In patients with non–ST-segment elevation MI, ACE inhibitors have not been shown to be of benefit in the acute setting. However, their use should be strongly considered.

DS9 Table 3–5

SE9 Table 3–3

plus

RX10 **Nitroglycerin** [C]: Relaxes smooth muscle of vessel media and reduces myocardial oxygen demand.

DS10 5–100 μg/min IV

SE10 Headaches, dizziness, and flushing. **Contraindicated** in patients with hypotension and hypertrophic obstructive cardiomyopathy.

Table 3-4. Summary of Intravenous Beta-Blockers

Generic (Brand) Name	Dose (IV)	Side Effects and Contraindications
Atenolol (Tenormin) [D]	5 mg every 5 minutes, repeated twice	See Table 3-3
Esmolol (Brevibloc) [C/D in second and third trimesters]	0.5 mg/kg followed with infusion at 0.05 mg/kg/min, increasing as needed to 0.2 mg/kg/min (titration to pain, blood pressure, or heart rate)	Serious side effects: hypotension, peripheral ischemia, bradycardia/asystole, dyspnea, bronchospasm, pulmonary edema, congestive heart failure, allergic reactions Common side effects: hypotension, headache, nausea, diaphoresis **Contraindicated** in patients with greater than first-degree heart block, bradycardia, cardiogenic shock, bronchial asthma, hypotension.
Metoprolol (Lopressor, Toprol —U.S.; Betaloc—Can.) [C/D in second and third trimesters]	5-mg bolus, repeated twice at intervals of 2 minutes	See Table 3-3
Propranolol (Inderal—U.S.; Detensol —Can.) [C/D in second and third trimesters]	1–5 mg given over 10 minutes	See Table 3-3

Table 3–5. Summary of Angiotensin-Converting Enzyme Inhibitors*

Generic (Brand) Name	Dose
Benazepril (Lotensin) [C/D in second and third trimesters]	10–40 mg PO qd
Captopril (Capoten) [C/D in second and third trimesters]	12.5–50 mg PO tid
Cilazapril (Inhibace)	1–5 mg PO qd
Enalapril (Vasotec) [C/D in second and third trimesters]	2.5–20 mg PO tid
Fosinopril (Monopril) [C/D in second and third trimesters]	10–40 mg PO qd
Lisinopril (Prinivil, Zestril) [C/D in second and third trimesters]	10–40 mg PO qd
Perindopril erbumine (Aceon—*U.S.*; Coversyl—*Can.*) [D]	2–8 mg PO qd
Quinapril (Accupril) [C/D in second and third trimesters]	10–40 mg PO qd
Trandolapril (Mavik) [C/D in second and third trimesters]	1–4 mg PO qd

*Side effects are listed in Table 3–3.

CARDIAC ARRHYTHMIAS

The treatment of cardiac arrhythmias is complex and varies depending on the clinical setting (**acute** versus **long term**). Thus, acute and long-term subheadings have been included in the TX section. **Many arrhythmias can be treated with a combination of different antiarrhythmic drugs.** Based on the predominant direct channel/ion effect of the antiarrhythmic medication, these drugs are divided into different classes (Table 3–6).

Atrial Fibrillation and Atrial Flutter

KY Most cases of atrial fibrillation are the result of reentry with multiple wavelets circulating in both atria. An alternate mechanism for atrial fibrillation is a single, rapidly firing focus that initiates and possibly even maintains atrial fibrillation. Such foci have been mapped in the pulmonary veins and, less commonly, in the left or right atrium. Atrial fibrillation is frequently seen in association with cardiovascular disorders such as valvular heart disease, coronary artery disease, hypertension, and cardiomyopathy. Although atrial fibrillation may occur in as many as 40% of patients after cardiac surgery, this is usually a self-limited problem. Transient noncardiac factors that can result in atrial fibrillation include hyperthyroidism, acute alcohol intoxication, cholinergic drugs, noncardiac surgery, and hypoxemia. "Lone atrial fibrillation" is defined as atrial fibrillation occurring in the absence of an identifiable cause. Typical atrial flutter (Type I) is a macroreentrant arrhythmia that is characterized by intra-atrial reentry. The circuit rotates in a counterclockwise direction in the right atrium and is maintained by a combination of anatomic and functional boundaries. Atypical atrial flutter (Type II) shares features of both atrial fibrillation and atrial flutter. It is usually found to be a transitional rhythm that degenerates into atrial fibrillation.

TX1 **Acute treatment:** The acute management of atrial flutter is similar to that of atrial fibrillation. The level of aggressiveness with which atrial fibrillation should be treated varies depending on the patient's condition. **Direct-current synchronized cardioversion, without delay, is indicated in the**

setting of hypotension, severe heart failure, or intractable chest pain. In most cases, the initial treatment consists of slowing of the ventricular rate and identifying and, when possible, correcting the underlying cardiac or noncardiac disorder. **Preexcited atrial fibrillation resulting from anterograde rapid conduction down an accessory pathway SHOULD NOT be treated with atrioventricular blocking agents** as they may enhance conduction down the accessory pathway and precipitate hemodynamic decompensation or ventricular fibrillation. **In this setting, intravenous procainamide is the most appropriate pharmacologic agent as it impairs conduction down the accessory pathway.** Intravenous digoxin is somewhat effective for slowing the ventricular rate, but its maximal effect is achieved only after several hours. **Intravenous calcium channel blockers and beta-blockers** produce more rapid rate control and are considered **first-line therapies.** Verapamil and diltiazem are similar in atrioventricular nodal blocking effects. However, diltiazem is used more commonly because it is less negatively inotropic than verapamil and is available for continuous infusion. Intravenous beta-blockers can also affect prompt rate control, especially with esmolol, an ultra–fast-acting agent offering the greatest control in both initiation and termination of therapy. Another option for rate control is intravenous amiodarone. Its use should be reserved for cases in which standard atrioventricular nodal blocking agents or even cardioversion have failed to control the arrhythmia.

RX1 Table 3–6

DS1 Table 3–6

SE1 Table 3–6

TX2 **Long-term treatment:** Attempts should be made to cardiovert atrial fibrillation by pharmacologic or electrical means. In the absence of spontaneous conversion, cardioversion is generally performed without regard for anticoagulation status only if the duration of the atrial fibrillation is known to be less than 48 hours. For patients with atrial fibrillation believed to be greater than 48 hours or of unclear duration, anticoagulation with warfarin adjusted to an international normalized ratio of 2–3 for 3 weeks before and 4 weeks after cardioversion is recommended. An alternative technique is cardioversion guided by transesophageal echocardiography. In this technique, multiplane transesophageal echocardiography that indicates the absence of thrombus is associated with an extremely low rate of thromboembolism after cardioversion, provided that short-term anticoagulant therapy is used before and during the procedure and that warfarin is prescribed for 4 weeks (international normalized ratio, 2–3) following cardioversion (Fig. 3–2). Patients with atypical atrial flutter (Type II) are considered to have a similar risk for stroke as patients with atrial fibrillation. Early drug therapy to restore sinus rhythm can be considered in patients in whom the arrhythmia has lasted less than 48 hours or who are receiving long-term warfarin therapy. Digoxin is not effective in converting atrial fibrillation to sinus rhythm, but antiarrhythmic therapy increases the likelihood of conversion to as much as 90%, if the drugs are administered early and in adequate doses. If pharmacologic therapy is contemplated, continuous electrocardiographic monitoring during the first 48–72 hours after the
(text continues on page 34)

Table 3–6. Established Antiarrhythmic Agents

Class	Description	Generic (Brand) Name	Dose
IA	Decreases the rate of rise of AP (Phase 0) Decreases conduction and increases refractoriness	Disopyramide (Norpace, Norpace CR—*U.S.*; Rythmoden—*Can.*) [C]	100–150 mg PO qid or 200–300 mg controlled-release formulation PO bid
		Procainamide (Procanbid, Pronestyl) [C]	100 mg IV q5min (not to exceed 50 mg/min) until 1 g is given followed by a perfusion at 2–6 mg/min
		(Pronestyl SR—*U.S.*; Procan SR—*Can.*) [C]	1,000–2,000 mg PO bid
		Quinidine (Cardioquin, Quinidex—*U.S.*; Biquin Durules—*Can.*) [C]	0.5–1.25 g PO bid
IB	Decreases conduction	Lidocaine (Anestacon, Lidoderm, Xylocaine—*U.S.*; Xylocard—*Can.*) [C]	50–100 mg IV bolus followed by an infusion at 1–2 mg/min
		Mexiletine (Mexitil) [C]	200–400 mg PO tid
IC	Decreases conduction and increases refractoriness	Flecainide (Tambocor) [C]	50–150 mg PO bid

Side Effects	Contraindications and Cautions
Serious side effects: hypotension, CHF, hypokalemia Common side effects: related to cholinergic blockade	**Contraindications:** cardiogenic shock, preexisting second- and third-degree heart block, congenital QT syndrome, sick sinus syndrome
Serious side effects: hypotension, atrial fibrillation or flutter, hypokalemia, potentially fatal blood dyscrasias Common side effects: GI intolerance, drug-induced lupus erythematosus	**Contraindications:** complete heart block, second-degree AV block, SLE, torsade de pointes, QT prolongation, myasthenia gravis
Serious side effects: neutropenia Common side effects: fever, GI intolerance, drug-induced lupus erythematosus	**Contraindications:** thrombocytopenia, thrombocytopenic purpura, myasthenia gravis, heart block greater than first degree, idioventricular conduction delays, concurrent use of quinolone antibiotics, amprenavir or ritonavir
Serious side effects: bradycardia, hypotension, heart block, cardiac arrhythmias, bronchospasm, allergic reactions Common side effects: dizziness, tremor, drug-induced lupus erythematosus	**Contraindications:** severe degrees of SA, AV, or intraventricular heart block
Serious side effects: cardiac arrhythmias, hypotension, CHF, electrolyte disturbances Common side effects: lightheadedness, dizziness, nervousness, incoordination, GI intolerance, tremor, ataxia	**Contraindications:** cardiogenic shock, second- and third-degree AV block
Serious side effects: cardiac arrhythmias, hypokalemia Common side effects: dizziness, dyspnea, visual disturbances, headache, fever, GI intolerance, tremor	**Contraindications:** preexisting second- or third-degree AV block or with right bundle branch block when associated with a left hemiblock, cardiogenic shock, coronary artery disease, concurrent use of ritonavir or amprenavir **Caution** in patients with hepatic impairment.

(continued)

Table 3–6. Established Antiarrhythmic Agents *(Continued)*

Class	Description	Generic (Brand) Name	Dose
IC		Propafenone (Rythmol) [C]	150–300 mg PO bid
II	Beta-adrenoreceptor antagonist	Esmolol (Brevibloc) [C/D in second and third trimesters]	0.5 mg/kg IV, repeat if necessary; follow with infusion at 0.05 mg/kg/min and increasing as needed up to 0.2 mg/kg/min
		Metoprolol (Lopressor, Toprol—*U.S.*; Betaloc—*Can.*) [C/D in second and third trimesters]	5 mg IV bolus, repeated twice at q2min intervals
		Propranolol (Inderal—*U.S.*; Detensol—*Can.*) [C/D in second and third trimesters]	1–5 mg IV infused over 10 minutes

Side Effects	Contraindications and Cautions
Serious side effects: cardiac arrhythmias, angina, CHF, hypotension, blood dyscrasias, renal failure, nephritic syndrome Common side effects: dizziness, fatigue, headache, ataxia, insomnia, anxiety, GI intolerance, tremor, arthralgia, blurred vision, dyspnea	**Contraindications:** SA, AV, and intraventricular heart block; sinus bradycardia; cardiogenic shock; uncompensated cardiac failure; hypotension; bronchospasm; uncorrected electrolyte abnormalities; concurrent use of amprenavir, cimetidine, metoprolol, propranolol, quinidine, and ritonavir **Caution** in patients with hepatic impairment.
Serious side effects: hypotension (which responds to drug discontinuation), cardiac arrhythmias, extravasation (which can cause skin necrosis) Common side effects: diaphoresis, peripheral ischemia, dizziness, somnolence, confusion, headache, agitation, fatigue	**Contraindications:** heart block greater than first degree, cardiogenic shock, asthma, uncompensated cardiac failure, hypotension
Serious side effects: cardiac arrhythmias, CHF, blood dyscrasias, bronchospasm, hepatitis Common side effects: drowsiness, insomnia, decreased sexual ability, edema, reduced peripheral circulation	**Contraindications:** sinus bradycardia, heart block greater than first degree, cardiogenic shock, uncompensated cardiac failure; avoid abrupt discontinuation in CAD
Serious side effects: cardiac arrhythmias, cardiogenic shock, blood dyscrasias, bronchospasm, pulmonary edema Common side effects: mental depression, lightheadedness, confusion, hallucinations, dizziness, insomnia, fatigue, alopecia, impotence, drug-induced lupus erythematosus	**Contraindications:** uncompensated CHF, cardiogenic shock, bradycardia, second- and third-degree heart block, pulmonary edema, asthma, COPD, Raynaud's disease; avoid abrupt discontinuation in CAD **Caution** in patients with concurrent use of beta-blockers verapamil or diltiazem; caution in patients with hepatic impairment.

(continued)

Table 3–6. Established Antiarrhythmic Agents *(Continued)*

Class	Description	Generic (Brand) Name	Dose
III	Increases duration of AP Increases absolute and effective refractory period	Amiodarone (Cordarone, Pacerone) [D]	800–1,600 mg/day PO in divided doses for 1–3 weeks followed by 400 mg PO bid for 1 month followed by 200–400 mg PO qd or 150 mg IV infused over 10 minutes (15 mg/min) followed by 540 mg IV infused over 18 hours (at 0.5 mg/min); after the first 24 hours, continue infusion at 0.5 mg/min (720 mg infused over 24 hours)
		Dofetilide (Tikosyn) [C]	0.5 mg PO bid
		Ibutilide (Corvert) [C]	For patients weighing 60 kg: 1 mg IV infused over 10 minutes For patients weighing < 60 kg: 0.01 mg/kg IV infused over 10 minutes Dose can be repeated once after 10 minutes following initial administration
		Sotalol (Betapace—U.S.; Sotacor—Can.) [B]	80–160 mg PO bid

Side Effects	Contraindications and Cautions
Serious side effects: hypotension, CHF, cardiac arrhythmias, myocardial depression, coagulation abnormalities, pulmonary toxicity, allergic reactions Common side effects: fever, fatigue, involuntary movements, incoordination, malaise, sleep disturbances, ataxia, dizziness, headache, photosensitivity, GI intolerance, noninfectious epididymitis, visual disturbances	**Contraindications:** severe sinus node dysfunction, second- and third-degree heart block, bradycardia **Caution** in patients with concurrent use of ritonavir, sparfloxacin, moxifloxacin, gatifloxacin; caution in patients with thyroid or liver disease.
Serious side effects: cardiac arrhythmias, hypertension Common side effects: headache, dizziness, insomnia, GI intolerance, dyspnea, cough, anxiety Adjust dose downward for patients with renal disease. **Hospitalization for initiation is mandatory.**	**Contraindications:** paroxysmal atrial fibrillation; congenital or acquired long QT syndromes; severe renal impairment; concurrent use with verapamil, cimetidine, trimethoprim (alone or in combination with sulfamethoxazole), ketoconazole, prochlorperazine or megestrol, amiodarone, or other drugs that prolong QT intervals (phenothiazines, bepridil, tricyclic antidepressants, sparfloxacin, gatifloxacin, moxifloxacin); hypokalemia or hypomagnesemia
Serious side effects: cardiac arrhythmias, renal failure, hypertension Common side effects: headache, palpitations	**Contraindications:** hypokalemia, hyperkalemia, hypomagnesemia, prolonged QT interval
Serious side effects: cardiac arrhythmias, electrolyte disturbances, CHF, hypotension Common side effects: confusion, anxiety, headache, insomnia, depression, decreased sexual ability, GI intolerance, paresthesia, visual problems, asthma	**Contraindications:** asthma; sinus bradycardia; second- and third-degree AV block; congenital or acquired long QT syndromes; cardiogenic shock; uncontrolled CHF; renal failure; concurrent use with gatifloxacin, moxifloxacin, or sparfloxacin

(continued)

Table 3-6. Established Antiarrhythmic Agents *(Continued)*

Class	Description	Generic (Brand) Name	Dose
IV	Decreases inward calcium^{2+} current	Diltiazem (Cardizem, Dilacor, Tiamate, Tiazac) [C]	IV formulation: 20 mg IV bolus followed, if necessary, by 25 mg IV bolus after 15 minutes from initial administration Maintenance infusion: 5–15 mg/hr Oral CR formulation: 180–300 mg PO qd
		Verapamil (Calan, Isoptin, Verelan) [C]	5–10 mg IV infused over 2–3 minutes; repeat in 30 minutes SR formulation: 120–240 mg PO qd–bid
Miscellaneous		Adenosine (Adenocard, Adenoscan) [C]	Must be administered within 1–2 seconds to be effective: 6 mg IV bolus followed, if necessary, by 12 mg IV bolus given 1–2 minutes after initial administration Daily dose: 0.125–0.5 mg IV
		Digoxin (Lanoxin) [C]	1–1.5 mg IV infused over 24 hours or 0.25–0.5 mg PO bid–tid
		Magnesium sulfate [B]	2 g IV infused over 1–2 minutes followed by an infusion of 3–20 mg/min

AP = action potential; AV = atrioventricular; CAD = coronary artery disease; CHF = congestive heart failure; CNS = central nervous system; COPD = chronic obstructive pulmonary disease; CR =

Side Effects	Contraindications and Cautions
Serious side effects: cardiac arrhythmias, blood dyscrasias, allergic reactions Common side effects: gingival hyperplasia, dizziness, headache, somnolence, insomnia, GI intolerance	**Contraindications:** sick sinus syndrome, second- or third-degree AV block, hypotension, acute MI, pulmonary congestion
Serious side effects: CHF, cardiac arrhythmias, angina, MI, bronchospasm; causes elevation in digoxin level Common side effects: gingival hyperplasia, dizziness, fatigue, headache, GI intolerance, dyspnea	**Contraindications:** severe left ventricular dysfunction, hypotension, cardiogenic shock, sick sinus syndrome, second- or third-degree AV block, atrial flutter or fibrillation, an accessory bypass tract (e.g., WPW, Lown-Ganong-Levine syndrome)
Serious side effects: cardiac arrhythmias, hypotension, bronchospasm, elevated intracranial pressure, hyperventilation Common side effects: palpitations, headache, dyspnea, diaphoresis, dizziness, paresthesia, numbness	**Contraindications:** asthma, second- or third-degree AV block, sick sinus syndrome, atrial flutter or fibrillation, ventricular tachycardia (note that adenosine is **not** effective in converting these arrhythmias to sinus rhythm)
Serious side effects: cardiac arrhythmias, blood dyscrasias, intestinal ischemia Common side effects: visual disturbances, headache, weakness, dizziness, confusion, anxiety, depression, delirium, hallucinations, fever, rash, edema, alopecia, GI intolerance, gynecomastia, sexual dysfunction, diaphoresis	**Contraindications:** hypersensitivity to cardiac glycosides, ventricular tachycardia or fibrillation, idiopathic hypertrophic subaortic stenosis, constrictive pericarditis, amyloid disease, second- or third-degree heart block, WPW syndrome, atrial fibrillation **Caution** in use in recent MI (within 6 months).
Serious side effects: hypotension and asystole, especially with rapid administration, CNS depression, complete heart block, respiratory paralysis Common side effects: diarrhea, blocked peripheral neuromuscular transmission	**Contraindications:** heart block, renal impairment, myocardial damage, hepatitis, Addison's disease **Toxicity (serum level > 4 mEq/L):** depressed deep tendon reflexes, respiratory depression **Treatment:** calcium gluconate (calcium 5–10 mEq) 1–2 g IV, and, in extreme cases, peritoneal dialysis or hemodialysis may be required

controlled release; GI = gastrointestinal; MI = myocardial infarction; SA = sinoatrial; SLE = systemic lupus erythematosus; SR = slow release; WPW = Wolff-Parkinson-White.

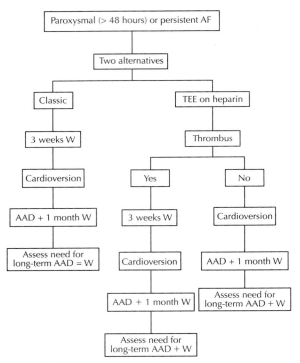

AF: atrial fibrillation, TEE: transesophageal echocardiogram, W: warfarin, AAD: antiarrhythmic drug.

FIGURE 3–2 Long-term therapy of atrial fibrillation.

initiation of antiarrhythmic therapy should be considered. Proarrhythmia is rarely seen in patients without structural heart disease. Ibutilide is the only intravenous agent labeled for acute conversion of atrial fibrillation. Oral loading of Class IC agents such as flecainide (300 mg) or propafenone (600 mg) is associated with high conversion rates for atrial fibrillation of recent (< 7 days) onset in patients without heart failure. Similar degrees of efficacy in maintaining sinus rhythm are observed with Class IA, Class IC, and Class III agents, although there is evidence that efficacy is superior with amiodarone than with other agents. Antiarrhythmic drug therapy seems to double the probability of maintaining sinus rhythm after cardioversion and should be started before electrical cardioversion to prevent the early recurrence of atrial fibrillation. The choice of antiarrhythmic drug for long-term maintenance of sinus rhythm depends on the presence or absence of left ventricular dysfunction and coronary artery disease (Table 3–7). Long-term antiarrhythmic drug therapy of atrial flutter is similar to that of atrial fibrillation. With Class IC agents, the atrial flutter rate may be slowed, thus facilitating conduction across the atrioventricular node. This may result in a ventricular rate that is faster than the 2:1 block rate seen before initiation of antiarrhythmic drug therapy and in a widening of the QRS owing to the rate-dependent effect of these drugs on ventricular muscle. Thus, atrioventricular blocking agents should also be administered to prevent rapid ventricular conduction when Class IC agents are used. Most typical atrial flutters (Type I) encountered in clinical practice are amenable to catheter mapping and ablation.

RX2 Table 3–6 and Table 3–7

DS2 Table 3–6

SE2 Table 3–6

Bradyarrhythmias

KY **Impairment of conduction** may range from delayed transmission of the atrial impulse to the ventricles **(first-degree atrioventricular block)** to intermittent failure of impulse transmission **(second-degree atrioventricular block)** to complete conduction failure **(third-degree atrioventricular block). Bradycardia** may also be caused by an absence of impulse generation within the sinus node or block of impulse conduction within perinodal atrial tissue owing to fibrosis or ischemia (Table 3–8).

Table 3–7. Long-term Therapy of Atrial Fibrillation

Generic (Brand) Name	Left Ventricular Function		Coronary Artery Disease or Previous Myocardial Infarction
	Normal	Reduced	
Amiodarone (Cordarone, Pacerone) [D]	Yes	Yes	Yes
Disopyramide (Norpace —U.S.; Rythmodan —Can.) [C]	Yes	No	No
Dofetilide (Tikosyn) [C]	Yes	Yes	Yes
Flecainide (Tambocor) [C]	Yes	No	No
Propafenone (Rythmol) [C]	Yes	No	No
Quinidine (Cardioquin, Quinaglute Dura-Tabs, Quinidex Extentabs —U.S.; Biquin Durules —Can.) [C]	Yes	No	No
Sotalol (Betapace—U.S.; Sotacor—Can.) [B]	Yes	No	Yes

TX Table 3–8

RX Table 3–6 and Table 3–8

DS Table 3–6 and Table 3–8

SE Table 3–6 and Table 3–8

Supraventricular Tachycardia

KY Supraventricular tachycardia is defined as any tachyarrhythmia that requires atrial or atrioventricular junctional tissue for its initiation and maintenance. Reentrant excitation caused by unidirectional conduction block in one region of the heart and slow conduction in another seems to be the mechanism of initiation of most cases of paroxysmal supraventricular tachycardia.

TX1 **Acute treatment:** If vagal maneuvers do not terminate a regular supraventricular tachycardia of recent onset, initial pharmacologic therapy should be directed toward blocking atrioventricular nodal conduction. Adenosine exerts effects that are apparent within 15–30 seconds (Fig. 3–3).

Table 3–8. Classification and Management of Heart Block

Classification of Heart Block	Etiology
First degree (PR interval longer than 0.2 seconds in adults or longer than 0.18 seconds in children)	Conduction disturbance at the level of the AV node. Narrow QRS: AV nodal delay Wide QRS: Infranodal delay
Second degree (Intermittent failure of the atrial impulse to be conducted to the ventricles)	
Type 1 (Wenckebach or Mobitz Type I)	Conduction disturbance at the level of the AV node. Gradual PR interval prolongation leading to failure of atrial impulse conduction to the ventricles. Narrow QRS: AV nodal delay Wide QRS: Infranodal delay
Type 2 (Mobitz Type II)	Abrupt failure of an atrial impulse (usually several atrial impulses) to be conducted to the ventricles. No change in PR interval duration before or following the pause.
Third degree	Complete failure of atrial impulse conduction to the ventricles. The cardiac rhythm depends on subsidiary pacemakers located within the His bundle (narrow QRS complex) or its more distal ramifications (wide QRS).

AV = atrioventricular.

However, because of its extremely short elimination half-life, its effects typically disappear within 10–20 seconds. The calcium channel blockers verapamil and diltiazem, when given intravenously, are also useful in terminating supraventricular tachycardia. Verapamil has a longer duration of action than adenosine. Although this may be an advantage in preventing the immediate recurrence of tachycardia, verapamil can cause hypotension. **Adenosine and calcium channel blockers should not be given to patients with preexcitation who have atrial fibrillation with an anterogradely conducting accessory pathway** since blocking atrioventricular nodal conduction will promote increased conduction down the accessory pathway, which leads to an increase in the ventricular rate and hemodynamic collapse.

RX1 Table 3–6

DS1 Table 3–6

SE1 Table 3–6

Treatment

Reversal of block following atropine, exercise. Drug effects are a common cause of this conduction disturbance (digoxin, beta-blockers, calcium channel blockers). Rarely requires implantation of a permanent pacemaker.

Reversal of block following atropine, exercise.

Drug effects are a common cause of conduction disturbance (digoxin, beta-blockers, calcium channel blockers).

May require implantation of a permanent pacemaker.

Usually associated with significant underlying conduction system disease (bundle branch block or bifascicular block) and has a greater propensity for the subsequent development of complete AV block.

Usually requires implantation of a permanent pacemaker.

In the setting of acute inferior wall myocardial infarction, AV block usually disappears, and its transient occurrence has no adverse long-term prognostic implication. In the setting of an anterior wall myocardial infarction, transient or fixed complete AV block is associated with a poor prognosis owing to the magnitude of ventricular damage. In congenital complete heart block, a permanent pacemaker is required when patients become symptomatic. Otherwise, all patients require implantation of a permanent pacemaker.

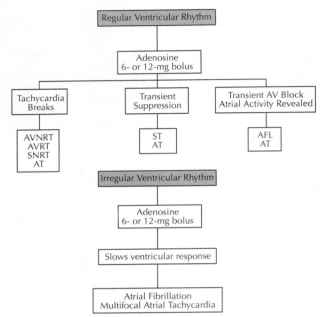

AV: atrioventricular, AVNRT: atrioventricular nodal reentrant tachycardia, AVRT:
Atrioventricular reentrant tachycardia, SNRT: sinus node reentrant tachycardia,
AT: atrial tachycardia, ST: sinus tachycardia, AFL: atrial flutter.

FIGURE 3–3 Narrow complex tachycardia.

TX2 **Long-term treatment:** Long-term therapy for patients with supraventricular tachycardia is shown in Table 3–9. Asymptomatic patients with
Wolff-Parkinson-White Syndrome have an incidence of sudden death of
about 0.1% per patient-year. Intervention may be appropriate for selected
asymptomatic persons in high-risk occupations.

RX2 Table 3–6 and Table 3–9

DS2 Table 3–6

SE2 Table 3–6

Ventricular Arrhythmias and Sudden Cardiac Death

KY **Ventricular tachycardia** is defined as at least three successive ventricular ectopic beats at a rate of 100 bpm or greater and a wide QRS complex (> 0.14 msec). Ventricular tachycardia is considered to be nonsustained if it lasts for more than 3 beats but less than 30 seconds and does

Table 3–9. **Long-term Therapy of Supraventricular Tachycardia**

Tachycardia	First Choice	Second Choice
Atrioventricular nodal reentrant tachycardia Atrioventricular reentrant tachycardia	Beta-blockers Calcium channel blockers Digoxin [C]	Radiofrequency catheter ablation
Multifocal atrial tachycardia	Calcium channel blockers Beta-blockers Digoxin [C]	—
Sinus node reentrant tachycardia	Beta-blockers Calcium channel blockers Digoxin [C] Flecainide [C] Propafenone [C] Sotalol [B]	Radiofrequency catheter ablation
Unifocal atrial tachycardia 　Reentrant	Flecainide [C] Propafenone [C] Sotalol [B]	Radiofrequency catheter ablation
Automatic	Beta-blockers Calcium channel blockers Digoxin [C]	Radiofreqency catheter ablation
Wolff-Parkinson-White Syndrome	Radiofrequency catheter ablation	Flecainide [C] Propafenone [C] Sotalol [B]

not require intervention for termination. Ventricular tachycardia lasting more than 30 seconds or requiring intervention for termination is defined as sustained. Ventricular tachycardia can be of uniform morphology (monomorphic) or of varying morphology on a beat-to-beat basis (polymorphic). **Sudden cardiac death** is heralded by the abrupt loss of consciousness and has been defined as unexpected natural death from a cardiac cause occurring over a short period, generally less than 1 hour from the onset of symptoms. The presence of premature ventricular contractions does not predict subsequent sudden cardiac death in patients without structural heart disease. In contrast, the presence of premature ventricular contractions or nonsustained ventricular tachycardia in patients with structural heart disease, especially those with substantially reduced left ventricular function or a myocardial scar, is associated with an increased risk of sudden cardiac death. Sustained ventricular tachycardia in association with chronic coronary artery disease and a healed MI with or without a left ventricular aneurysm is the most common ventricular tachycardia encountered. The underlying mechanism is reentry facilitated by an area of slow conduction and streaks of fibrosis that provide anatomic obstacles.

TX1 **Acute treatment:** The level of aggressiveness with which ventricular tachycardia should be treated depends on the patient's symptoms and hemodynamic implications of the arrhythmia. Patients who are hemodynamically unstable, in pulmonary edema, or in unstable angina should be promptly cardioverted back to sinus rhythm with a **direct-current, synchronized shock. A thorough search for acute reversible arrhythmogenic triggers** such as electrolyte abnormalities, hypoxemia, drug toxicity (e.g., tricyclic antidepressants, phenothiazines, digoxin, antiarrhythmic drugs, amphetamines, phencyclidine, alcohol ingestion or withdrawal), metabolic disorders (hypomagnesemia, hypocalcemia, hypokalemia), and ischemia should be initiated. Adenosine may be administered to differentiate ventricular tachycardia from other causes of a wide complex tachycardia (Fig. 3–4). **First-line therapy for hemodynamically stable ventricular tachycardia is the administration of lidocaine or procainamide.** Lidocaine is more effective in acute myocardial ischemia, whereas procainamide seems to be more effective for chronic paroxysmal scar–related ventricular tachycardia. If unsuccessful in slowing or converting the arrhythmia to normal sinus rhythm, intravenous amiodarone can be used, or the patient should be cardioverted electrically. Rarely, patients may present with incessant, sustained ventricular tachycardia that fails to respond to intravenous antiarrhythmic therapy and, if cardioverted, tends to recur after a few sinus beats. Factors associated with refractory ventricular tachycardia include electrolyte abnormalities (especially hypomagnesemia), digitalis toxicity, acute myocardial ischemia, reperfusion arrhythmias, proarrhythmia, or torsade de pointes. **Magnesium sulfate** may be effective in suppressing the arrhythmia even if the serum magnesium level is within the normal range. **Intravenous beta-blockers** and **amiodarone** may also be required. **Overdrive pacing** may also be effective in terminating and suppressing the arrhythmia.

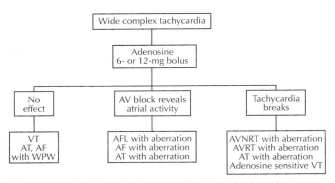

AV: atrioventricular, VT: ventricular tachycardia, AT: atrial tachycardia, AF: atrial fibrillation, WPW: Wolff-Parkinson White syndrome, AFL: atrial flutter, AVNRT: atrioventricular nodal reentrant tachycardia, AVRT: atrioventicular reentrant tachycardia.

FIGURE 3–4 Wide complex tachycardia.

RX1 Table 3–6

DS1 Table 3–6

SE1 Table 3–6

TX2 **Long-term treatment:** Antiarrhythmic therapy with d,1-sotalol, amiodarone, and implantable cardioverter defibrillators are treatments applied to nonsustained ventricular tachycardia (Fig. 3–5), sustained ventricular tachycardia (Fig. 3–6), and aborted sudden cardiac death (Fig. 3–7). In patients receiving an implantable cardioverter defibrillator, a significant proportion will also require concomitant antiarrhythmic drug therapy to reduce the frequency of ventricular arrhythmias that trigger shock therapy, alter the rate of the ventricular tachycardia to enhance antitachycardia pacing efficacy, or suppress supraventricular arrhythmias.

RX2 Table 3–6, Table 3–10, and Table 3–11

DS2 Table 3–6

SE2 Table 3–6

CHRONIC ISCHEMIC HEART DISEASE

KY Vascular endothelial injury is a major inciting event in the formation of atherosclerosis. The earliest manifestation of atherosclerosis is endothelial dysfunction, and it reflects a functional defect rather than a physical one. Over time, repetitive injury leads to the accumulation of lipids and macrophages and eventually the genesis of an atherosclerotic plaque. Abnormal stimulation from damaged endothelial cells leads to the migration and

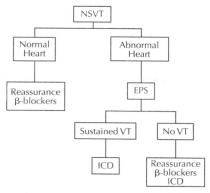

NSVT: nonsustained ventricular tachycardia, EPS: electrophysiologic study, VT: ventricular tachycardia, ICD: implantable cardioverter defibrillator.

FIGURE 3–5 Long-term therapy of non-sustained ventricular arrhythmias (NSVT).

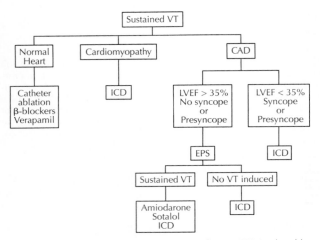

VT: ventricular tachycardia, CAD: coronary artery disease, ICD: implantable cardioverter defibrillator, LVEF: left ventricular ejection fraction, EPS: electrophysiological study.

FIGURE 3–6 Long-term therapy of ventricular arrhythmias.

proliferation of smooth muscle cells along the intima. The resulting lesion consists of a fibrointimal cap with a lipid-rich core. Continued injury to the intima may lead to plaque rupture, thrombus formation, and initiation of an acute coronary syndrome. Major risk factors for coronary artery disease include advanced age, male sex, a family history of premature coronary artery disease, smoking, diabetes mellitus, hypertension, and hyperlipidemia.

TX Pharmacotherapy of angina alleviates symptoms by either increasing the myocardial oxygen supply or decreasing the myocardial oxygen demand (Fig. 3–8). **All patients with coronary heart disease should have**

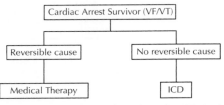

VF: ventricular fibrillation, VT: ventricular tachycardia, ICD: implantable cardioverter defibrillator.

FIGURE 3–7 Long-term therapy of ventricular arrhythmias.

Table 3–10. Summary of Angiotensin Receptor Blockers

Generic (Brand) Name	Dose	Side Effects and Contraindications
Losartan (Cozaar) [C/D in second and third trimesters]	50–100 mg PO qd	Serious side effects: angioedema, hypotension
Valsartan (Diovan) [C/D in second and third trimesters]	40–160 mg PO tid	Common side effect: dizziness **Contraindications:** hyperaldosteronism, hyperkalemia, pregnancy, renal artery stenosis **Caution** in patients with chronic renal failure.

aggressive treatment of their cardiac risk factors. Drugs available for the treatment of chronic ischemic heart disease are shown in Table 3–3. For patients with chronic coronary artery disease whose symptoms do not improve with medical therapy or those considered at high risk for future cardiac events, revascularization therapy, whether bypass surgery or angioplasty, should be strongly considered (Fig. 3–9).

RX1 **Acetylsalicylic acid (aspirin)** [C/D in third trimester]: **Has been shown to prevent future coronary events in patients who have suffered an MI.** Its use is advocated for all patients with established symptomatic coronary artery disease.

DS1 Table 3–3

SE1 Table 3–3

or

RX2 **Clopidogrel** (Plavix) [B]: Effective substitute in patients intolerant or allergic to acetylsalicylic acid.

DS2 Table 3–3

Table 3–11. Summary of Beta-Blockers Used in Heart Failure

Generic (Brand) Name	Dose	Side Effects and Contraindications
Carvedilol (Coreg) [C/D in second and third trimesters]	3.125–25 mg PO bid	Serious side effects: heart failure, bronchospasm
Bisoprolol (Zebeta—*U.S.*; Monocor—*Can.*) [C/D in second and third trimesters]	1.25–10 mg PO qd	Common side effects: fatigue, impotence, decreased libido, nightmares, depression **Contraindicated** in patients with asthma, decompensated heart failure, significant
Metoprolol (Lopressor, Toprol—*U.S.*; Betaloc —*Can.*) [C/D in second and third trimesters]	25–100 mg PO qd	heart block, bradycardia, and hypotension.

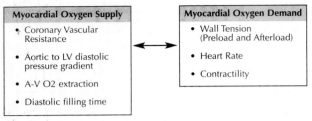

LV: left ventricle, A-V O2: arterio-venous oxygen.

FIGURE 3–8 Determinants of cardiac ischemia; balance between myocardial oxygen supply and demand.

SE2 Table 3–3

with or without

RX3 Ramipril (Altace) [C/D in second and third trimesters]: an ACE inhibitor found to decrease future cardiac events in patients with established cardiovascular disease.

DS3 Table 3–3

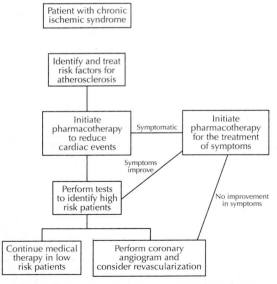

FIGURE 3–9 Management of chronic ischemic heart disease.

SE3 Table 3–3

with or without

RX4 **Beta-blockers:** These agents decrease myocardial oxygen demand by decreasing heart rate, myocardial wall tension, and myocardial contractility. These agents are essential therapy in patients with symptomatic stable coronary artery disease, particularly if they also suffer from hypertension.

DS4 Table 3–3

SE4 Table 3–3

with or without

RX5 **Nitrates:** Vasodilators that act primarily on smooth muscle cells of the media in capacitance vessels. This vasodilation of the venous vasculature (preload) leads to a reduction in left ventricular wall tension that in turn diminishes myocardial oxygen demand. To a lesser extent, nitrates also relieve angina by improving myocardial oxygen supply by dilating coronary arteries. However, with prolonged exposure, tolerance to their effects usually develops. Nitrates are the most commonly used agents in the treatment of angina. Nitrates are available as short-acting preparations for the relief of pain from acute anginal episodes and as longer-acting preparations for angina prevention.

DS5 Table 3–3

SE5 Table 3–3

with or without

RX6 **Calcium channel blockers:** Not all calcium channel blockers improve symptoms of angina by the same mechanism. Verapamil and diltiazem decrease myocardial oxygen demand by decreasing heart rate and contractility with lesser affects on afterload reduction. Nifedipine and amlodipine act primarily as afterload reducing agents and may also improve myocardial oxygen supply by causing coronary vasodilation.

DS6 Table 3–3

SE6 Table 3–3

HEART FAILURE

KY Heart failure is the result of an inability of the heart to effectively pump blood at the body's required metabolic needs or to do so at only a higher filling pressure. The cascade of events leading to overt heart failure is initiated by myocyte injury. This leads to cardiac remodeling and a reduction in ventricular systolic function. Chronic congestive heart failure is a clinical syndrome characterized by signs and symptoms of volume overload as well as reduced exercise tolerance. Patients with congestive heart failure present with exertional dyspnea, fatigue, orthopnea, paroxysmal nocturnal dyspnea, and leg swelling. Heart failure severity may be assessed using the New York Heart Association functional classification. This classification is useful for predicting patient survival and therefore dictates patient therapy (Table 3–12).

Table 3–12. The New York Heart Association Functional Classification

Class	Symptoms	2-Year Mortality Rate
I	No limitation of physical activity Minimally symptomatic	10%
II	Slight limitation of physical activity No symptoms at rest Regular physical activity results in fatigue, palpitations, dyspnea, or anginal pain	20%
III	Marked limitation of physical activity No symptoms at rest Less than regular physical activity causes fatigue, palpitations, dyspnea, or anginal pain	30%–40%
IV	Inability to perform any physical activity Symptoms at rest Any physical activity worsens symptoms, including dyspnea and anginal pain	40%–50%

TX **The most important initial step in the management heart failure is to establish the cause and to correct the underlying disease before more myocardial injury and remodeling occurs.** In the case of coronary artery disease, this would require control of ischemic risk factors and often leads to consideration for coronary angiography and coronary revascularization. The goals of drug therapy in heart failure are to improve patient symptoms and to prolong survival. Heart failure medications achieve these goals by increasing contractility, decreasing preload, decreasing afterload, decreasing the incidence of life-threatening arrhythmias, and interfering with cardiac remodeling. **Most calcium channel blockers are contraindicated in patients with heart failure because they reduce survival and exacerbate symptoms.** The only agents with equivalent results compared with placebo were amlodipine and felodipine. Currently, calcium channel blockers should only be used to treat resistant hypertension in patients with heart failure whose blood pressure is not controlled by ACE inhibitors and beta-blockers.

RX1 **Angiotensin-converting enzyme (ACE) inhibitors:** Should be considered as **first-line therapy in all patients with heart failure.** They are potent vasodilators of both the arterial and venous vasculature and as such improve both the pulmonary congestion and the reduced cardiac output seen in heart failure. Renal blood flow is also augmented by ACE inhibitors, which, in turn, leads to less sodium and water retention. Independent from their effects on hemodynamics, ACE inhibitors impede remodeling owing to their antihypertrophic properties. The ACE inhibitors are also anti-ischemic agents. Consequently, preventing a future MI would also prevent further deterioration in ventricular function. **Five ACE inhibitors have been approved for the treatment of heart failure: captopril, enalapril, lisinopril, quinapril, and ramipril.**

DS1 Table 3–3 and Table 3–5

SE1 Table 3–3 and Table 3–5

or

RX2 **Angiotensin receptor blockers: Considered second-line agents,** especially when patients are intolerant to ACE inhibitors. Angiotensin receptor blockers impede angiotensin II, a potent vasoconstrictor and the signaling molecule for aldosterone secretion. In contrast to ACE inhibitors, these agents do not influence the bradykinin pathway believed to be responsible for dry cough.

DS2 Table 3–10

SE2 Table 3–10

with or without

RX3 **Beta-blockers:** To improve symptoms and survival in patients with heart failure. Believed to block excessive and most likely myocyte toxic levels of norepinephrine as well as reduce the frequency of malignant arrhythmias. Current recommendations include the use of beta-blockers in patients with class II or III heart failure. Discontinue therapy if the patient's condition deteriorates.

DS3 Table 3–11

SE3 Table 3–11

with or without

RX4 **Digoxin** (Lanoxin) [C]: A positive inotropic agent that has been shown to improve cardiac output and lower filling pressure. **Improves symptoms but not survival.** It is recommended in all patients with congestive heart failure with atrial fibrillation and for patients whose symptoms are not controlled with ACE inhibitor monotherapy.

DS4 0.0625 mg PO every other day to 0.25 mg PO qd

SE4 Digoxin toxicity can induce arrhythmias, which can be treated with lidocaine or phenytoin. **Contraindicated in patients with ventricular fibrillation.** The recommended dose for digoxin decreases with advanced age and is **contraindicated in patients with advanced renal failure.** Dose should be adjusted downward in patients who are taking verapamil, amiodarone, quinidine, or propafenone.

with or without

RX5 **Furosemide** (Lasix) [C]: A loop diuretic that inhibits sodium reabsorption in the ascending loop of Henle. It improves the pulmonary congestion seen in patients with heart failure, but studies have failed to show an impact on morbidity and mortality rates. Its use should be reserved for patients whose congestive symptoms do not respond to ACE inhibitor and digoxin therapy.

DS5 20–120 mg PO 1–2 times/day

SE5 Volume depletion and hypokalemia.

with or without

RX6 **Metolazone** (Zaroxolyn) [B–D]: This thiazide diuretic prevents reabsorption of sodium in the distal nephron that potentiates the effects of furosemide. When the dose of furosemide exceeds 120 mg qd, then the addition of metolazone should be considered.

DS6 2.5–10 mg PO one-half hour before the dose of furosemide

SE6 The volume status and the serum electrolytes should be carefully monitored.

or

RX7 **Ethacrynic acid** (Edecrin) [B]: A loop diuretic that inhibits sodium reabsorption in the ascending loop of Henle. In patients who are allergic to furosemide, ethacrynic acid is a suitable alternative loop diuretic.

DS7 50–200 mg PO 1–2 times/day

SE7 Volume depletion and hypokalemia.

or

RX8 **Spironolactone** (Aldactone) [D]: Spironolactone is a potassium-sparing diuretic that has been shown to be of benefit in patients with advanced

Table 3–13. Pharmacologic Treatment of Hyperlipidemia

Class	Generic (Brand) Name	Dose
Bile acid resins	Cholestyramine resin (Questran) [C]	4 g PO bid–qid (maximum 24 g/day)
	Colestipol (Colestid) [C]	5 g PO qd–tid (maximum 30 g/day)
Fibrates	Bezafibrate (Bezalip)*	400 mg PO qd
	Fenofibrate (Tricor—*U.S.*; Lipidil—*Can.*)* [C]	100–200 mg PO qd
	Gemfibrozil (Lopid) [C]	600 mg PO bid
HMG-CoA reductase inhibitors (statins)	Atorvastatin (Lipitor) [X]	10–80 mg PO qhs
	Fluvastatin (Lescol) [X]	10–40 mg PO qhs
	Lovastatin (Mevacor) [X]	10–40 mg PO qhs
	Pravastatin (Pravachol) [X]	10–40 mg PO qhs
	Simvastatin (Zocor) [X]	10–40 mg PO qhs
Nicotinic acid	Niacin (Niacor, Niaspan, Nicolar, Nicotinex) PO [A/C at doses > 6 g/day	Start with 250 mg PO qd, then increase to 1–2 g tid (maximum 6 g/day)

LDL = low-density lipoprotein; VLDL = very low-density lipoprotein; HDL = high-density lipoprotein; HMG-CoA = hydroxymethyl glutaryl coenzyme A; CK = creatine kinase.
*Available in Canada.

heart failure. It reduces mortality rates by 25% in class III and IV heart failure. **Its use should only be considered in patients with advanced heart failure who remain symptomatic despite aggressive treatment of their condition with the drug therapy described previously.**

DS8 25 mg PO qd

SE8 Patients should be warned of possible gynecomastia (1%–2%). Spironolactone is **contraindicated in patients with hyperkalemia. Potassium levels should be monitored carefully, particularly when spironolactone is used in combination with ACE inhibitor therapy.**

with

RX9 **Warfarin** (Coumadin) [D]: Chronic anticoagulation is recommended for patients with heart failure in atrial fibrillation as well as those with systolic dysfunction and a previous cardioembolic event.

DS9 See Ch 9 Hematology.

SE9 See Ch 9 Hematology.

Mechanism of Action	Side Effects and Contraindications
Increases bile acid secretion Increases hepatic LDL receptors Reduces LDL by 15%	Serious side effect: fecal impaction Common side effects: gastrointestinal complaints **Contraindication:** biliary obstruction
Decreases VLDL synthesis Increases VLDL hydrolysis Reduces triglycerides by 30% Reduces LDL by 10% Increases HDL by 10%	Serious side effects: myelosuppression, hepatitis, myositis (particularly with concomitant statin administration) Common side effects: gastrointestinal complaints **Caution** with impaired renal or liver function and with concomitant statin therapy.
Inhibits cholesterol production Increases LDL receptors Reduces LDL 25%–50% Increases HDL 5%–10%	Serious side effects: rhabdomyolysis and hepatotoxicity (serial CK and liver enzyme testing recommended), myositis Common side effects: gastrointestinal complaints, myalgias, muscle weakness **Contraindications:** active liver disease, pregnancy, lactating patients
Increases HDL production Decreases production and increases clearance of LDL and VLDL particles Raises HDL by 15% Lowers triglycerides by 20% Lowers LDL by 30%	Common side effects: flushing (may be prevented with aspirin 325 mg PO 1 hour before each dose of niacin), pruritus, hepatitis, peptic ulcers, hyperglycemia **Contraindications:** active liver disease, active peptic ulcer **Caution** in patients with diabetes mellitus.

HYPERLIPIDEMIA

KY Dietary lipids can be divided into cholesterol and triglycerides. Metabolized in the gut and transported to blood, they become associated with hydrophilic proteins owing to their insolubility in aqueous solutions. The resultant product is termed a lipoprotein. There are **four types of circulating lipoproteins:** high-density lipoproteins (HDLs), low-density lipoproteins (LDLs), very low-density lipoproteins (VLDLs), and chylomicrons. Both HDLs and LDLs are mainly involved in cholesterol metabolism, whereas VLDLs and chylomicrons are involved in triglyceride metabolism. **Any alteration in the production or elimination of these lipoproteins has been established as a major risk factor for the development of coronary artery disease.**

TX Secondary causes of hyperlipidemia should be sought and ruled out, including familial dyslipidemias, diabetes mellitus, thyroid disease, renal disease, excessive alcohol consumption, liver disease, pregnancy, and medications (e.g., diuretics). Patients with hyperlipidemia should be on a low-fat, low-cholesterol diet consisting of less than 30% of total calories being derived from total fat and less than 200 mg of cholesterol daily. They should also be involved in regular aerobic exercise, and patients who smoke should be advised to quit. Less than 20% of patients with coronary artery disease will achieve established cholesterol-lowering guidelines without pharmacotherapy. Thus, a combination of both pharmacologic and nonpharmacologic therapy is required in most patients at risk for or with established coronary artery disease. **The four classes of drug therapy for hyperlipidemia include** hydroxymethyl glutaryl coenzyme A reductase inhibitors (statins), fibric acid derivatives (fibrates), bile acid resins (resins), and nicotinic acid (niacin) (Table 3–13 on page 49). **The choice of a particular class of lipid-lowering agent depends on the patient's cholesterol profile.** In general, patients with elevated LDL levels benefit from initiation of a statin. Patients with elevated triglyceride levels and moderately elevated LDL levels may benefit more from fibrate therapy. Finally, niacin could be considered first-line therapy in patients with low HDL levels. In some instances, combination therapy may be necessary to achieve recommended target cholesterol levels.

RX Table 3–13

DS Table 3–13

SE Table 3–13

4

Dermatology

ARNON M. KATZ

This chapter focuses on the most commonly encountered dermatologic conditions. The treatment of sexually transmitted diseases is covered in Ch 8 Gynecology and Ch 22 Urology. Malignancies are not discussed here because treatment usually involves surgical resection.

ABSCESSES, FURUNCLES, AND CARBUNCLES

KY Individuals who carry *Staphylococcus aureus* have a higher probability of developing abscesses, furuncles, or carbuncles. In addition, people with diabetes, obesity, or poor hygiene habits are more likely to carry *S. aureus* in their nares, axillae, perineum, or bowel. In such contexts, furunculosis may be recurrent.

TX Surgical drainage is usually adequate treatment. To achieve healing, topical or systemic antibiotics that target *S. aureus* may be necessary.

RX **Cloxacillin sodium** (Cloxapen) [B]

DS 250–500 mg PO qid for 7–10 days

SE Nausea, diarrhea, and abdominal pain; **hypersensitivity,** including immediate and delayed **allergic reactions; antibiotic-associated pseudomembranous colitis;** and **interstitial nephritis** that does not seem to be dose related and can be reversible on discontinuation of drug. **Hematologic disorders** (eosinophilia, hemolytic anemia, agranulocytosis, neutropenia, leukopenia, granulocytopenia, thrombocytopenia, and bone marrow suppression) and **hepatotoxicity** have also been described.

CANDIDIASIS (CANDIDAL PARONYCHIA, INTERTRIGO, MUCOSAL CANDIDIASIS, VULVITIS)

KY *Candida albicans* is a part of the normal flora of the oral mucosa and the gastrointestinal tract, but it may develop into a disease condition (candidiasis) under certain circumstances. Factors that predispose patients to candidiasis include immunosuppression, a wet local environment, heat, and diabetes mellitus.

TX For **cutaneous candidiasis:** a topical imidazole cream, such as ketoconazole or clotrimazole.
For **mucosal candidiasis:** fluconazole or itraconazole. For **vulvitis:** intravaginal clotrimazole.

RX1 **Clotrimazole (topical)** [B]

DS1 Apply cream to affected area bid for 1–4 weeks.

SE1 See DERMATOPHYTE INFECTIONS.

or

RX2 **Clotrimazole (vaginal)** (Gyne-Lotrimin, Gynix—*U.S.*; Canesten Topical—*Can.*) [C]

DS2 Intravaginal application of cream: 1% concentration, insert 1 applicatorful qd for 7 days; 2% concentration, insert 1 applicatorful qd for 3 days. Intravaginal tablet: insert 1 mg qd for 7 days, or 500 mg single dose.

SE2 Local erythema, blistering, peeling, edema, pruritus, and urticaria have been reported.

or

RX3 **Fluconazole** (Diflucan) [C]: Interferes with the activity of cytochrome P-450, decreasing the principal sterol in fungal cell membrane (ergosterol) and inhibiting cell membrane formation.

DS3 150 mg PO qd; treatment should be continued until clinical parameters and laboratory tests indicate that an active fungal infection has been cured or has subsided.

SE3 Exfoliative skin disorders and hepatic necrosis.

or

RX4 **Itraconazole** (Sporanox) [C]

DS4 100 mg PO qd; treatment should be continued until clinical parameters and laboratory tests indicate that an active fungal infection has been cured or has subsided.

SE4 See DERMATOPHYTE INFECTIONS.

or

RX5 **Ketoconazole cream** (Nizoral cream) [C]

DS5 Apply cream to affected area qd–bid for 2–4 weeks.

SE5 Local skin irritation and pruritus.

CARBUNCLES

See ABSCESSES, FURUNCLES, AND CARBUNCLES.

CELLULITIS AND ERYSIPELAS

See Ch 10 Infections Diseases.

DERMATOPHYTE INFECTIONS

KY The common organisms that cause dermatophyte infections are ***Trichophyton*** (e.g., *Trichophyton rubrum*), ***Microsporum,*** and ***Epidermophyton* spp**. Dermatophytes live within the keratinized stratum corneum compartment of the epidermis; they do not invade the dermis. **Conditions that**

increase the likelihood of dermatophyte infections include underlying conditions such as sweating, occlusion, atopy, and systemic corticosteroid use. To identify the infection, one may use the Wood's lamp (long-wave [365-nm] UVA). Definitive diagnosis requires microscopic examination and identification of hyphae or spores on skin scraping.

TX Dermatophyte infections of the skin can usually be successfully treated with **topical antifungal agents** such as **imidazoles** or **allylamines.** Examples of imidazoles include ketoconazole and clotrimazole; examples of allylamines include terbinafine. Infections of scalp (tinea capitis) and nails (tinea unguium) require **systemic therapy** because topical penetration is usually inadequate.

RX1 **Clotrimazole** (Lotrimin—*U.S.*; Clotrimaderm—*Can.*) [B]: Damages the permeability barrier in the cell membrane of fungi and inhibits ergosterol biosynthesis, an essential constituent of fungal cell membranes.

DS1 Apply cream to the affected area bid for 1–4 weeks.

SE1 Local erythema, blistering, peeling, edema, pruritus, and urticaria have been reported.

or

RX2 **Griseofulvin** (Fulvicin) [C]: Solely used to treat superficial fungal infections.

DS2 20–25 mg/kg PO (tinea capitis); absorption is enhanced when ingested with a fatty meal. The duration of treatment depends on the site of infection and should be determined by serial fungal cultures.

SE2 Hepatotoxicity, headache, neutropenia, and the potentiation of the effects of alcohol.

or

RX3 **Itraconazole** (Sporanox) [C]: Inhibits the P-450–dependent synthesis of ergosterol, a vital component of fungal and yeast cell membranes.

DS3 For **tinea of the skin:** 100 mg/day PO; as **pulse therapy for nail involvement:** 200 mg PO bid for 1 week/month.

SE3 **Do not administer itraconazole concurrently with terfenadine; serious cardiovascular side effects, including death, ventricular tachycardia, and torsades de pointes, have been reported,** probably as a result of increased terfenadine levels caused by itraconazole. **Other concomitant drugs to avoid include astemizole, cisapride, midazolam, triazolam, erythromycin, and lovastatin and other hydroxymethyl glutaryl coenzyme A reductase inhibitors. Contraindicated in patients with congestive heart failure.**

or

RX4 **Ketoconazole cream** (Nizoral cream) [C]

DS4 Apply cream qd for 2–4 weeks.

SE4 Local skin irritation and pruritus.

or

RX5 **Terbinafine cream** (Lamisil cream) [B]: This allylamine has a broad spectrum of antifungal activity. It interferes with fungal sterol biosynthesis by inhibition of squalene epoxidase in the fungal cell membrane, causing an intracellular accumulation of squalene and resulting in fungal cell death.

DS5 Apply cream bid for 1–2 weeks.

SE5 Local skin irritation, pruritus, contact dermatitis.

ECZEMATOUS DERMATITIS

Atopic Dermatitis ("Eczema")

KY The etiology is as yet unknown. There is often a family or personal history of atopy (e.g., asthma or environmental allergies). Various indices point to an immunologic cause (e.g., peripheral eosinophilia, increased IgE, defective cell-mediated immunity, altered CD4:CD8 ratios, and increased interleukin 4 [IL-4], all of which may result from TH_1). A significant portion of childhood atopic dermatitis will remit over time.

TX Topical treatment requires frequent application (e.g., tid–qid dosing). The treatments include **topical corticosteroids.** For severe cases of atopic dermatitis, systemic **steroids,** such as prednisone, are indicated. For refractory cases, **immunosuppressive agents,** such as azathioprine (Imuran) or cyclosporine (Sandimmune), should be considered.

RX1 **Azathioprine** (Imuran) [D]: The exact mechanism by which this drug suppresses the immunoinflammatory response is not known. Azathioprine is considered a slow-acting drug, and effects may persist after the drug has been discontinued.

DS1 1 mg/kg/day PO

SE1 **Severe leukopenia and thrombocytopenia are dose related. Serious infections—including bacterial, viral, fungal, and protozoal infections—are a constant hazard for patients receiving chronic immunosuppression.**

or

RX2 **Cyclosporine** (Neoral, Sandimmune) [C]: This immunosuppressive agent has specific effects on T-cell proliferation and function. It inhibits the activation cascade, leading to decreased production of IL-2, IL-4, and interferon γ (IFN-γ). Its actions subsequently cause inhibition of T-helper and T-cytotoxic cells, without effects on T-suppressor cells.

DS2 5–6 mg/kg PO q12–24hr

SE2 Hypertension, nephrotoxicity, and hepatotoxicity. Hypertrichosis, gingival hyperplasia, tremor, pancreatitis, hyperglycemia, and hyperkalemia have been described. Patients should be warned of the possibility of gynecomastia. Long-term toxicity is associated with biliary calculi.

RX3 **Systemic corticosteroids** (e.g., prednisone) [B]: These drugs diffuse freely across the plasma membrane of a cell and then bind, with relatively high affinity, to glucocorticoid receptors that are present in the cytoplasm. The direct effects on gene activation, inhibition of proliferation, arachidonic acid metabolism, and cytokine synthesis (IL-1, IL-2, IFN-γ decreased) can then occur.

DS3 1 mg/kg/day PO in a tapering schedule usually over 2–3 weeks

SE3 **Systemic corticosteroids have multiple significant toxicities** (hypertension, fluid retention, psychologic effects, pituitary suppression, peptic ulcer disease, fatty liver, lipid profile abnormalities, osteoporosis, osteonecrosis, cataracts, and more). **Absolute contraindications** include systemic fungal infection and untreated tuberculosis. **Relative contraindications** include acute or chronic infections, pregnancy, diabetes mellitus, hypertension, peptic ulcer, osteoporosis, psychotic tendencies, renal insufficiency, and congestive heart failure.

or

RX4 **Topical corticosteroids:** Potent anti-inflammatory agents.

DS4 See Table 4–1. Apply to affected area bid for 1–4 weeks; strong topical steroids can be used to control severe flares but should not be used for long periods to avoid side effects.

SE4 **Topical corticosteroids can have multiple side effects on the skin,** including atrophy, striae, telangiectasia, purpura, impaired wound healing, folliculitis, acne, susceptibility to infection, hypertrichosis, and hypopigmentation.

or

RX5 **Topical tacrolimus** (Prograf, Protopic) [C]: Immunosuppressant agents used in patients not responsive to conventional therapy.

DS5 Apply 0.02–0.1% bid

SE5 Skin burning, pruritis, erythema, peripheral edema, and allergic reaction.

Table 4–1. Relative Potency of Topical Corticosteroids

Potency Level	Generic (Brand) Name
Extremely potent	Betamethasone 0.05% (Diprolene) [C]
	Clobetasol 0.05% (Temovate—*U.S.*; Dermovate—*Can.*) [C]
	Halobetasol 0.05% (Ultravate) [C]
Very potent	Desoximetasone 0.25% (Topicort) [C]
	Fluocinonide 0.05% (Lidex) [C]
	Halcinonide 0.1% (Halog) [C]
Potent	Amcinonide 0.1% (Cyclocort) [C]
	Betamethasone 0.1% (Betatrex—*U.S.*; Betnovate—*Can.*) [C]
	Fluocinolone 0.025% (Synalar—*U.S.*; Lidemol—*Can.*) [C]
	Mometasone furoate 0.1% (Elocon) [C]
Moderately potent (nonfluorinated)	Desonide 0.05% (Tridesilon—*U.S.*; Desocort—*Can.*) [C]
	Hydrocortisone 0.2% (Westcort) [C]
Least potent	Hydrocortisone 0.5%, 1%, 2.5% [C]

Contact Dermatitis

KY This broad and complex topic encompasses thousands of known contactants and their common sources.

TX Treatment is usually simple once the diagnosis is made: patients should **eliminate and avoid the cause** and treat the dermatitis with **topical corticosteroids** (the potency will depend on the severity of the eruption and its regional distribution). Severe cases (e.g., widespread poison ivy dermatitis) may require **systemic corticosteroids.**

RX1 **Systemic corticosteroids** [B] (e.g., prednisone): See Atopic Dermatitis ("Eczema").

DS1 0.5–1 mg/kg/day PO in a tapering schedule usually over 2–3 weeks

SE1 **Systemic corticosteroids have multiple significant toxicities, including Absolute Contraindications and Relative Contraindications. See Atopic Dermatitis ("Eczema").** Note Cautions.

or

RX2 **Topical corticosteroids:** See Atopic Dermatitis ("Eczema").

DS2 See Atopic Dermatitis ("Eczema").

SE2 **Topical corticosteroids can have multiple side effects on the skin.** See Atopic Dermatitis ("Eczema").

ERYTHRASMA

KY Erythrasma is caused by the bacterium *Corynebacterium minutissimum* and usually appears with red, scaly patches in the inguinal folds. The diagnosis can be confirmed by observing a coral-red fluorescence on Wood's light examination.

TX This dermatosis can be **treated topically** with **imidazole antifungals** (e.g., ketoconazole), **ciclopirox olamine** (Loprox), or **clindamycin** (Cleocin T—*U.S.*; Dalacin T—*Can.*).

RX1 **Ciclopirox** (Loprox) [B]: A synthetic broad-spectrum antifungal agent that inhibits the growth of pathogenic dermatophytes, yeasts, and *Malessezia furfur*. Its mode of action is presumed to be through the depletion of essential substrates or ions causing mediated growth inhibition or death of fungal cells.

DS1 Cream or lotion applied bid for a minimum of 4 weeks

SE1 Local pruritus.

or

RX2 Clindamycin (Cleocin T—*U.S.*; Dalacin T—*Can.*) [B]

DS2 Apply bid for 8–12 weeks

SE2 Contains an alcohol base, which can cause burning and irritation of the eye.

or

RX3 **Ketoconazole** (Nizoral cream) [C]: This topical antifungal impairs the synthesis of ergosterol, a component of fungal and yeast cell membranes.

DS3 Apply cream qd for 2–4 weeks

SE3 Local skin irritation.

FURUNCLES

See ABSCESSES, FURUNCLES, AND CARBUNCLES.

HERPES SIMPLEX

KY Two serotypes exist: **HSV-1** has a predilection for facial-oral infection (about 80% of cases) and **HSV-2** has a predilection for genital infection (about 80% of cases). **Infection is acquired via direct contact.**

TX Antiviral treatment is indicated for a primary (i.e., first-episode) genital infection, prophylaxis for frequently recurrent orolabial or genital infection, recurrent HSV-associated erythema multiforme, or if the patient is immunocompromised.

RX1 **Acyclovir** (Zovirax) [B]: An antiviral agent that inhibits viral DNA polymerase.

DS1 200 mg PO 5 times/day for 7–10 days; 400 mg PO bid for prophylaxis; 400 mg PO qid or 5 mg/kg IV q8hr in the immunocompromised patient

SE1 Headache, rash, and paresthesia.

or

RX2 **Famciclovir** (Famvir) [B]

DS2 250 mg PO bid for 7 days

SE2 Headache, fever, dizziness, somnolence, and pruritus.

or

RX3 **Valacyclovir** (Valtrex) [B]

DS3 500 mg PO bid for 7 days

SE3 Headache and rash.

HERPES ZOSTER (SHINGLES)

KY This is **a reactivation of the varicella-zoster virus infection** (after a primary varicella infection). The virus can remain dormant in the dorsal root sensory ganglia for years until decreased immunity from immunosuppression or advanced age allows its reactivation in a dermatomal distribution.

TX Specific treatment with **antiviral agents** should be started within 72 hours of onset of symptoms for best results. **In severely immunocompromised patients, intravenous antiviral administration should be considered.** Control of postherpetic neuralgia presents a challenge; the following treatments can be tried: antihistamines, analgesics, tricyclic antidepressants, or topical capsaicin 0.025% (Zostrix) applied tid–qid. (Capsaicin, derived from hot chili peppers, induces the release of substance P from neurons in the skin and blocks the reuptake of substance P back into those neurons.)

RX1 **Acyclovir** (Zovirax) [B]: An antiviral agent that inhibits viral DNA polymerase.

DS1 800 mg PO qid, or 12.4 mg/kg IV tid in the severely immunocompromised patient

SE1 Headache, rash, and paresthesia.

or

RX2 **Famciclovir** (Famvir) [B]

DS2 500 mg PO tid for 7 days

SE2 Headache, fever, dizziness, somnolence, and pruritus.

or

RX3 **Valacyclovir** (Valtrex) [B]

DS3 1 g PO tid for 7 days

SE3 Headache and rash.

IMPETIGO

KY *Staphylococcus aureus* and **group A beta-hemolytic** *Streptococcus pyogenes* are the main pathogens of impetigo. Conditions that contribute to colonization include warm temperature, high humidity, and underlying skin diseases (e.g., atopic dermatitis).

TX Treatment: **topical antibiotics,** such as fusidic acid or mupirocin; **systemic antibiotics,** including cephalexin, cloxacillin, and erythromycin are alternative treatment options.

RX1 **Cephalexin (Keflex)** [B]: Inhibits bacterial cell wall synthesis.

DS1 250–1,000 mg q6hr PO for 7–10 days

SE1 Diarrhea, rash, colitis, and hypersensitivity reactions.

or

RX2 **Cloxacillin** (Cloxapen—*U.S.*; Tegopen—*Can.*) [B]: A penicillinase-resistant, acid-resistant, semisynthetic penicillin, it acts through the inhibition of biosynthesis of cell wall mucopeptides.

DS2 250–500 mg PO qid for 7–10 days

SE2 **Hypersensitivity, allergic reactions, antibiotic-associated pseudomembranous colitis, and other serious side effects.** See ABSCESSES, FURUNCLES, AND CARBUNCLES.

RX3 **Erythromycin** [B]: This drug exerts its antibacterial action by binding with the 50S ribosomal subunit of the organism, inhibiting peptide bond formation and protein synthesis within the cell.

DS3 1 g/day PO for 7–10 days

SE3 Abdominal cramping and discomfort, diarrhea, and pancreatitis. Erythromycin can cause **elevated serum levels of the following drugs** when administered concomitantly: theophylline, carbamazepine, digoxin, phenytoin, oral anticoagulants, and cyclosporine.

or

RX4 **Fusidic acid** (Fucidin): A conformation steroid antibiotic that is active against staphylococci and streptococci species.

DS4 Fusidic acid 2% ointment or cream tid–qid

SE4 Hypersensitivity. Local itching, burning, striae, skin atrophy, atrophy of subcutaneous tissue, telangiectasia, hypertrichosis, change in pigmentation, and secondary infection. If applied to the face, acne, rosacea, or perioral dermatitis can occur. Safety during pregnancy has not been established.

or

RX5 **Mupirocin** (Bactroban) [B]: A metabolite of *Pseudomonas fluorescens* that binds to bacterial isoleucyl-tRNA synthetase. It is active against staphylococci and streptococci species and methicillin-resistant *S. aureus*.

DS5 Mupirocin 2% ointment tid for 7–10 days

SE5 Hypersensitivity and local itching, burning, and erythema.

ULCERS

Ulcer treatments include the following principles: treat the underlying disease process, treat the local wound using the principles of moist interactive wound healing, treat the secondary infections, and prevent further outbreaks.

Arterial Ulcers

KY **Arterial insufficiency** is the main cause of arterial ulcers. Patients may have large-vessel disease such as arteriosclerosis. Patients with small-vessel disease, such as diabetes mellitus, may also present with ischemic or gangrenous ulcers.

TX If the ankle-brachial pressure ratio is < 0.6, the **blood supply may be insufficient for adequate healing.** The wound may be painted with povidone-iodine to prevent further secondary infection; **debridement may worsen the ulcer.** Otherwise, the patient's wound may heal, provided that proper local wound care is undertaken. A topical vasodilator, such as a nitroglycerin patch, may be useful if used locally. Pentoxifylline may be used adjuvantly.

RX1 **Povidone-Iodine** (Betadine, topical) [D]: This solution is bactericidal, trichomonacidal, fungicidal, and virucidal.

DS1 Apply to affected area as needed for treatment and prevention of microbial infections.

SE1 Local hypersensitivity reactions.

with or without

RX2 **Pentoxifylline** (Trental) [C]: A xanthine derivative that belongs to a group of vasoactive drugs that improve peripheral blood flow, thus enhancing peripheral tissue oxygenation.

DS2 400 mg PO bid<en]]–tid for up to 2 months

SE2 **Contraindicated in patients with myocardial infarction or severe coronary artery disease.** Flushing and dyspepsia have been reported.

Neuropathic Ulcers

KY Neuropathic ulcers are often secondary to pressure or trauma. People with diabetes exhibit the most common examples of neuropathic ulcers. With the loss of sensory, motor, and autonomic function, the diabetic neuropathic foot is susceptible to infection, trauma, and ischemia.

TX The treatment of neuropathic ulcers involves **pressure off-loading.** Debridement of callus around the ulcer usually reduces the local pressure. Proper footwear with inserts, equipment for sitting, and beds must be evaluated and optimized to reduce pressure on the wound. The ulcer should be protected within a moist environment. **Becaplermin** may be a useful therapeutic agent in some cases.

RX **Becaplermin** 0.01% (Regranex) [C]: A recombinant platelet-derived growth factor. It has biological activity similar to that of naturally occurring platelet-derived growth factor, which includes promoting the chemotactic recruitment and proliferation of cells involved in wound repair.

DS Apply topically as a continuous thin layer to the ulcerated area once daily. The sites of application should be **covered with a dressing to maintain a moist wound-healing environment.** Before the next application, the wound should be rinsed with saline to remove residual gel. Treatment should be repeated daily for 10–20 weeks.

SE Erythema, ulcer infection, tunneling of ulcer, exuberant granulation tissue, and local pain.

Venous Ulcers

KY **Venous insufficiency is common** in patients with poorly functioning venous valvular systems. Poor venous pumping results in venous hypertension and the pooling of fluid in the lower extremities. The specific cause of ulcers is still controversial and may involve increased fibrosis of the venules. In Doppler studies, an ankle-brachial pressure ratio > 0.8 indicates venous insufficiency. Ratios between 0.6 and 0.8 are classified as mixed arterial-venous disease.

TX **The goal of treatment is to decrease the edema of the extremities.** High-pressure compression stockings (20–30 and 50–60 mm Hg pressure) are an efficient method to achieve adequate control of edema. **Topical or oral antibiotics** may be prescribed according to the clinical signs of infection. In cases of mixed venous-arterial disease, modified compression is necessary if the patient cannot tolerate the high-pressure compression.

RX1 **Cloxacillin** (Cloxapen—*U.S.*; Tegopen—*Can.*) [B]

DS1 See ABSCESSES, FURUNCLES, AND CARBUNCLES.

SE1 See ABSCESSES, FURUNCLES, AND CARBUNCLES.
with or without

or

RX2 **Cefazolin** (Ancef) [B]: This cephalosporin antibiotic exerts its bactericidal action through inhibition of bacterial cell wall synthesis.

DS2 1 g IV q8hr

SE2 Diarrhea, oral candidiasis, hypersensitivity reactions, pseudomembranous colitis, nephropathy, and cytopenia.

RX3 Ciprofloxacin (Ciloxan, Cipro) [C]: A fluoroquinolone antibiotic that inhibits DNA-gyrase in susceptible organisms.

DS3 500 mg PO bid

SE3 Headache, nausea, diarrhea, vomiting, acute renal failure, pseudomembranous colitis, and allergic reaction.

5

Endocrinology

IVY M. FETTES

Endocrinology refers to the study of hormones, including steroid, thyroid, and peptide hormones. Hormone synthesis, action, and responsiveness are extensively regulated by the body. The most common causes of endocrine disorders are **hyperfunction,** resulting in hormonal excess, and **hypofunction,** resulting in hormonal deficiency. Syndromes of hormone excess may also result from administration of exogenous hormones. Hormone resistance, or decreased sensitivity to hormones, is basic in the development of type 2 diabetes mellitus (DM). Treatment of hormone deficiency states such as hypothyroidism, Addison's disease, or type 1 DM involves replacement of the deficient hormone. Hormones are often given for other purposes (e.g., glucocorticoids to suppress inflammation or an immune response; estrogen, progesterone, or both for contraception; and tamoxifen for breast cancer). Hormone excess states may be treated by decreasing production or blocking or altering hormone action by pharmacologic means. When appropriate, surgery or radiotherapy is directed to the cause of the excess.

This chapter focuses on the pharmacologic treatment of endocrine disorders caused by hormone excess or deficiency, with the full realization that therapies may change as we expand our understanding of endocrinology and that some of the recommended medications may not be approved or available in certain countries.

ADRENAL DISORDERS

Adrenocortical Insufficiency

KY Adrenocortical insufficiency is the most commonly recognized adrenal disorder. **Primary adrenal insufficiency,** or Addison's disease, is usually the result of an autoimmune disorder and is often associated with other endocrine and nonendocrine autoimmune disorders. Infections such as tuberculosis and human immunodeficiency virus (HIV), adrenal hemorrhage, and metastatic and infiltrative diseases are also important considerations. **Secondary adrenal insufficiency** is usually caused by glucocorticoid therapy but may also be caused by hypothalamic or pituitary disorders. (See **ANTERIOR PITUITARY DISORDERS.**) Adrenocortical insufficiency may be presented as **acute adrenal crisis,** and this is **a life-threatening medical emergency.** It usually occurs in patients with adrenal insufficiency who are exposed to infection, trauma, surgery, or dehydration.

TX **Acute adrenal crisis:** Intravenous hydrocortisone and adequate fluid replacement. **Primary adrenal insufficiency:** Chronic replacement consisting of both glucocorticoid and mineralocorticoid replacement. **Secondary adrenal insufficiency:** Glucocorticoid replacement only. Oral steroids are used for replacement, with the lowest possible dose required to control signs and symptoms and avoid over-replacement. Usually higher doses of glucocorticoid are required for primary adrenal failure than for secondary failure. The glucocorticoid is given bid, two-thirds in the morning and one-third in the late afternoon. The mineralocorticoid is given qd in the morning.

For acute adrenal crisis:

RX Hydrocortisone [C]: A glucocorticoid with some mineralocorticoid activity. It has both metabolic and anti-inflammatory actions.

DS 100 mg IV q8hr, to mimic the 200–400 mg/day cortisol produced during stress in someone with normal adrenal function

SE **Without treatment for acute adrenal crisis, shock, coma, and death may occur.** With treatment, symptoms usually resolve. Hydrocortisone can cause insomnia, nervousness, hirsutism, DM, and cataracts. Rarely, hypertension, seizures, hypokalemia, hyperglycemia, peptic ulcer, immunosuppression, and hypersensitivity reactions occur.

For chronic replacement for primary or secondary adrenal insufficiency:

RX1 Cortone acetate (Cortone) [D]

DS1 25–37.5 mg PO given in divided daily doses, two-thirds in the morning and one-third in the late afternoon.

SE1 **Over-replacement** could result in **bone loss** and symptoms of **hypercortisolism.**

or

RX2 Prednisone (Deltasone) [B]

DS2 5–7.5 mg PO given in divided daily doses

SE2 Same as for cortisone acetate.

or

RX3 Hydrocortisone [C]

DS3 20–30 mg PO given in divided daily doses

SE3 See RX for acute adrenal crisis.

For chronic replacement for primary insufficiency: add mineralocorticoid replacement:

RX Fludrocortisone (Florinef) [C]

DS 0.05–2 mg PO qd

SE **Over-replacement** could result in **hypertension** and **hypokalemia.**

Cushing's Syndrome

KY Cushing's syndrome is the result of **chronic glucocorticoid excess, usually iatrogenic.** Spontaneous Cushing's syndrome may be caused by increased adrenocorticotropic hormone (ACTH) secretion from the pituitary (Cushing's disease) or an ectopic source or adrenal neoplasms or nodular hyperplasia. Therapy for Cushing's disease usually involves surgery, radiation, or both, and therapy for the ectopic ACTH syndrome is directed at the primary tumor. Non–ACTH-dependent adrenal adenomas and nodular hyperplasia are treated surgically. Surgical cure is rare for adrenal carcinoma because it has often metastasized by the time of diagnosis.

TX Adrenal carcinoma: The drug of choice is **mitotane,** but this drug is not readily available.

RX Mitotane (Lysodren) [C]: An adrenal cytotoxic agent that causes adrenal inhibition without cellular destruction. It acts by modifying the peripheral metabolism of steroids and by directly suppressing the adrenal cortex.

DS 6–12 g/day PO in 3–4 doses

SE Diarrhea, nausea, vomiting, depression, and somnolence are common dose-limiting side effects.

Pheochromocytoma

KY A pheochromocytoma is a tumor that develops from the adrenal medulla with unregulated growth and secretion. Endocrine hypertension may be the result of pheochromocytoma with increased catecholamine production.

TX The treatment is **surgical excision of the tumor. Preparation for surgery with medical therapy greatly decreases the risks. If persistent hypertension is present, alpha-adrenergic antagonists such as long-acting phenoxybenzamine or shorter-acting prazosin are used** (see Ch 11 Nephrology). If there is tachycardia or an arrhythmia, a beta-adrenergic blocker such as **propranolol** can be added (see Ch 3 Cardiology). The alpha-blocker is always initiated before the beta-blocker. For benign tumors, these drugs are used preoperatively, but for metastatic or inoperable disease they can be used chronically.

RX1 Phenoxybenzamine (Dibenzyline) [C]: Produces long-acting alpha-adrenergic blockade of postganglionic synapses in both smooth muscle and exocrine glands.

DS1 60–80 mg/day or more may be required to normalize blood pressure. The initiation dose is usually 20–40 mg/day, with dosage increments every 1–2 days to avoid postural hypotension.

SE1 Postural hypotension, tachycardia, confusion, and gastrointestinal (GI) upset.

and/or

RX2 Prazosin (Minipress) [C]: Competitive inhibitor of alpha-adrenergic receptors, producing vasodilatation of veins and arterioles and decreasing overall peripheral resistance and blood pressure.

DS2 Prazosin 3–20 mg/day in divided doses 3–4 times/day

SE2 Headache, weakness, palpitations, edema, orthostatic hypotension, syncope, and urinary frequency. Rarely, angina, bradycardia, tachycardia, pancreatitis, and allergic reaction.

Primary Aldosteronism

KY Aldosteronism is an adrenocortical disorder caused by excessive secretion of aldosterone. Endocrine hypertension may be caused by primary aldosteronism, with renin-independent overproduction of aldosterone.

TX Primary aldosteronism is usually caused by unilateral adenoma, but it may be caused by hyperplasia or, more rarely, glucocorticoid remediable disease or carcinoma. Treatment for a unilateral adenoma is surgical excision, and preoperative medical therapy is advised to normalize blood pressure and serum potassium. **Spironolactone** is usually used; however, **potassium-sparing diuretics** or **calcium channel blockers** can also be used.

RX **Spironolactone** (Aldactone) [D]: A specific antagonist of aldosterone, it acts primarily through competitive binding of receptors at the aldosterone-dependent, sodium-potassium exchange site in the distal convoluted renal tubule. Increased amounts of sodium and water are excreted, and potassium loss is minimized. Thus, **spironolactone acts both as a diuretic and as an antihypertensive drug.**

DS 100–300 mg/day

SE Epigastric discomfort, skin rash, and dizziness. If used long term in men it may cause gynecomastia and impotence because it also blocks the androgen receptor.

CALCIUM DISORDERS AND OSTEOPOROSIS

The human skeleton contains 99.5% of the body's calcium. About 50% of total serum calcium is ionized, and it is the ionized calcium that is regulated by parathyroid hormone (PTH) and vitamin D.

Hypercalcemia

KY Hypercalcemia is usually the result of either hyperparathyroidism or malignancy. Other causes include granulomatous disease, drugs, various endocrine disorders, and immobilization.

TX **Rehydration with saline is the first step in the treatment of hypercalcemia.** An **antiresorptive agent,** usually a bisphosphonate, is then added. The bisphosphonate of choice is **pamidronate.** Synthetic salmon calcitonin can also be used, but it is not as potent at reducing calcium levels, and most patients become refractory to calcitonin within a few days. **High-dose glucocorticoids** may be used for conditions that are steroid responsive, such as vitamin A or D intoxication, sarcoidosis, and multiple myeloma.

RX **Pamidronate** (Aredia) [C]: A bisphosphonate that strongly binds to bone and slows down the resorption of bone. Used to reduce the amount of calcium in the blood, it is also used in other conditions with increased bone turnover or pain.

DS 60–90 mg by IV infusion over 4–24 hours

SE Transient fever, myalgia, increased serum creatinine. The hypocalcemic effect may persist for 1–6 weeks.

Hypocalcemia

KY Hypocalcemia may be caused by deficiencies of PTH (usually surgically induced) or vitamin D (usually malabsorption), blood transfusions, or acute pancreatitis.

TX Treatment depends on whether the hypocalcemia is **acute** or **chronic** (Table 5–1).

RX Table 5–1

DS Table 5–1

SE For calcitriol, monitor the patient for symptoms of hypercalcemia.

Table 5–1. Treatment of Hypocalcemia

Hypo-calcemia	Generic (Brand) Name	Dose
Acute	Calcium chloride (Calciject)* [C]	500–1,000 mg (7–14 mEq)/dose repeated q4–6hr (**PEDS:**—2.7–5.0 mg/kg/dose q4–6hr)
	Calcium gluceptate* [C]	500–1,100 mg/dose IM or 1,100–4,400 mg (90–360 mg calcium) IV infusion slowly at ≤ 2 mL/min (**PEDS:**—200–500 mg [16.4–41 mg calcium]/kg/day IM divided q6hr)
	Calcium gluconate* [C]	2–15 g/24 hr as continuous IV infusion or in 4 divided doses IV
	Additional infusion of calcium chloride or gluconate** and	0.2–2.0 mg/kg/hr IV
	1, 25 (OH)₂ vitamin D or calcitriol (Calcijex, Rocaltrol) [C]	0.25–0.20 µg/day PO
Chronic	Oral calcium lactate (Calcimax) [C]	To provide 1.5–3.0 g elemental calcium/day
	Vitamin D₂ (ergocalciferol) (Calciferol, Drisdol—*U.S.;* Ostoforte, Radiostol—*Can.*) [A/C depending on dose] or Vitamin D₃ (cholecalciferol) (Delta-D—*U.S.;* D-tabs—*Can.*) (onset of action is 1 month) [C]	**For hypoparathyroidism:** 0.625–5 mg/day (25,000–200,000 U/day) **For malabsorption:** 0.25–7.5 mg/day (10,000–300,000 U/day)
	1, 25 (OH)₂ vitamin D (calcitriol) (Calcijex, Rocaltrol) [C]	**For patients with renal failure:** 0.5–2.0 µg/day PO (individual dosage to maintain calcium levels of 9–10 mg/dL)

*If creatine clearance is < 25 mL/min, dosage adjustments depend on serum calcium levels.
**Calcium chloride is 3× more potent than calcium gluconate.

Osteoporosis

KY Osteoporosis is a skeletal disorder characterized by low bone mass and microarchitectural disruption, leading to enhanced bone fragility and an increase in fracture risk. Osteoporosis can be **primary,** as in post-menopausal women or with aging, or **secondary** to drugs or clinical disorders (e.g., hyperthyroidism, hyperparathyroidism).

TX An adequate intake of calcium and vitamin D is necessary for building bone but may not be sufficient for maintaining bone. Treatment with calcium and vitamin D reduces fracture risk in older adults. Decreased sunlight exposure particularly in northern latitudes and in people in nursing homes justifies an increase in vitamin D intake to 800 units. Pharmacologic therapies for prevention and treatment of osteoporosis include antiresorptive agents, with a much greater effect on suppressing bone resorption than increasing bone formation. Bisphosphonates (alendronate, risedronate, etidronate), raloxifene, estrogen, and calcitonin improve bone mineral density. (Fracture reduction is much greater with alendronate, risedronate, and raloxifene.) Combination of antiresorptive agents is used judiciously and in the future may be replaced by combinations or cycles of bone-forming agents (such as PTH) and antiresorptive agents.

RX Table 5–2

DS Table 5–2

SE Bisphosphonates have to be taken on an empty stomach. The side effects of bisphosphonates are mainly GI, including dyspepsia, regurgitation, flatulence, and diarrhea. The major side effects of raloxifene are hot flashes and leg cramps. There is **an increased risk of thromboembolism with both raloxifene and estrogen replacement** therapies. Although facial flushing, nausea, and diarrhea may occur with the SC administration of calcitonin, the intranasal preparation usually has no side effects and is very well tolerated.

DIABETES MELLITUS

Diabetes mellitus is a hyperglycemic disorder that may be classified into two major groups: **type 1 DM,** caused by pancreatic islet beta cell destruction, and **type 2 DM,** caused by insulin resistance and impaired insulin secretion.

Type 1 Diabetes Mellitus

KY **Type 1 DM requires insulin replacement.** It is usually autoimmune in nature and is the most common cause of DM in children and lean young adults. People with type 1 DM are prone to **ketoacidosis** if they have inadequate insulin for their needs. Self-monitoring of blood glucose is important for safety, flexibility, and control.

TX There are **four major types of insulin for use in type 1 DM:** ultra–short-acting insulin (lispro or aspart insulin), short-acting insulin (regular), intermediate-acting insulin (NPH or lente), and long-acting insulin (ultralente). Most of the insulin in use is human insulin produced by

Table 5–2. Treatment of Osteoporosis

Generic (Brand) Name	Dose	Side Effects
Calcium carbonate (Amitone, Biocal, Caltrate, Os-Cal, Tums, Calcite) [C]	1–1.5 g/day PO	Headache, constipation, laxative effect, acid rebound, nausea, vomiting, anorexia, abdominal pain, flatulence. Milk-alkali syndrome with very high chronic dosing or renal-failure (headache, nausea, irritability, and weakness or alkalosis, hypercalcemia, renal impairment). Calcium carbonate absorption is impaired in achlorhydria.
Vitamin D$_2$ (ergocalciferol) (Calciferol, Drisdol—*U.S.*; Ostoforte, Radiostol—*Can.*) [A/C depending on dose]	400–800 U/day PO	Hypercalcemia. Adequate dietary (supplemental) calcium is necessary for clinical response to vitamin D. Avoid use with renal function impairment and secondary hyperparathyroidism.
Alendronate (Fosamax) [C]	Prevention: 5 mg/day PO Treatment: 10 mg/day PO or 70 mg/week PO	Dyspepsia, regurgitation, esophagitis after regurgitation, flatulence, diarrhea
Risedronate (Actonel) [C]	5 mg/day PO	
Etidronate (Didronel)	400 mg/day PO for 2 weeks every 3 months	
Raloxifene (Evista) [X]	60 mg/day PO	Hot flashes, leg cramps, thromboembolism
Salmon calcitonin (Calcimar, Miacalcin—*U.S.*; Caltine—*Can.*) [C]	200 U/day intranasally or 100 U/day SC	Flushing, nausea, diarrhea with injectable form
Estrogen replacement [X]	A wide variety of estrogens, alone or with progesterone, may be used for the prevention and treatment of osteoporosis.	Nausea, bloating, breast tenderness and enlargement, thromboembolism, increased risk of breast cancer with prolonged use

recombinant DNA techniques. Regular insulin is currently the only insulin available for pulmonary inhalation. Pancreatic islet cell transplantation is investigational at present.

RX Insulin (Table 5–3)

DS The insulin regimen most commonly recommended involves **multiple (3–4) daily SC injections of a combination of ultra–short- or short-acting insulin and intermediate-acting insulin.** Regular insulin should be given 20–30 minutes before a meal, whereas lispro or insulin aspart can be given 5–15 minutes before a meal. A typical initial program is as follows:

- Before breakfast: a combination of an intermediate-acting insulin such as NPH and either lispro or regular insulin
- Before the evening meal: ultra-short or regular insulin
- At bedtime: NPH

The **total daily dose of SC insulin** is usually in the range of 0.3–0.5 U/kg body weight, with two-thirds given in the morning and one-third in the evening, and two-thirds as intermediate- or long-acting insulin and one-third as short- or ultra–short-acting insulin.

A portable, battery-operated **continuous SC insulin infusion** pump may also be used. Short- or ultra–short-acting insulins are used in the pump, which is programmed to deliver various concentrations of insulin throughout the 24-hour day. Boluses are given by pump before meals.

SE Inadequate insulin therapy results in **hyperglycemia,** with the possibility of acute complications such as **ketoacidosis** and chronic complications such as **nephropathy** and **retinopathy.** The patient should be taught to adjust the dosage of insulin in response to self–glucose monitoring, meal content, exercise, and illness.

Type 2 Diabetes Mellitus

KY **Type 2 DM** is the most common type of DM and can present with variable degrees of insulin deficiency and resistance.

TX Most patients with type 2 DM are obese adults, and **a healthy weight-reducing diet is the first therapeutic step.** When diet alone does not control the DM, an **oral antihyperglycemic or hypoglycemic agent** is added. Various combinations of oral agents, oral agents and insulin, or insulin alone can be used. Because of the different mechanisms of these agents, they can be complementary to each other and to insulin. Choice of the ini-

Table 5–3. Bioavailability of Commonly Used Insulins

Insulin Type	Insulin Action		
	Onset	Peak	Duration
Ultra–short-acting: lispro (Humalog) [B] and insulin aspart (NovoLog) [C]	5–15 minutes	1–1.5 hr	3–4 hr
Short-acting: regular (Velosulin)	15–30 minutes	1–3 hr	5–7 hr
Intermediate-acting: NPH and lente	2–4 hr	8–10 hr	18–24 hr
Long-acting: ultralente (Ultralente)	4–5 hr	8–14 hr	25–36 hr

tial drug depends on the degree of obesity and insulin resistance—where **insulin sensitizers** (biguanides and thiazolidinediones) are useful—and the degree of hyperglycemia—where **insulin secretagogues** (sulfonylureas and meglitinides) or **insulin** may be required to restore an acceptable glycemic status.

Except for the thiazolidinediones, which may be given once daily, the oral agents are given 2–3 times/day. The insulin secretagogues, short- or ultra–short-acting insulin alone or in combination with an intermediate-acting insulin should be given before meals. Intermediate-acting insulin alone may be used at bedtime to help prevent fasting hyperglycemia (in contrast to type 1 DM, where bid injections of short- and intermediate-acting insulins often result in nocturnal hypoglycemia, this is not usually a problem in type 2 DM).

A variety of premixed insulin preparations with combinations of short- or ultra–short-acting insulin and intermediate-acting insulin are available for twice daily therapy. Two commonly used combinations are (1) a mix of 30% regular and 70% NPH and (2) a mix of 25% lispro and 75% intermediate insulin. The short- and ultra–short-acting insulins, NPH, and the premixes are all available in vials for syringe needle administration and in cartridges for insulin pen needle administration. Short-acting insulin for inhalation, where available, is another option.

Owing to insulin resistance, the doses of insulin are usually higher (> 0.5 U/kg) in type 2 DM than in type 1 DM.

RX Type 2 DM oral antihyperglycemic agents and insulin (Table 5–4).

DS Table 5–4

SE Table 5–4

Hyperglycemic Emergencies in Adults (Diabetic Ketoacidosis and Hyperosmolar Hyperglycemic State)

KY **Diabetic ketoacidosis (DKA):** hyperglycemia (caused by insulin deficiency), dehydration, and ketoacidosis. **Hyperosmolar hyperglycemic state (HHS):** hyperosmolarity without ketoacidosis. The glucose levels are usually higher (often > 30 mmol/L) and the fluid deficit greater (≥ 9 L).

TX After initial evaluation of the patient with DKA or HHS, IV fluid replacement with 0.9% normal saline should begin. A small bolus of regular insulin is given IV, and an infusion of regular insulin is started. The glucose levels should be checked hourly and the infusion adjusted as necessary to obtain a steady decline of glucose level—in the range of 50–70 mg/dL/hr. Potassium is added to the IV fluid if the serum potassium level is < 3.3 mEq/L. Potassium should not be given if the serum level is > 5.5 mEq/L. Potassium replacement is continued as required to maintain a normal serum potassium level. Bicarbonate may be diluted in water and infused over 1 hour if the pH is < 7.0. The IV fluid replacement may be switched from 0.9% saline to 0.45% sodium chloride (NaCl) and 5% dextrose when the glucose has decreased to a level of approximately 250 mg/dL. Intravenous insulin is continued until the glucose level has reached approximately 250 mg/dL for HHS or 180 mg/dL for DKA. Patients with

Table 5–4. Commonly Used Oral Drugs for Type 2 Diabetes Mellitus

Class	Generic (Brand) Name	Dose*	Side Effects
Drugs that Increase Insulin Secretion (Insulin Secretagogues)			
Sulfonylureas	Glyburide (DiaBeta) [C]	1.25–20 mg/day before meals	Hypoglycemia. Sulfonylureas are associated with poorer outcomes after myocardial infarction.
	Glyburide, micronized	1.5–12 mg/day	
	Glipizide (Glucotrol) [C]	2.5–25 mg/day	
	Glipizide GITS*	5–10 mg/day	
	Glimepiride (Amaryl) [C]	1–8 mg/day	
Meglitinides	Repaglinide (Prandin—*U.S.*; Gluconorm—*Can.*) [C]	0.5–4 mg/day before meals	Hypoglycemia. It is not yet established whether repaglinide is associated with poorer outcomes after myocardial infarction.
	Nateglinide (Starlix) [C]	120 mg before meals	
Drugs that Reduce Insulin Resistance (Insulin Sensitizers)			
Biguanides	Metformin (Glucophage) [B]	1,500–2,000 mg/day in divided doses	GI complaints, including anorexia, nausea, and diarrhea. Lactic acidosis is a low risk. **Contraindicated in patients with renal impairment.**
	Metformin, extended action (Glucophage XR)	500–2000 mg/day	
Thiazolidinediones	Pioglitazone (Actos) [C]	15–40 mg/day	Fluid retention. **Contraindicated in patients with hepatic impairment or congestive heart failure.**
	Rosiglitazone (Avandia) [C]	4–8 mg/day	

(continued)

Table 5–4. Commonly Used Oral Drugs for Type 2 Diabetes Mellitus *(Continued)*

Class	Generic (Brand) Name	Dose*	Side Effects
Drugs that Delay the Digestion of Complex Carbohydrates			
	Acarbose (Precose—*U.S.*; Prandase—*Can.*) [B]	25–100 mg at the start of each meal	GI complaints, including flatulence, diarrhea, and abdominal pain.
	Miglitol (Glyset) [B]	25–50 mg at the start of each meal	
Insulin Preparations* (see Table 5–3)	Ultra-short-acting: lispro, insulin aspart		
	Short-acting: regular		
	Intermediate-acting: NPH, lente		
	Long-acting: ultralente		
	Premixed short-acting/NPH in the following ratios: 10/90, 20/80, 30/70, 40/60, 50/50		
	Premixed ultra-short-acting/ NPH in the following ratio: 25/75		

GITS = gastrointestinal therapeutic system.

*Except for the thiazolidinediones, which may be taken once daily, the oral agents are taken 2–3 times daily.

type 1 DM can then be switched to SC insulin if they are otherwise well and able to eat and drink.

RX Multistep treatment approach as described in **TX** and **DS**.

DS Doses for regimen are as follows:

- Initiate 0.9% NaCl IV at 1 L/hr.
- Regular insulin IV bolus 0.15 U/kg.
- Regular insulin IV infusion 0.1 U/kg/hr.
- Add potassium IV infusion 40 mEq/hr if serum potassium is < 3.3 mEq/L.
- Add bicarbonate 50 mmol in 200-mL water IV infusion if pH < 7.0.
- Monitor hourly glucose levels until glucose reaches 180–250 mg/dL and then q2–4hr until stable. Adjust infusions of NaCl, insulin, and potassium as required.
- Switch from 0.9% NaCl to 0.45% NaCl and 5% dextrose for hydration when glucose level reaches 250 mg/dL.

SE Hypokalemia and hypoglycemia.

Hypoglycemia

KY Hypoglycemia can occur with oral hypoglycemic agents such as the sulfonylureas or meglitinides or with insulin.

TX The manifestations of hypoglycemia are relieved with glucose administration.

RX Glucose

DS In the **conscious** patient who is able to swallow, fruit juice (e.g., orange juice), sugar-containing beverages, glucose tablets, or carbohydrate-containing foods can be taken. Two teaspoons of honey, syrup, or sugar could also be used. If the patient is **semiconscious or unconscious** and at home, glucagon 1 mg IM can be given by a friend or family member. If trained personnel and IV glucose are available, 50 mL of 50% glucose solution can be given over 3–5 minutes. If neither glucagon nor IV glucose is available, syrup, honey, or a glucose gel can be rubbed into the oral mucosa.

SE No significant side effects.

GONADAL DISORDERS

Female Gonadal Disorders

KY Most ovarian disorders are seen in postpubertal adults and include **problems of estrogen deficiency** caused by one of the following: menopause; hypothalamic or pituitary disease; or androgen excess, usually resulting from polycystic ovarian syndrome (PCOS). This section focuses on PCOS, a disorder characterized by menstrual dysfunction, hyperandrogenism, insulin resistance, and the variable expression of these problems. (For treatment of estrogen deficiency resulting from hypothalamic or pituitary disease, see **ANTERIOR PITUITARY DISORDERS**.)

TX The treatment chosen for PCOS depends on the problems of concern, which may include hirsutism, acne, alopecia, irregular menstruation, infertility, obesity, type 2 DM, and hyperlipidemia. Most commonly, patients will seek help for symptoms of **hyperandrogenism,** and the medical therapy will involve drugs to decrease androgen production, reduce androgen action, or both. These drugs include hormonal oral contraceptives, insulin sensitizers, androgen blockers, and local cosmetic therapies. **Combination therapy is more effective than any single therapy.** Menstrual irregularities are usually treated with oral contraceptives or cyclic progestin. Ovulation induction is usually with clomiphene citrate. Insulin sensitizers such as metformin and the thiazolidinediones are investigational for assistance with ovulation induction. The gonadotropins and pulsatile gonadotropin-releasing hormone (GnRH) are less commonly used for ovulation induction as they are not usually required.

RX Table 5–5

DS Table 5–5

SE Table 5–5. Oral contraceptives are contraindicated for women with blood clotting disorders or who are heavy smokers (see Ch 8 Gynecology). **Metformin is contraindicated in patients with renal insufficiency.** Use of spironolactone alone may result in irregular uterine bleeding. **Flutamide may cause hepatotoxicity** and for that reason is not commonly used. Nausea and fluid retention may occur with initial doses of an oral contraceptive. The presence of prolactin-secreting microadenomas, or DM without vascular disease, is not a contraindication to the oral contraceptive. Multiple births are uncommon ($\leq 10\%$) with clomiphene.

Male Gonadal Disorders

KY **Male hypogonadism** may be caused by gonadal abnormalities, hypothalamic or pituitary disorders, or defects in androgen action with partial or complete androgen insensitivity. The most common cause of male hypogonadism is **Klinefelter's syndrome,** which occurs in 1 in 500 male births and is characterized by an extra X chromosome, azoospermia, and low circulating testosterone levels. **Cryptorchidism** occurs in about 5% of males at birth, but only 0.75% of adult males are cryptorchid. There is a high incidence of infertility and inguinal hernia in these males, and there is an increased risk of malignancy with intra-abdominal testis. Other causes of **infertility** in adult males include varicocele, mumps, gonococcal orchitis, irradiation, uremia, alcoholism, antineoplastic drugs, systemic illness, and endocrine disease. Adult Leydig cell failure with testosterone deficiency may occur with aging (andropause). **Erectile dysfunction** may be the result of psychogenic causes (e.g., depression) or organic causes, including DM, hypertension, aging, and androgen deficiency from a variety of causes.

TX Androgen deficiency caused by gonadal abnormalities may be treated with testosterone replacement. The treatment of erectile dysfunction depends on the underlying cause (see Ch 22 Urology).

Table 5-5. Pharmacologic Treatment of Hyperandrogenism Caused by Polycystic Ovarian Syndrome

Generic (Brand) Name	Dose	Side Effects
Drugs to Block Androgen Action		
Cyproterone acetate (progestin with antiandrogenic activity), Diane-35 (available in Canada and Europe)	50–100 mg/day for first 7–10 days of oral contraceptive cycle or 2 mg/day for 21 consecutive days/month as progestational with 30 μg estradiol	For all drugs listed: irregular menses, dizziness depression. Flutamide may cause hepatotoxicity. Additionally: Cyproterone can also cause fluid retention and
Finasteride (Propecia, Proscar) [X]	5 mg/day	
Flutamide (Eulexin—*U.S.*; Euflex—*Can.*) [D]	250 mg bid	
Spironolactone (Aldactone) [D]	50–200 mg/day	
Drugs to Decrease Androgen Production (also see Ch 8 Gynecology)		
Oral contraceptives [X]	Estradiol: 20–35 μg with variable doses and types of progestin depending on formulation used	
Metformin (Glucophage) [B]	500 mg tid or 850 mg bid	Nausea and diarrhea. **Metformin is contraindicated in patients with renal insufficiency.**
Drugs to Regulate Menses (also see Ch 8 Gynecology)		
Oral contraceptives [X]	Combination estrogen/progesterone, or progestin alone Cyclic progestins (medroprogesterone) 5–10 mg/day PO for 5–12 days every month	Nausea, fluid retention, **thromboembolism**

Nausea, fluid retention, **thromboembolism**

(continued)

Table 5–5. Pharmacologic Treatment of Hyperandrogenism Caused by Polycystic Ovarian Syndrome *(Continued)*

Generic (Brand) Name	Dose	Side Effects
Drugs to Induce Ovulation (also see Ch 8 Gynecology)		
Clomiphene citrate (Clomid, Milophene, Serophene) [X]	50–150 mg for 5 consecutive days	Most common side effects of clomiphene: hot flashes, headache Others: abdominal discomfort, ovarian enlargement. Visual blurring may occur and resolves after discontinuation of drug. Note: Multiple births are uncommon ($\leq$ 10%) with clomiphene.
Oral contraceptives: Combination estrogen/progesterone, or progestin alone	Various formulations available	Nausea, fluid retention, **thromboembolism**
Cyclic progestins (medroxy-progesterone acetate)	5–10 mg/day PO for 5–12 consecutive days every month	

RX Table 5–6. Androgen deficiency in males may be treated with a variety of testosterone preparations and routes, including intramuscular, oral, subdermal, and transdermal administration.

DS Table 5–6

SE Table 5–6. **Carcinoma of the prostate or breast and obstructive prostate hypertrophy are contraindications to the use of androgens.** Serum prostate-specific antigen should be monitored.

HYPERSECRETORY SYNDROMES

Growth Hormone–Secreting Adenomas

KY Excessive secretion of **growth hormone** (GH) can be caused by **GH-secreting adenomas.** The persistent hypersecretion of GH stimulates the hepatic secretion of **insulin-like growth factor** I (IGF-I), which causes most of the clinical manifestations of **acromegaly.**

TX The primary treatment for GH-secreting tumors is surgical excision, with adjunctive medical therapy, both before and after surgery. Currently, the medical therapy of choice is the long-acting **synthetic somatostatin analogs,** which lower both GH and IGF-I levels.

RX **Octreotide LAR** (Sandostatin) [B]: Simulates natural somatostatin and decreases GH and IGF-I in acromegaly. The drug also inhibits the release of serotonin and the secretion of gastrin, vasoactive intestinal peptide, insulin, glucagon, secretin, and motilin and pancreatic peptide.

DS 10–30 mg IM monthly

SE The most common side effects are GI. Cholelithiasis may occur. There may be dose-related pain at the injection site.

Hyperprolactinemia

KY Hyperprolactinemia is the most common pituitary disorder, and prolactinomas are the most common pituitary tumors. The mainstay of treatment is medical therapy with **oral dopamine agonists.**

TX The clinical manifestations of hyperprolactinemia from prolactinomas respond quickly to the dopamine agonists **bromocriptine** and **cabergoline.** Bromocriptine has to be given in divided doses, usually twice daily, whereas cabergoline can be given once or twice weekly. There are fewer side effects with cabergoline, and it seems to be more efficacious in lowering prolactin levels.

RX1 **Bromocriptine** (Parlodel) [B]: **This semisynthetic ergot alkaloid derivative is a dopamine receptor agonist.** It activates postsynaptic dopamine receptors in the tuberoinfundibular and nigrostriatal pathways.

DS1 2.5–5.0 mg bid, but the drug should be initiated with a dose of 1.25 mg at bedtime and gradually titrated to normalize prolactin levels with a minimum of side effects.

Table 5-6. Drugs for Male Hypogonadism

Generic (Brand) Name	Dose	Side Effects
Testosterone Replacement Strategies		
Testosterone cypionate (Depo-Testosterone), testosterone enanthate (Delatestryl, Testro), or testosterone propionate	100 mg IM q1wk, or 150–200 mg IM q2wk, or 200–300 mg IM q3wk, or 300–400 mg IM q4wk	Testosterone levels variable with dosage intervals, acne, priapism, and aggressive behavior are dose-related side effects.
Testosterone undecanoate	40–80 mg PO bid	
Testosterone patch, scrotal or nonscrotal (Androderm, Testoderm)	2.5–5 mg/day	Skin reactions
Testosterone gel (AndroGel)	5–10 g/day applied to upper arms	
Testosterone pellet (Testopel)	4 × 200 mg (800 mg) subdermal implantation q4–6mo	Pain at the injection site, extrusion of pellets
Erectile Dysfunction (also see Ch 22 Urology)		
Prostaglandin E₁ [alprostadil] (Caverject, Edex, Muse pellet, Prostin VR)	Injection: 2–20 μg intracavernosal injection (erection lasts 30–60 minutes) Pellets: 125–1000 μg pellets intraurethral	Penile and urethral pain, hypotension, dizziness. **Avoid in CHF.**
Sildenafil (Viagra)	50–100 mg PO 2 hours before sexual activity (starting dose: 50 mg)	Headache, hypotension, dizziness. **Should not be prescribed to patients taking nitrates or nitric oxide donor drugs because the combination could cause fatal hypotension. Avoid in CHF.**

CHF = congestive heart failure.

SE1 The most common side effects of bromocriptine are nausea, headache, and dizziness. Constipation and nasal congestion may also occur. The **dopamine agonists are generally not used during pregnancy unless there is a macroadenoma with risk of enlargement.**

RX2 **Cabergoline** (Dostinex) [B]: Prolactin secretion by the anterior pituitary gland is predominantly controlled by hypothalamic inhibition through the release of dopamine. Cabergoline is a long-acting dopamine receptor agonist with a high affinity for D2 receptors.

DS2 0.25–0.5 mg once or twice weekly

SE2 The **dopamine agonists are generally not used during pregnancy** unless there is a macroadenoma with risk of enlargement.

OSTEOPOROSIS

See CALCIUM DISORDERS AND OSTEOPOROSIS.

ANTERIOR PITUITARY DISORDERS

Hypopituitarism

KV **Hypopituitarism may be caused by destruction of the anterior pituitary or by a deficiency of hypothalamic stimulation.** The causes include invasion by intracranial space–occupying lesions, for example, tumors, and treatment of these lesions with surgery or radiation; infiltrative diseases; infarction; head trauma; autoimmune lymphocytic hypophysitis; and infection. **There may be loss of one or more pituitary hormones.** The usual order of loss is GH, luteinizing hormone (LH), follicle-stimulating hormone (FSH), thyroid-stimulating hormone (TSH), ACTH, and, finally, prolactin. In general, the symptoms of hypopituitarism are similar to those of primary target gland failure. However, in primary failure, the LH, FSH, TSH, and ACTH will be elevated, whereas they are low or normal in hypopituitarism.

TX **Secondary adrenal insufficiency:** Treat with a **glucocorticoid before treatment of any other hormone deficiency.** Unlike primary adrenal insufficiency, mineralocorticoid replacement is not usually required. The minimum effective dose of an oral glucocorticoid should be given for maintenance. The dose is usually divided, with two-thirds given in the morning and one-third in the late afternoon. The dose is increased by 2–3 times during stress and given parenterally for major stress.

Secondary hypogonadism: Treatment involves **replacement of sex steroids** and, as required, restoration of fertility with **pulsatile GnRH** for hypothalamic disorders and **gonadotropins for pituitary disorders.** Sex steroid replacement includes estrogen and progesterone for women and testosterone for men.

Secondary hypothyroidism: Treatment is identical to that for primary hypothyroidism, with levothyroxine (T4). However, the dosage adjustments are monitored with measurement of free thyroxine levels rather than TSH levels.

Growth hormone deficiency: Diagnosis is based on the failure of GH response to provocative stimuli. The treatment of adult GH deficiency is controversial. Only recombinant GH is used owing to the risk of prion contamination of cadaveric pituitary tissue. Two forms are available: **somatropin,** which is a 191–amino acid natural sequence form of GH, and **somatrem,** which is a 192–amino acid methionyl form.

RX Table 5–7

DS Table 5–7

SE Table 5–7

POSTERIOR PITUITARY DISORDERS

Diabetes Insipidus

KY **Antidiuretic hormone (ADH)** or arginine vasopressin is synthesized in the hypothalamus and secreted by the posterior pituitary. When ADH is present, water is resorbed by the kidneys; with a deficiency or absence of ADH, resorption of water decreases, leading to polyuria. Central or neurogenic diabetes insipidus (DI) is caused by the failure of the posterior pituitary to secrete adequate amounts of ADH. This failure is usually caused by compression or damage of the pituitary stalk or damage to the regions of the hypothalamus involved in the synthesis of ADH. Diabetes insipidus may be partial or complete; it is usually transient after pituitary surgery and **may be either transient or permanent** after head trauma. Levels of ADH are low in central DI (unlike in nephrogenic DI, in which ADH levels are normal or elevated and the DI is caused by renal unresponsiveness to ADH). During pregnancy, increased vasopressinase secretions by the placenta may enhance the destruction of ADH and cause gestational DI.

TX **Central DI responds quickly to replacement with ADH. Desmopressin acetate, a synthetic analog of vasopressin, is the drug of choice.** The route and frequency of administration (mouth, nose, or subcutaneously) will depend on the clinical situation and patient preference. The SC route is used for acute postoperative or post–head trauma DI. Oncedaily dosing at bedtime may be adequate to control polyuria and polydipsia in partial DI, but more frequent dosing will be required for complete DI.

RX **Desmopressin acetate** (DDAVP, Octostim, Stimate) [B]: A two–amino acid substitute of ADH that has a potent antidiuretic action (enhances absorption of water in the kidneys by increasing the cellular permeability of the collecting ducts) without vasopressor activity.

DS 1–2 µg SC qd–bid, or 10 µg intranasally bid, or 5–20 µg by nasal catheter qd–bid, or 0.1–0.2 mg PO bid–tid

SE Flushing, headache, nausea, nasal congestion, and pain at the injection site occur in less than 10% of patients. Fluid balance must be monitored in the acute situation. Overhydration should be avoided.

Table 5–7. Treatment Strategies in Hypopituitarism

Generic (Brand) Name, Sex, or Age	Dose (PO) or Replacement Therapy	Contraindications and Cautions
Secondary Adrenal Insufficiency		
Cortisone acetate (Cortone) [D]	25–37.5 mg/day	Iatrogenic hypercortisolism may occur if the dose used is higher than the patient requires.
Prednisone (Deltasone) [B]	5–7.5 mg/day	
Hydrocortisone [C]	20–30 mg/day	
Secondary Hypothyroidism		
Levothyroxine (T4) (Synthroid—*U.S.*; Eltroxin—*Can.*) [A]	1–2 μg/kg/day (mean dose of 0.125 mg/day)	Iatrogenic hyperthyroidism may occur if the dose used is higher than the patient requires.

Secondary hypogonadism Women*	Oral estradiol 1–2 mg/day
	Conjugated oral estrogen 0.3–1.25 mg/day
	Transdermal estradiol 50–100 μg/day
	Medroxyprogesterone
	  Cyclical therapy: 5–10 mg/day for 12 days/month
	  Continuous therapy: 2.5–5 mg/day
	Micronized progesterone
	  Cyclical therapy: 200–300 mg/day for 12 days/month
	  Continuous therapy: 100 mg/day
	Combination estradiol 5 mg + norethindrone 1 mg qd
	Combination conjugated estrogen 0.625 mg
	  + medroxyprogesterone 2.5–5 mg/day
	Combination transdermal estradiol 0.05 mg
	  + norethindrone 150–250 mg/day
		Contraindicated in patients with thrombophlebitis and abnormal blood clotting, liver or heart disease, breast or untreated uterine cancer, abnormal vaginal bleeding, and pregnancy. **Side effects:** thromboembolism, myocardial infarction, stroke, hypertension, headache, depression, anxiety, chloasma, melasma, cholestatic jaundice, increased triglycerides. Nausea, bloating, and breast tenderness may occur with initiation of therapy.

(continued)

*If uterus intact, estrogen and progesterone are used. If uterus absent, estrogen alone is used.

81

Table 5-7. Treatment Strategies in Hypopituitarism *(Continued)*

Generic (Brand) Name, Sex, or Age	Dose (PO) or Replacement Therapy	Contraindications and Cautions
Secondary hypogonadism Men	Testosterone cypionate, enanthate, or propionate 100 mg IM q1wk, or 150–200 mg IM q2wk, or 200–300 mg IM q3wk, or 300–400 mg IM q4wk Testosterone patch, scrotal or nonscrotal, 2.5–5 mg/day Testosterone gel 5–10 g/day Testosterone undecanoate 40–80 mg PO bid Testosterone pellets 4×200 mg (800 mg) q4–6mo by subdermal implantation	**Contraindications** include carcinoma of the breast or prostate and prostatic hypertrophy with obstruction. **Side effects:** Gynecomastia may develop with initiation of therapy. Acne and alopecia may occur with increasing dosage. Aggressive behavior and sleeplessness may occur with supraphysiologic levels of testosterone. Abuse or overuse of androgens can cause testicular atrophy and oligospermia. Premature fusions of epiphysis occur if androgens are used in adolescents before age 13 years.
Growth Hormone Deficiency Children	Somatropin or somatrem 0.3 mg/kg/week in six or seven divided doses	**Contraindicated** in patients with active malignancy, intracranial hypertension, and proliferative retinopathy.
Adults	Somatropin or somatrem 0.075 mg/kg/day, usually with initiation at 0.15 mg/day and titration up to $\leq$ 1 mg/day to normalize IGF-1 levels	**Side effects:** Fluid retention and mild elevation in glucose levels may occur; growth hormone replacement does not seem to increase the recurrence rates of pituitary tumors or craniopharyngiomas that existed before therapy was initiated.

Syndrome of Inappropriate Secretion of ADH

KY The syndrome of inappropriate secretion of ADH (SIADH) is the increased secretion of ADH, which can cause water retention and hyponatremia. Causes include increased secretion of ADH from neoplasms in the posterior pituitary, bronchogenic carcinoma, pulmonary tuberculosis, lymphoma, and sarcoma. The SIADH can also be caused by central nervous system disorders such as trauma or infection and deficiencies of thyroid hormone or cortisone. Additional causes include HIV infection and drugs that increase the release of ADH (e.g., vincristine and cyclophosphamide).

TX **The acute treatment of SIADH involves fluid restriction** and occasionally hypertonic saline and loop diuretics. **Long-term therapy** should involve the underlying cause. Drugs such as demeclocycline, which decreases the renal responsiveness to ADH, are not commonly used owing to nephrotoxicity. The use of lithium for the same purpose is limited by the proximity of the therapeutic and toxic dosages.

RX **Demeclocycline** (Declomycin) [D]: A tetracycline antibiotic that inhibits the action of ADH in chronic SIADH.

DS 900–1,200 mg qd on an empty stomach

SE Photosensitivity, nausea, diarrhea. Dosage adjustments are required for renal or hepatic impairment and, **in general, demeclocycline should be avoided in patients with renal or hepatic dysfunction.**

THYROID DISORDERS

Thyroid function is regulated by hypothalamic thyrotropin-releasing hormone, pituitary TSH, TSH receptor autoantibodies, the iodine supply, and pituitary and peripheral deiodinases. The follicular cells of the thyroid gland secrete tetraiodothyronine (thyroxine, T_4) and lesser amounts of triiodothyronine (T_3). The most common thyroid disorders are **hyperthyroidism** or **thyrotoxicosis,** which results from an excess of T_4 and T_3, and **hypothyroidism,** which is caused by deficiency of T_4. Thyroid enlargement, either diffuse or nodular, may or may not be associated with thyroid dysfunction. Patients with thyroid cancer, which is rare, usually present with a solitary nodule and normal thyroid hormone levels.

Hyperthyroidism and Thyrotoxicosis

KY **Thyrotoxicosis** is usually caused by hyperactivity of the thyroid gland (hyperthyroidism) from Graves' disease. Other causes of **hyperthyroidism** include toxic nodules and subacute thyroiditis. Less commonly, thyrotoxicosis is caused by overdosage of thyroid hormone, ectopic secretion of thyroid hormone, for example, from struma ovarii, a TSH-secreting pituitary tumor, hydatiform mole, or pituitary resistance to thyroid hormones.

TX During the acute phase of thyrotoxicosis beta-adrenergic blocking drugs can provide symptomatic relief of tachycardia and tremor. If there are no contraindications, propranolol 10–40 mg PO q6hr can be used. More specific therapies will vary with the cause of the thyrotoxicosis. For

Graves' hyperthyroidism and toxic nodules, there are three major treatment options: antithyroid drugs, radioiodine, and surgery. The **initial treatment for Graves' hyperthyroidism is often an antithyroid drug** to block the synthesis of thyroid hormone, either propylthiouracil or methimazole. The duration of therapy required for remission of Graves' hyperthyroidism is extremely variable, ranging from 6 months to more than 15 years. After rendering a patient with one or more toxic nodules euthyroid with an antithyroid drug, more definitive therapy with **radioiodine** or **surgery** is used. Radioiodine is the preferred definitive therapy for a nonpregnant adult with Graves' hyperthyroidism, particularly if there is a concern about the cardiovascular risks of recurrence.

RX1 **Methimazole** (Tapazole) [D]: Antithyroid agent that inhibits the synthesis of thyroid hormones by blocking the oxidation of iodine and the combination of iodine with tyrosine to form T4 and T3.

DX1 30–40 mg qd as a single dose every morning or as a split dose q8hr

SE1 A mild allergic reaction with a **rash** (5% of patients) may be treated with antihistamines. **Agranulocytosis,** which usually involves a sore throat and fever and occurs in approximately 0.5% of patients, is an indication for **immediate cessation of the antithyroid drug. Hepatotoxicity,** although rare, is also an indication for **cessation of the drug.** Hypothyroidism in a patient who takes antithyroid drugs can be readily treated by a dosage adjustment, whereas hypothyroidism after radioiodine is typically permanent.

RX2 **Propylthiouracil** (PTU, Propyl-Thyracil) [D]: Antithyroid agent with the same mechanism of action as methimazole.

DS2 100–150 mg PO q8hr

SE2 Same as for methimazole.

Hypothyroidism

KY Hypothyroidism is usually caused by primary thyroid failure from Hashimoto's thyroiditis, postradioiodine therapy or thyroid surgery, or subacute thyroiditis. Iodine deficiency or excess, goitrogens such as lithium, and hypopituitarism are much less common causes. Hypothalamic dysfunction and peripheral resistance are rare causes of hypothyroidism. The symptoms reflect a slowing down of metabolic processes and are usually reversible with therapy.

TX The treatment for hypothyroidism is replacement with T4. The half-life of T4 is about 7 days, so it need only be given once daily, preferably on arising in the morning. Since T_4 can be converted to T_4 within the cells, additional therapy with T_3 is not usually required.

RX Levothyroxine (Synthroid) [A]: The exact mechanism of action is not known; however, thyroid hormone is thought to exert its metabolic effects through the control of DNA transcription and protein synthesis.

DS For adults, T4 0.05–0.2 mg/day with a mean dose of 0.125 mg/day. The doses are higher for infants and children and pregnant women and lower for older adults. For replacement therapy, 1–2 μg/kg/day is used in adults, with higher doses for suppression of nodules or cancer. In a healthy young adult you may start with the full replacement dose. In older adults, particularly those with known cardiac disease, the rule is to "start low and go slow." The usual starting dose for such a patient would be 0.025 mg/day. The dosage can be adjusted every 4–6 weeks until the levels of TSH and free T4 are normalized for replacement therapy. If angina pectoris or a cardiac arrhythmia develops during the period of dosage increment, the dosage should be immediately reduced and then more slowly adjusted until equilibrium has been reached. For suppression therapy, the dosage is adjusted to suppress the TSH level but maintain the free T4 in the normal range.

SE Any side effects are usually caused by overdosage and include palpitations, tremor, and insomnia. Osteoporosis may occur in estrogen-deficient postmenopausal women who are chronically over-replaced with T4. Note that changes in thyroid function can alter the requirements of the antidiabetic agents digoxin and warfarin.

6

Gastroenterology

GABOR KANDEL, CLIFFORD M. OTTAWAY

CIRRHOSIS COMPLICATIONS

The major **life-threatening complications** of cirrhosis, including variceal bleeding, ascites, and encephalopathy, are caused more by the circulatory disturbances of portal hypertension than by hepatocyte dysfunction. The most catastrophic complication of cirrhosis is upper gastrointestinal (GI) tract bleeding from varices, which has a mortality rate approaching 30%. The basis for pharmacologic therapy developed from the observation that variceal hemorrhage develops only if the portal pressure (the pressure difference between the portal vein and systemic circulation) is greater than 12 mm Hg.

Ascites

KV Fluid accumulates in the peritoneal cavity in cirrhosis because of two factors: (1) kidney retention of fluid caused by avid distal tubular sodium resorption secondary to poorly understood mechanisms and (2) abnormal partitioning of extracellular fluid more into the peritoneal cavity than into the vascular space because of high portal pressure plus low serum oncotic pressure (from the hypoalbuminemia of chronic liver disease) pushing fluid out of the vascular space. The ascites of portal hypertension is characterized by a serum-ascites albumin gradient (albumin concentration in serum minus albumin concentration in ascitic fluid) greater than or equal to 1.1 g/dL (in other ascitic forming conditions, such as peritoneal carcinomatosis, the serum-ascitic albumin gradient is higher). All patients with new-onset ascites should have a diagnostic paracentesis, and the ascitic fluid should be routinely examined for albumin, cell count, culture, and cytology. If **portal hypertension** (including cirrhosis) is the underlying etiology of ascites, a search should be made to identify a precipitating cause. **Common precipitants are increase in alcohol intake and increase in dietary sodium, hepatoma, and sepsis.**

TX The cornerstone of treating cirrhotic ascites is dietary sodium restriction to 44 mEq/day in hospitalized patients and 88 mEq/day in ambulatory patients. Achieving a negative sodium balance will be beneficial if the urine sodium excretion is greater than 50 mEq/day, indicating early mobilizable ascites. Otherwise, **diuretics** need to be added for the ascitic fluid to be decreased at an acceptable rate. **Spironolactone is the diuretic of choice** because it directly antagonizes the increased distal tubular resorption of sodium, which occurs in the setting of cirrhosis. In patients not responding to medical therapy, adherence to sodium restriction should be verified, and nonsteroidal anti-inflammatory drugs (NSAIDs) should be discontinued as these drugs can impair renal excretion of sodium. If the ascites continues to persist, then therapeutic paracentesis is indicated; direct removal of 4–6 L of ascitic fluid. **Intravenous albumin** is often concomitantly given at a dose of 6–8 g/L of ascitic fluid removed. Ascites almost always recurs after paracentesis, so diuretics should be prescribed after the procedure. True refractory ascites occurs in less than 10% of cirrhotic ascites. It can be treated by a peritoneovenous shunt, transjugular intrahepatic portosystemic shunt (TIPS), or by liver transplantation.

RX1 **Spironolactone** (Aldactone) [D]: Potassium-sparing diuretic.

DS1 Starting dose: 100 mg PO qd increased gradually to 400 mg PO qd, with a goal weight loss of 0.5 kg/day

SE1 **Hyperkalemia is a possible side effect and a contraindication.** Patients should be warned of the possibility of gynecomastia.

with or without

RX2 **Furosemide** (Lasix) [C]: A loop diuretic that inhibits sodium resorption in the ascending loop of Henle.

DS2 40 mg PO qd

SE2 Volume depletion and hypokalemia.

Esophagogastric Varices

KY Gastroesophageal variceal bleeding presents with hematemesis, melena, or hematochezia, the same as upper GI tract bleeding from any cause but characteristically more massive. The first step in management is **resuscitation,** which in cirrhosis includes endotracheal intubation if there is a decreased level of consciousness or difficulty in protecting the airway, as occurs in encephalopathy. Often, in addition to red blood cell transfusion, plasma and platelets need to be transfused to correct the coagulation disturbances of end-stage liver disease. **Caution is advised in administering fluid volume, especially blood products, to bleeding cirrhotic patients since replacing all of the blood lost leads to rebound of portal pressure above baseline.** Endoscopy is the mainstay of definitive therapy to determine the site of bleeding and ligate or inject varices causing bleeding. Uncontrollable variceal bleeding is an indication for a TIPS.

TX1 **Acute variceal bleeding: Intravenous somatostatin or its longer-acting synthetic analog octreotide** may control variceal bleeding. Both of these agents selectively vasoconstrict the splanchnic circulation both by direct action on vascular smooth muscle and by inhibition of the release of vasodilatory hormones such as glucagon. **Such pharmacologic treatment is best given in conjunction with endoscopic therapy** and continued for 5 days after the bleeding event. **Intravenous vasopressin** also lowers portal pressure and has some effect in decreasing variceal bleeding, but it has more side effects and is less effective than octreotide. Upper GI bleeding in cirrhosis predisposes to bacterial infections, especially spontaneous bacterial peritonitis (infection of ascitic fluid), and **antibiotic prophylaxis is considered standard care. Norfloxacin** can be given orally or through a nasogastric tube. Alternatively, **cefazolin** can be administered intravenously.

RX1a **Somatostatin:** Produced by paracrine cells in the GI tract. Inhibits serotonin release and secretion of gastrin, vasoactive intestinal peptide (VIP), insulin, glucagon, secretin, motilin, and pancreatic polypeptide. It also inhibits growth hormone release and exerts neural control.

DS1a Bolus of 250 μg IV followed by 250 μg/hr continuous infusion

SE1a Sinus bradycardia, hyperglycemia, diarrhea, abdominal discomfort, constipation, nausea, edema, headache, vertigo, hypoglycemia, hypothyroid, and hypertensive crisis.

or

RX1b **Octreotide** (Sandostatin) [B]: Synthetic analog of somatostatin.

DS1b Bolus of 50 μg IV followed by 50–100 μg/hr continuous infusion

SE1b Same as for somatostatin.

with or without

RX1c **Vasopressin** (Pitressin—*U.S.*; Pressyn—*Can.*) [B]: Increases cyclic adenosine monophosphate, which increases water permeability at the renal tubule, which results in decreased urine volume and increased osmolality. Vasopressin directly stimulates GI tract smooth muscle, causing peristalsis.

DS1c Bolus of 20 U in 100 mL of D-5-W continuous infusion over 15 minutes, followed by 0.2–0.4 U/min infusion

SE1c Hypertension, cardiac arrhythmias, venous thrombosis, and vasoconstriction, which can lead to myocardial and intestinal infarction.

with

RX1d **Norfloxacin** (Chibroxin, Noroxin) [C]

DS1d 400 mg PO bid for 7 days after bleed

SE1d Headache, GI upset, acute renal failure, seizures, and allergic reactions.

or

RX1e **Cefazolin** (Ancef, Kefzol) [B]

DS1e 1 g IV bid for 7 days after bleeding event

SE1e GI upset, pseudomembranous colitis, seizures, and allergic reactions.

TX2 **Prevention of recurrent bleeding:** To lower the recurrence rate of variceal bleeding, continuing endoscopic ligation approximately every 2 to 3 weeks until the varices are completely obliterated has proven effective. **Nonselective beta blockade is also indicated both as an adjunct** to endoscopic therapy and by itself if repeated endoscopies cannot be done. Beta-blockers lower portal pressure, and addition of the potent vasodilator **isosorbide mononitrate** may decrease the recurrent variceal bleeding rate to a lower rate than beta-blockers alone; however, there is as yet insufficient evidence to recommend such combination treatment routinely.

RX2a **Propranolol** (Inderal) [C/D in the second and third trimesters]: Nonselective beta-blocker.

DS2a Starting dose: 40 mg PO bid, adjusted as necessary until either the wedged hepatic vein pressure gradient falls below 12 mm Hg or the resting pulse decreases by 25% to a minimum of 55 bpm (although pulse rate can only roughly approximate wedged hepatic vein pressure).

SE2a Fatigue, impotence, decreased libido, depression, heart failure, and bronchospasm. **Contraindicated** in patients with asthma, heart failure, heart block, bradycardia, and hypotension.

or

RX2b **Nadolol** (Corgard) [C]: Nonselective beta-blocker.

DS2b 40 mg PO qd

SE2b Same as for propranolol.

with or without

RX2c **Isosorbide mononitrate** (Imdur, ISMO) [C]: Vasodilator.

DS2c Starting dose: 20 mg PO qd; increase gradually over 2 weeks to 40 mg PO bid

SE2c Headaches, dizziness, and flushing. **Contraindicated** in patients with hypotension and hypertrophic obstructive cardiomyopathy. The incidence of hypotension and adverse cardiovascular events can be increased with concomitant sildenafil (Viagra) administration.

TX3 **Prevention of first variceal hemorrhage:** Oral beta-blockers used as described in the paragraph on prevention of recurrent bleeding lower the risk of bleeding from asymptomatic large varices from 25% to 15% in 2 years.

RX3 Beta-blockers (nadolol or propranolol)

DS3 See the Prevention of recurrent bleeding paragraph.

SE3 See the Prevention of recurrent bleeding paragraph.

Hepatic Encephalopathy

KY Hepatic encephalopathy is a neuropsychiatric syndrome that develops in the presence of liver disease or portal hypertension. In acute hepatic failure, cerebral edema plays a critical role. However, in the more common chronic type of hepatic encephalopathy ("portosystemic encephalopathy") related to portal hypertension rather than hepatocyte destruction, **pathogenesis has been attributed to ammonia generated by bowel bacteria entering the brain because of impaired hepatic extraction,** preventing the normal metabolism of ammonia into urea. High serum concentrations of aromatic amino acids, false neurotransmitters, and short-chain fatty acids may also contribute. Characteristic features of hepatic encephalopathy include an insidious, gradual onset; early development of a reversal in the day-night cycle; and changes in alertness, behavior, and intellect, followed by a progressive decrease in level of consciousness and asterixis in the absence of focal neurologic signs. Once the diagnosis has been established, a search is indicated for precipitating causes, especially GI bleed, drugs such as diuretics and sedatives, sepsis, renal failure, and hepatoma.

TX After treating both the underlying and precipitating causes, daily protein intake should be reduced to 20–80 g/day depending on severity. The most commonly used drug is lactulose, which acidifies the gut luminal contents so that **less ammonia** is absorbed across the bowel epithelium, and less ammonia-producing bacteria grows in the gut lumen. If lactulose does not resolve the encephalopathy, neomycin can be added, but care is required to ensure that renal failure and auditory problems do not develop. In refractory cases, bromocriptine can be added to lactulose; **bromocriptine** is not useful when given alone.

RX1 **Lactulose** (Cholac, Chronulac, Constilac, Constulose, Duphalac, Enulose, Evalose, Kristalose—*U.S.*; Acilac, Laxilose—*Can.*) [B]: A synthetic, nonabsorbable disaccharide metabolized by bowel bacteria into lactic and acetic acids.

DS1 Starting dose: 40 g (60 mL) qd, adjusted gradually to the dose that produces three to four soft-bowel movements daily

SE1 Intolerable diarrhea, dehydration, and electrolyte losses (e.g., hypernatremia).

with or without

RX2 **Bromocriptine** (Parlodel) [B]: Semisynthetic ergot alkaloid derivative and dopamine receptor agonist.

DS2 Starting dose: 2.5 mg PO qd, increasing gradually over 2 weeks to 15 mg PO qd

SE2 Headaches, GI upset, hypotension, cardiac arrhythmias, alopecia, insomnia, paranoia, and visual hallucinations.

with

RX3 **Neomycin** (Mycifradin—*U.S.*; Myciguent—*Can.*) [C]: Aminoglycoside that interferes with bacterial protein synthesis.

DS3 1 g PO tid

SE3 Nephrotoxicity and ototoxicity when administered chronically.

Spontaneous Bacterial Peritonitis

KY Spontaneous bacterial peritonitis is **bacterial infection of preexisting ascites,** which usually occurs in the setting of alcoholic cirrhosis. It is commonly caused by *Escherichia coli*, *Bacteroides fragilis*, streptococci, or *Klebsiella*. Paracentesis is diagnostic and is established by an ascitic fluid neutrophil concentration of > 250 cells/μL.

TX **Treatment is guided by culture results if available; otherwise, cefotaxime** (or another third-generation cephalosporin) **or amoxicillin** can be administered. If the infection is community acquired and the patient is stable, without renal dysfunction or encephalopathy, oral ofloxacin can be prescribed. **Aminoglycosides should not be used** because of the high incidence of nephrotoxicity in liver disease.

RX1 **Cefotaxime** (Claforan) [B]

DS1 2 g IV q8hr until the ascitic neutrophil concentration falls below 250 cells/μL

SE1 GI upset, nephrotoxicity, seizure, and allergic reactions

or

RX2 **Amoxicillin** (Amoxil) [B]

DS2 1 g IV q8hr

SE2 GI upset, hematologic dyscrasias, hepatitis, and allergic reactions. Increased incidence of developing rash in patients with infectious mononucleosis taking amoxicillin. Decreased doses required with renal impairment.

or

RX3 **Ofloxacin** (Floxin) [C]

DS3 400 mg PO bid

SE3 GI upset, headache, seizure, tendinitis and tendon rupture, and allergic reactions

DIARRHEA: ACUTE AND INFECTIOUS

KY A practical classification of diarrhea of < 10 days' duration (acute) is **inflammatory** versus **noninflammatory.** Acute diarrhea developing in a hospital is most often caused by medications, only rarely by an infection other than *Clostridium difficile*.

TX1 **Fluid and electrolyte replacement:** Management of hyponatremia and hypokalemia are discussed in Ch 11 Nephrology.

TX2 **Symptomatic treatment:** Agents are available for relief of acute diarrhea.

RX2a **Bismuth** (Bismatrol, Pepto-Bismol) [C/D in the third trimester]: Antisecretory and antimicrobial agent.

DS2a Effective regimen is 524 mg PO q30min for eight doses. High-dose treatment up to 4.2 g/day PO has also been shown to reduce stool frequency successfully.

SE2a Darkening of stool and tongue. **Do not use in young patients with influenza or chickenpox** because of risk of Reye syndrome.

or

RX2b **Loperamide** (Imodium) [B]: Inhibits peristalsis of the intestinal muscle.

DS2b Doses up to 4 mg PO qid, regularly or prn

SE2b Abdominal cramping. **Contraindicated** in the presence of bowel mucosal inflammation (inflammatory diarrhea) to prevent toxic megacolon and prolongation of the disease.

TX3 **Antibiotics: Only selected bacterial enteric infections require specific therapy with antibiotics.** Stool culture results are instrumental in choosing the proper treatment for the cause of the diarrhea. Because of the inherent delay of stool culture techniques, antibiotics are given at the time of patient presentation to optimize the benefit of these antimicrobials. Empiric use of ciprofloxacin for 3–5 days in adults with acute diarrhea, especially if it is inflammatory, decreases the duration of the disease, some-times even when a pathogen is not found.

RX3 **Ciprofloxacin** (Ciloxan, Cipro) [C]

DS3 500 mg PO bid for 3–5 days

SE3 GI upset, headache, hypersensitivity, renal damage, and tendon inflammation or rupture. **Contraindicated** in patients with *C. difficile* infection.

TX4 *Clostridium difficile* infection: This infection is caused by previous antibiotic administration, and the most important step in treatment is the cessation of the inciting antibiotic. First-line treatment is metronidazole and alternatively vancomycin.

RX4a **Metronidazole** (Flagyl) [B/X in the first trimester]

DS4a 250 mg PO qid

SE4a Headache, ataxia, seizures, disulfiram-type reactions, pancreatitis, and hypersensitivity reactions.

RX4b **Vancomycin** (Lyphocin, Vancocin, Vancoled) [C]

DS4a 125 mg PO qid

SE4a Bitter taste, GI upset, chills, fever, eosinophilia, thrombocytopenia, ototoxicity, renal failure, hypotension, and allergic reactions.

GASTROESOPHAGEAL REFLUX DISEASE

KY Usually, gastric acid moves from the stomach forward to the duode-num, where it is neutralized by bicarbonate. Reflux refers to the abnormal retrograde movement of acid from the stomach to the esophagus, most often caused by inappropriate relaxations of the lower esophageal sphinc-ter. In addition to the cardinal symptoms of **heartburn** and **acid regurgi-tation,** reflux has also been recently shown to cause **wheezing, laryngitis, and even aspiration pneumonia.** The most accurate test for reflux is 24-hour esophageal pH monitoring. Reflux can cause esophagitis (esophageal mucosal inflammation), which can lead to stricture, bleeding, and **colum-nar metaplasia of the esophageal squamous mucosa (Barrett's esopha-gus),** now considered a premalignant condition.

TX Since **effective drugs are not currently available to reverse the abnormality** in control of lower esophageal sphincter pressure, medical management consists chiefly of **suppressing gastric acid production. Pro-ton pump inhibitors (PPIs)** (Table 6–1) are the most effective drugs in this regard, and are now considered the medical treatment of choice for severe reflux. **Less potent medications are also available,** including histamine H_2 antagonists, dopamine antagonists, antacids, and alginic acid (Table 6–2); these are becoming less popular with time since the PPIs are now considered to be virtually free of significant side effects.

RX Proton pump inhibitors. Absence of reflux symptoms is considered a suitable goal for maintenance therapy. Follow-up studies have shown that the theoretical concerns of proton pump–induced long-term gastric

Table 6–1. Proton Pump Inhibitors

Generic (Brand) Name	Dose (PO)	Theoretical Advantages	Side Effects
Esomeprazole (Nexium) [B]	40 mg qd	Most potent	Allergic reactions, GI upset, headache; long-term effects unknown
Lansoprazole* (Prevacid) [B]	30 mg qd–bid	Rapid onset of action	Allergic reactions, GI upset
Omeprazole* (Prilosec—U.S.; Losec—Can.) [C]	20 mg qd–bid	Longest time on the market	Allergic reactions, dizziness, GI upset, headache
Pantoprazole (Protonix—U.S.; Panto, Pantoloc—Can.) [B]	40 mg qd–bid	Less interaction with other drugs	Allergic reactions, chest pain, GI upset, hyperglycemia, migraine, pruritus, rash; long-term effects unknown

GI = gastrointestinal.

*Theoretical concerns include an increased incidence of gastric malignancies, enteric infections, and low vitamin B_{12} levels with long-term use.

acid suppression causing gastric malignancies, enteric infections, and low vitamin B_{12} levels (gastric acid is required to liberate protein-bound vitamin B_{12} into an absorbable state) are minimal even after 10 years of regular omeprazole therapy. Only minimal differences exist between the various commercially available PPIs.

DS Table 6–1

SE Table 6–1. Theoretical concerns that long-term use of PPIs causes gastric malignancies, enteric infections, and low vitamin B_{12} levels.

HEMORRHOIDS

KY Hemorrhoids are the tissue cushions lining the anal canal. External hemorrhoids are dilated veins distal to the dentate line. Skin tags are redundant skin at the anal verge resulting from previously thrombosed external hemorrhoids. Internal hemorrhoids are congested vascular cushions above the dentate line.

TX Treatment is aimed at relieving vascular congestion and decreasing straining to pass stool. The combination of increased fiber intake and increased water intake facilitates evacuation. Regular exercise improves colonic motility. Creams and ointments can relieve the symptoms of external hemorrhoids. Suppositories are more useful for internal hemorrhoids.

RX Table 6–3

DS Table 6–3

SE Table 6–3

Table 6-2. Alternative Drugs for Gastroesophageal Reflux Disease

Generic (Brand) Name	Dose (PO)	Side Effects and Cautions
Antacids [C] Aluminum hydroxide (Amphojel—*U.S.*; Basaljel—*Can.*) [C]	Depends on preparation that is used 600 mg 5–6 times/day between meals qhs	Well tolerated Constipation, phosphatemia; aluminum intoxication and osteomalacia may occur in patients with uremia
Calcium carbonate [C]	1,000–1,300 mg/day in 4–6 divided doses	Well tolerated
Aluminum hydroxide and magnesium carbonate (Gaviscon)	Aluminum hydroxide 160 mg and magnesium carbonate 105 mg (sodium 1.3 mEq/5 mL) qid prn	GI upset
Histamine H$_2$ antagonists Cimetidine (Tagamet—*U.S.*; Peptol—*Can.*) [B] Ranitidine (Zantac) [B] Nizatidine (Axid) [C] Famotidine (Mylanta, Pepcid) [B]	300 mg qid 300 mg qhs 300 mg qhs 20 mg qhs	GI upset, headache; rarely, arrhythmias, blood dyscrasias, bronchospasm, hypersensitivity
Dopamine antagonists Domperidone Metoclopramide (Reglan—*U.S.*; Maxeran—*Can.*) [B]	10 mg qid 10 mg qid	Drowsiness, extrapyramidal movements, including incapacitating dystonias, galactorrhea Side effects resolve when drug is discontinued. **Contraindicated** in GI obstruction, perforation, or hemorrhage; pheochromocytoma; and seizure disorder

GI = gastrointestinal.

Table 6–3. Pharmacologic Treatment of Hemorrhoids

Treatment Options	Dose	Side Effects and Cautions
Fiber	Best sources are foods: cereals, grains, legumes, and fruit. Psyllium [B] products or bran are alternates.	25–30 g PO qd	Often causes bloating and gas in first 2 weeks of therapy. **Contraindicated** in patients with partial or complete obstruction.
Stool softeners	Docusate (Colace) [C]	100–300 mg/day PO in 1–4 divided doses	GI obstructions Hypokalemia can occur in overdose.
Suppositories and cream	Pramoxine (Anusol, Tronolane, Tronothane) [C] Mesalamine (Asacol, Canasa, Pentasa, Rowasa—*U.S.*; Mesasal, Salofalk—*Can.*) [B]	1–2 times/day Can be used with or without 1% hydrocortisone. Bedtime insertion is most effective if maintained while sleeping.	Seepage can occur. Very little absorption of steroid occurs.
Water		1.5–2 L/day	Increased urinary frequency usually accommodates in 1–2 weeks

GI = gastrointestinal.

HEPATITIS

Alcoholic Hepatitis

KY The toxicity of carbon chain alcohols associated with liver disease have been recognized for centuries, and alcoholic hepatitis (AH) occurs in up to half of all heavy alcohol users. The characteristic hepatic features are a steatohepatitis in which liver cell injury occurs in the presence of a neutrophilic inflammatory response and pericellular fibrosis. AH is a precursor to alcoholic cirrhosis, but the two diseases can occur concomitantly. Clinically, patients with AH present with nonspecific symptoms, and physical findings may include hepatosplenomegaly, jaundice, ascites, and encephalopathy. The patient may also have signs of chronic liver disease (spider angiomata, Dupuytren's contractures, gynecomastia, testicular atrophy, etc.). Laboratory results include moderately elevated aspartate transaminase (AST) and alanine transaminase (ALT) (with AST > ALT), hyperbilirubinemia, coagulopathy, and, in severe cases, azotemia.

TX The first principles of treating AH include **complete abstinence, supportive care, and rehabilitation** of the patient. **It is also important to recognize the patient who is severely ill with AH.** Moderately ill patients respond to initial therapy, but the in-hospital mortality rate with severe illness is up to 50%. Corticosteroids are of some benefit in a subset of patients with severe AH (Table 6–4). **Pentoxifylline** has been shown to decrease in-hospital mortality rates and to decrease the occurrence of hepatorenal syndrome in patients with severe AH (Table 6–4).

RX Table 6–4

DS Table 6–4

SE Table 6–4

Hepatitis B Virus

KY Hepatitis B virus (HBV) infection is **acquired through exposure to blood or body secretions from infected individuals.** Following acute HBV infection, some individuals become chronically infected. Less than 10% of immunocompetent adults will experience chronic HBV after infection, but up to 90% of infants exposed to HBV will become chronically infected. In chronic HBV infection, patients in whom active viral replication continues are at risk for cirrhosis and hepatocellular carcinoma. The activity of the virus and the impact of the infection on the liver of the patient need to be evaluated before antiviral therapy. Patients with normal ALT and AST levels do not benefit from current antiviral treatments, and patients with decompensated liver disease do poorly with antiviral therapy.

TX Treatment for **acute HBV infection** is supportive. Therapy for **chronic HBV infection** is aimed at patients with ALT and AST elevations (for at least 3 months) and active viral replication and includes **interferon alpha** or **lamivudine.**

RX Table 6–5

DS Table 6–5

SE Table 6–5

Table 6-4. Treatment Options for Alcoholic Hepatitis

Clinical Situation	Generic (Brand) Name	Dose	Side Effects and Cautions
Severe AH, with coagulopathy, encephalopathy in the absence of advanced cirrhosis, jaundice	Prednisolone (Prednisol, Prelone) [C]	20–40 mg/day PO/IM/IV in single or divided doses for 30 days	AVN, acne, adrenal suppression, anxiety, cataracts, dyspepsia, glaucoma, hypersensitivity reactions, hypertension, insomnia, osteoporosis, poor wound healing **Use with caution** in patients with seizure disorders, cardiac disease, diabetes. **Contraindicated** in patients with infections.
Severe AH with jaundice, coagulopathy, and one or more of the following: encephalopathy, leukocytosis $> 12,000/mm^3$, tender hepatomegaly, no evidence of advanced cirrhosis	Pentoxifylline (Trental) [C]	400 mg PO tid for 28 days	Abdominal pain, diarrhea, headache, nausea, skin rash, vomiting **Contraindicated** in patients with active bacterial infection.

AH = alcoholic hepatitis; AVN = avascular necrosis.

Table 6–5. Treatment Options for Hepatitis B Virus

Generic (Brand) Name	Dose	Side Effects and Cautions
Interferon alfa-2b (Intron A) [C]	10 MU IM/SC 3 times/ week or 5 MU IM/SC qd for 16 weeks	Alopecia, fatigue, fever, headache, leucopenia, myalgia, nausea, thrombocytopenia, thyroid dysfunction **Contraindications:** Liver diseases, severe psychiatric disorders
Lamivudine (Epivir—*U.S.*; 3TC—*Can.*) [C]	100 mg PO qd for 12 months	Fatigue, headache, nausea **Caution:** Check HIV status. Coinfection requires more complex antiviral therapy.

HIV = human immunodeficiency virus.

Hepatitis C Virus

KY Hepatitis C virus (HCV) infection is usually acquired through parenteral exposure to infected blood products. HCV is less easily transmitted through sexual activity than is HBV. Acute HCV infection is rarely recognized. Clinical recognition of HCV infection comes with detection of antibodies to HCV, which can become reactive within 2–3 weeks. Chronic HCV is the most common outcome of HCV infection, and up to 20% of infected persons can progress to cirrhosis and are at risk for hepatocellular carcinoma.

TX The current standard of care for patients with HCV is interferon alpha in combination with ribavirin (Table 6–6). Treatment with interferon alpha alone may be useful for patients in whom ribavirin is contraindicated. Patients with normal ALT levels and low HCV RNA levels

Table 6–6. Treatment Options for Hepatitis C Virus

Generic (Brand) Name	Dose	Side Effects and Cautions
Interferon alfa-2b (Intron A) [C]	3 MU IM/SC 3 times/week	See Table 6–5
Ribavirin (Rebetol, Virazole) [X]	500 mg PO bid* (Note: if body weight is > 75 kg: 600 mg PO bid)	Dyspnea, hemolytic anemia, insomnia, pruritus **Caution:** Check HIV status. Coinfection requires more complex antiviral therapy. **Contraindications:** Anemia, coronary artery disease

HIV = human immunodeficiency virus.

*Patients with hepatitis C virus genotype 1, high pretreatment levels of hepatitis C virus RNA ($> 2 \times 10^6$ copies/mL) or established hepatic fibrosis or cirrhosis benefit from treatment for 48 weeks; otherwise, 24 weeks of combined treatment is optimal.

do not benefit from treatment. Patients should be advised that continued use of alcohol can enhance progression of HCV infection. Patients with HCV should be vaccinated against hepatitis A and HBV (see Ch 18 Pediatrics).

RX Table 6–6

DS Table 6–6

SE Table 6–6

INFLAMMATORY BOWEL DISEASE

Ulcerative colitis (UC) and **Crohn's disease (CD)** are the two main forms of **idiopathic inflammatory bowel disease.** UC is limited to the colon and rectum, is continuous, and involves ulceration of the mucosal layer. In contrast, CD can affect the entire GI tract, and the inflammation is patchy and usually involves both the mucosal and deeper layers of the intestinal wall. The causes of UC and CD are not yet known.

Crohn's Disease

KY The manifestations of CD depend on the site of involvement, severity, and the extent to which inflammation, fibrostenosis, or fistulae interfere with normal gut function. A working scale of CD activity has been proposed by the American College of Gastroenterology (Table 6–7).

TX1 **Induction of remission.**

RX1 Table 6–8

DS1 Table 6–8

SE1 Table 6–8

TX2 **Maintenance of remission:** Once remission is achieved, approximately 50% of patients with CD will experience a relapse during the next

Table 6–7. American College of Gastroenterology Criteria for Severity of Crohn's Disease

Clinical Features	Severity of Crohn's Disease
Ambulatory, adequate nutrition/hydration with oral diet, no abdominal mass or tenderness, no obstruction, no toxic signs or symptoms	Mild to moderate
Low-grade fever, weight loss, abdominal pain, abdominal tenderness, anemia, obstructive signs or symptoms	Moderate to severe
Symptoms as above despite oral corticosteroids Cachexia, high fever, frank obstruction, abscess, peritoneal signs	Severe or fulminant

Table 6–8. Treatment Options for Inducing Remission in CD

Clinical Situation	Treatment Options	
Mild to moderate ileocolonic or colonic CD	Oral 5'ASA	Sulfasalazine [B/D at term] Mesalamine [B]
Mild to moderate ileocolonic or colonic CD or perianal fistulae	Antibiotics	Metronidazole (Flagyl) [B] Ciprofloxacin (Ciloxan, Cipro) [C] Clarithromycin (Biaxin) [C]
Moderate to severe CD activity	Oral corticosteroids	Prednisone [B] Prednisolone [C]
		Budesonide (Entocort) [C]
	Methotrexate (Folex, Rheumatrex) [D]	
Moderate to severe CD activity despite treatment with conventional agents, or intolerant to conventional agents	Infliximab (Remicade) [B]	
Fistulizing CD	Infliximab (Remicade) [B]	
Severe CD activity	Intravenous corticosteroids	Methylprednisolone (Solu-Medrol) [C]

CD = Crohn's disease; 5'ASA = 5'aminosalicylate; AVN = avascular necrosis; CHF = congestive heart failure.

12–18 months. Continued treatment with conventional corcticosteroids offers no benefit in maintaining remission, but several other alternatives exist (Table 6–9).

RX2 Table 6–9

DS2 Table 6–9

SE2 Table 6–9

TX3 Maintenance of remission after surgical resection in CD: This refers to the special situation in which a patient achieves remission through surgical resection of affected bowel rather than through medical induction. The natural history of this situation is different, but a

Dose	Side Effects and Cautions
4 g/day PO in divided doses	Table 6–12
4 g/day PO in divided doses	
500 mg PO bid	Hypersensitivity. **Ciprofloxacin should not be used in children** because of potential interference with cartilage development
40 mg/day PO	Table 6–12
9 mg/day PO (effective for ileal, ileal-cecal, and ascending-colon CD)	AVN, acne, allergic reactions, alopecia, headache, hypertension, infection, easy bruising, edema, fat redistribution, osteoporosis, psychosis, striae
25 mg/week IM	Hepatic fibrosis, myelosuppression, teratogenesis
5 mg/kg IV initially and then (if no response) a second dose 4 weeks later	Delayed hypersensitivity reactions with repeat infusions Development of autoimmune markers Increased risk of lymphoma Increased incidence of fatal outcome and hospitalization in CHF patients taking infliximab
5 mg/kg IV initially and then 2 and 6 weeks later	Increased risk of serious infections
1 mg/kg IV in single dose	Steroids should be **used with caution** in patients who have or may have an abscess.

few therapeutic options have been shown to prolong remission (Table 6–10).

RX3 Table 6–10

DS3 Table 6–10

SE3 Table 6–10

Ulcerative Colitis

KY Patients with active UC experience diarrhea, with or without blood, bowel urgency, and rectal tenesmus, and clinical recognition of the severity of UC is important (Table 6–11).

Table 6–9. Treatment Options for Maintaining Remission in CD

Generic (Brand) Name	Dose	Side Effects and Cautions
Oral 5'ASA Azathioprine (Imuran) [D]	2–3 g/day PO 1.5–2 mg/kg/day provides benefit for 2–4 years (optimal length of treatment unknown)	Table 6–8 Leukopenia, pancytopenia, hepatotoxicity Occasionally, a flulike syndrome of malaise, myalgia, and arthralgia Theoretical risk of lymphomas **CBC and tests of liver enzymes** should be performed weekly in the first 4–6 weeks and then monthly thereafter for as long as therapy continues. Allopurinol is an inhibitor of xanthine oxidase, and **azathioprine doses should be reduced** by at least half if allopurinol treatment is required for hyperuricemia.
Methotrexate [D]	15 mg/kg/week IM	Table 6–8
Budesonide (Entocort) [C]	6 mg PO qd for up to 1 year	Table 6–12. Note that side effects from long-term use are unknown.
Infliximab (Remicade) [B]	5 mg/kg IV q8wk (optimal number treatments unknown).	Table 6–8. Note that side effects from long-term use are unknown.

5'ASA = 5'aminosalicylate.

TX1 **Induction of remission:** The choice of drug and route of delivery depends on the extent and severity of the UC (Table 6–12).

RX1 Table 6–12

DS1 Table 6–12

Table 6–10. Treatment Options for Remission After Surgical Resection in Crohn's Disease

Generic (Brand) Name	Dose	Side Effects
5'ASA (only marginal benefit in isolated small-bowel disease)	2–3 g PO qd	Table 6–8
Azathioprine (Imuran) [D]	Table 6–9	Table 6–9
Metronidazole (Flagyl) [B]	20 mg/kg/day PO in divided doses q8hr started within 1 week of surgery and continued for 3 months	Table 6–8

5'ASA = 5'aminosalicylate.

Table 6–11. Criteria for Severity of Ulcerative Colitis

Clinical Features	Severity*
BM ≤ 4/day with or without blood Systemic disturbance = 0 ESR < 30 mm/hr	Mild
BM > 6/day with blood Resting HR > 90 bpm Temperature > 37.5°C Hb < 105 g/L ESR > 30 mm/hr	Severe

BM = bowel movement; ESR = erythrocyte sedimentation rate; HR = heart rate; Hb = hemoglobin.

*Moderate is between mild and severe.

Reprinted with permission from Truelove SC, Witts LJ. Cortisone in ulcerative colitis: final report on therapeutic trial. BMJ 1955;2:1041–1048.

SE1 Table 6–12. **Caution is needed in the case of toxic megacolon,** an extreme form of severe UC in which the clinical manifestations of severe UC (Table 6–11) are accompanied by colonic dilatation, demonstrated by a colonic diameter > 6 cm on plain abdominal radiograph, and systemic toxicity. Patients with this syndrome need care by gastroenterologic and colorectal surgical consultants jointly and are in **danger.** Treatment with **intravenous corticosteroids** should be initiated. Patients who do not show clinical improvement within 48–72 hours are likely to require urgent subtotal colectomy.

TX2 **Maintenance of remission:** This is best achieved with either continued 5'aminosalicylate (5'ASA) therapy or with azathioprine. Corticosteroids are not of benefit in maintaining remission of UC.

RX2a Oral or topical 5'ASA (Table 6–12).

DS2a Usual maintenance dose is 2–3 g/day PO in divided doses. Patients can be instructed to increase their medication immediately if they develop increased colitis symptoms.

SE2a Table 6–12

or

RX2b **Azathioprine:** Optional treatment in patients who have had frequent or severe attacks of UC or are intolerant to 5'ASA.

DS2b If thiopurine methyltransferase (TMTase) activity levels are available, patients with normal activity of this enzyme can be treated with **doses of azathioprine 1.5–2 mg/kg PO qd.** Patients with intermediate activities should be treated with half the usual dose. **Patients with no TMTase activity should not receive this drug.** If TMTase activity cannot be measured, an alternative strategy is to start treatment at half the dosage for at least 4 weeks because patients with low levels respond adversely within that time frame. After 4 weeks, normal dosing can be undertaken.

Table 6–12. Treatment Options for Inducing Remission in UC

Severity	Treatment Options	
Mild to moderate distal UC	Topical 5'ASA Oral 5'ASA	Sulfasalazine (Azulfidine, EN-Tabs—*U.S.*; Salazopyrin—*Can.*) [B/D at term]
		Olsalazine (Dipentum) [C]
		Mesalamine (Asacol, Canasa, Pentasa, Rowasa; Mesasal, Quintasa—*U.S.;* Salofalk—*Can.*) [B]
Mild to moderate distal UC not responding to 5'ASA	Topical steroids	CIR-budesonide (Entocort) enema [C]
		Hydrocortisone enema (Cortenema) [C]
		Hydrocortisone foam (Cortifoam) [C]
Moderate UC extending to the splenic flexure	Oral 5'ASA	See above
Severe UC	Oral corticosteroids	Prednisone* [B]
	Intravenous cortico-steroids (used in patients unresponsive to oral corticosteroids)	Methylprednisolone (Solu-Medrol) [C]
	Intravenous cyclosporine (used in patients unre-sponsive to IV corticosteroids)	Cyclosporine (Sandimmune) [C]

UC = ulcerative colitis; 5'ASA = 5'aminosalicylate; GI = gastrointestinal; GU = genitourinary; CIR = controlled ileal-release; PR = per rectum; AVN = avascular necrosis.

*Prednisone can be tapered at approximately 5 mg/day/week; at doses of 10–15 mg/day, it can be tapered at 2.5 mg/day/week.

Dose	Side Effects and Cautions
1–4 g/day	Anal irritation
2–6 g/day PO in divided doses	GI upset, headache, hemolytic anemia, photo-sensitivity, reversible oligospermia, urticaria **Use with caution** in patients with renal or hepatic impairment, blood dyscrasias, and severe allergies or asthma. **Contraindicated** in patients with hyper-sensitivity to sulfa drugs or salicylates; porphyria; GI or GU obstruction; in children < 2 years.
1–3 g/day PO in divided doses	Depression, diarrhea, fatigue, headache, rash; rarely, blood dyscrasia, hepatitis, cirrhosis, jaundice **Contraindicated** in patients with hypersensitivity to sulfa drugs or salicylates.
2–6 g/day PO in divided doses	May cause an acute intolerance syndrome and drug should be discontinued. GI upset, chest pain, edema; rarely, pericarditis, pancreatitis, blood dyscrasias, renal impairment. **Use with caution** in patients with renal or hepatic impairment. **Contraindicated** in patients with hypersensitivity to sulfa drugs or salicylates.
2 mg/100 mL PR qhs	Anal irritation and potentially the side effects listed in Table 6–8.
100 mg/60 mL PR qhs	Anal irritation and potentially the side effects listed for oral corticosteroids
80 mg/6.5 mL PR qhs	
See above	See above
Doses up to 40 mg/day PO (clinical improvement may take up to 3 weeks) 1 mg/kg IV (once the patient is improving, oral prednisone at an equivalent dose can be substituted)*	Acne, increased appetite, mood disruption, sleep disturbance, swelling Long-term use increases risk of diabetes mellitus, myopathy, abdominal striae, easy bruising, bone mineral loss,† and AVN.‡
Continuous infusion starting at 4 mg/kg/day for up to 7 days (dosage needs to be adjusted to achieve and maintain serum concentration at 100–300 mg/mL)	Hypertension and renal insufficiency—usually transient, but can persist after drug cessation. Hypertrichosis, paresthesia Seizures can occur during infusion, and low serum cholesterol is thought to be a risk factor for this event.

†Prednisone and prednisolone (Solu-Medrol) predictably lead to bone mineral loss, and patients should be offered treatment to offset this with bisphosphonates, calcium, and vitamin D supplementation (see Ch 5 Endocrinology, the Osteoporosis section).

‡AVN can occur at any dosage and at any time during treatment; patients taking corticosteroids are advised to seek medical attention when knee or hip pain is experienced.

SE2b Leukopenia, pancytopenia, pancreatic irritation, and occasionally a flulike syndrome of malaise, myalgia, and arthralgia. Complete blood cell count and liver enzymes should be tested weekly in the first 4–6 weeks and then monthly thereafter for as long as the patient continues therapy. **Theoretical risk of lymphomas.** Allopurinol is an inhibitor of xanthine oxidase, and **azathioprine dosages should be reduced by at least half if allopurinol treatment is required for hyperuricemia.**

Other Forms of Idiopathic Inflammatory Bowel Disease

KY There are two forms of colitis that lead to nonbloody, loose, watery stools: collagenous colitis and lymphocytic colitis. In these conditions, the colonic mucosa is endoscopically normal, but histologic examination reveals either a thickened layer of collagen beneath the epithelium (collagenous colitis) or an infiltrate of lymphocytes in the lamina propria beneath the epithelial band. The etiology of these conditions is unknown.

TX Treatment is aimed at controlling the diarrhea and at eliminating aggravating factors such as lactose, caffeine, and NSAIDS.

RX **Bismuth** [C/D in the third trimester]: See DIARRHEA: ACUTE AND INFECTIOUS.

DS 524 mg PO qid for 8 weeks

SE See DIARRHEA: ACUTE AND INFECTIOUS.

PEPTIC ULCER

KY Peptic ulcer means a hole in the lining of the stomach or duodenum, most commonly caused by either *Helicobacter pylori* infection in the stomach (diagnosed by serology, urea breath test, or endoscopic gastric biopsy) or NSAIDs. **Cancer should always be ruled out by biopsy in gastric ulcer.** Far less common causes are Zollinger-Ellison syndrome, viruses such as cytomegalovirus, ischemia, and CD. Idiopathic peptic ulcer is being increasingly recognized.

TX Pharmaceuticals are only rarely sufficient in the presence of complications such as bleeding, perforation, and obstruction. Use of NSAIDs should be discontinued, if possible; otherwise, a PPI (Table 6–1) should be coadministered. *Helicobacter pylori* infection should be treated (Table 6–13).

RX Table 6–13 describes treatment options for *H. pylori*.

DS Table 6–13

SE If diarrhea develops during combination therapy for *H. pylori* infection, the treatment should be discontinued immediately to lower the risk of **life-threatening *C. difficile* colitis** (see DIARRHEA: ACUTE AND INFECTIOUS). Vomiting is more likely to be caused by the drugs, so treatment should be discontinued.

Table 6–13. Treatment of *Helicobacter pylori*

Recommended regimen: if no penicillin allergy, 2-week course of:
Proton pump inhibitor (double dose)
Omeprazole 20 mg PO bid or lansoprazole 30 mg PO bid
plus
Clarithromycin 250 mg PO bid
plus
Amoxicillin 1 g PO bid

Alternative regimen: 2-week course of:
Proton pump inhibitor (double dose)
Omeprazole 20 mg PO bid or lansoprazole 30 mg PO bid
plus
Clarithromycin 250 mg PO bid
plus
Metronidazole 500 mg PO bid

Alternative regimen: 2-week course of:
Bismuth (Pepto-Bismol) 524 mg PO qid
plus
Metronidazole 250 mg PO qid
plus
Tetracycline 500 mg PO qid

If preferred regimen fails: 2-week course of:
Proton pump inhibitor (double dose)
Omeprazole 20 mg PO bid or lansoprazole 30 mg PO bid
plus
Bismuth (Pepto-Bismol) 524 mg PO qid
plus
Tetracycline 500 mg PO qid
plus
Metronidazole 500 mg PO tid or clarithromycin 500 mg PO tid (whichever of
these two drugs was **not** given with the first course of treatment)

UPPER GI TRACT BLEEDING

KY Bleeding from proximal to the ligament of Trietz. The two most common causes include peptic ulcer and varices.

TX The optimal approach to bleeding from proximal to the ligament of Trietz involves resuscitation, transfusions, and endoscopy for accurate diagnosis and therapeutic intervention. However, effective **adjuvant pharmaceutical therapy** is now available for the two most common causes of upper GI tract bleeding: peptic ulcer and varices (Table 6–14) Since both of these drugs are usually safe, they can be used empirically, that is, before endoscopy to treat a suspected cause of bleeding. Once the patient is eating, **intravenous pantoprazole** can be replaced by any of the **oral PPIs** (Table 6–1).

RX Table 6–14
DS Table 6–14
SE Table 6–14

Table 6-14. Treatment of UGI Bleeding

Generic (Brand) Name	Dose	Mechanism of Action	Indication	Side Effects and Cautions
Octreotide (Sandostatin) [B]	50 μg IV over 20 minutes, followed by 50 μg/hr for 24–72 hours	Direct splanchnic vasoconstriction decreases azygous and thus variceal blood flow	Acute variceal bleeding	GI upset, hyperglycemia, sinus bradycardia **Use with caution** in patients with renal impairment.
Nonselective beta-blockers				
Propranolol (Inderal) [C]	40 mg PO qd, then titrating to 25% fall in resting pulse	Decrease portal pressure by (1) decreasing cardiac output, (2) allowing adrenergic vasoconstriction to be unopposed, thus constricting splanchnic vessels	Prevention of repeated variceal bleed or primary prevention of a first bleeding episode if varices are large or have stigmata of hemorrhage	Depression, fatigue, impotence, decreased libido, nightmares; rarely, heart failure, bronchospasm **Contraindicated** in patients with asthma, decompensated heart failure, significant heart block, bradycardia, and hypotension. **Avoid concomitant use with either verapamil or diltiazem**, which can cause heart block.
Nadolol (Corgard) [C]	20 mg PO qd, then titrating to 25% fall in resting pulse			
Pantoprazole (Protonix—U.S.; Panto, Pantoloc—Can.) [B]	80 mg IV over 30 minutes, then 8 mg/hr	Decreases gastric acid to stabilize clot, heal ulcer	Bleeding peptic ulcer	Table 6–1

GI = gastrointestinal.

108

7

Geriatrics

RAJIN MEHTA

The aging population provides an interesting challenge for the clinician, particularly in the field of clinical pharmacology. Multisystem disease increases the complexity of care plans, and "atypical" disease presentation is extremely common. Unfortunately, these challenges may result in the elderly being both overtreated for some conditions and undertreated for others. This chapter highlights some of the consequences of aging and discusses common geriatric syndromes, with particular reference to therapeutics.

PHARMACOKINETIC CHANGES WITH AGE

The effects of age on drug pharmacokinetics include changes in absorption, distribution, metabolism, and excretion. These changes are summarized in Table 7–1. Although there are many changes, two important considerations should be kept in mind. **First, change in renal drug excretion resulting from an inevitable decline in renal function is the most important pharmacokinetic change in the elderly.** Therefore, drugs that are cleared renally will have higher plasma concentrations, and dosages should be adjusted to account for this. Serum creatinine may not be a good marker for renal function in the elderly as it may remain relatively normal owing to a smaller muscle mass despite declining renal function. As renal function may have declined by 30%–50% by age 80 years, the actual creatinine clearance may be estimated by using the Cockcroft and Gault formula:

For men: Cl_{creat} (ml/min) = (140 − age) × (weight in kg) ÷
serum creatinine (in mg/dL) × 72
For women: Cl_{creat} (ml/min) = [(140 − age) × (weight in kg) ÷
serum creatinine (in mg/dL) × 72] × 0.85

Second, given the decrease in homeostatic reserve as individuals age, superimposed illnesses, even minor ones, may have significant effects on these changes. For example, malnutrition and dehydration may greatly exacerbate change in distribution, metabolism, and excretion.

PHARMACODYNAMIC CHANGES WITH AGE

The impact of aging on the physiologic and biochemical effects of drugs as well as the mechanisms of action are not clearly delineated. Generalizations are difficult as responses vary widely. However, most changes cited in the literature and routinely seen suggest an increased sensitivity to medications. Some common examples include the increased sedative effects and memory impairment with benzodiazepines, greater analgesic effects with morphine, and greater hypotensive effects (particularly postural hypotension) with antihypertensives. The most frequently cited examples of decreased sensitivity

Table 7–1. Age-Related Changes in Pharmacokinetics

Parameter	Change	Significance
Absorption	Increase in gastric pH	Likely minimal
	Decrease in intestinal blood flow	Likely minimal
	Mild decrease in motility	Possibly minimal delay in absorption of certain drugs (e.g., analgesics) resulting in delayed onset of effect
Distribution	**Body composition**	
	Decrease in total body water and lean body mass	Decrease in volume of distribution of water-soluble drugs; lower loading doses should be used (e.g., digoxin, lithium, alcohol)
	Increase in total fat content	Increase in volume of distribution, and duration of action, of lipid-soluble drugs (e.g., diazepam has a much greater/larger toxic effect)
	Altered protein binding	
	Decrease in serum albumin (which is significantly worsened by chronic disease or malnutrition)	May interfere with interpretation of drug levels, especially those that are highly protein bound (e.g., phenytoin level may be low or normal but free level may be normal or high)
	Increase in alpha-acid glycoprotein	Increase in binding and possibly decrease in clearance (e.g., lidocaine)
Excretion*	Decrease in excretion	Increase in serum level of drugs or active metabolites that are renally excreted (e.g., angiotensin-converting enzyme inhibitors, aminoglycosides, digoxin, lithium)
	Decrease in renal concentrating ability	
Metabolism	Decrease in liver mass and blood flow	Decrease in metabolism with higher serum levels of drugs metabolized in the liver (e.g., acetaminophen, theophylline, codeine)
		Increase in oral bioavailability for drugs with significant first-pass metabolism (e.g., morphine, propanolol, lidocaine, nifedipine)
	Decrease in oxidative metabolism (no change in conjugation and acetylation)	Increase in drug levels (e.g., diazepam)

*Excretion is the most important change.

are diminished response to isoproterenol to increase heart rate and to propranolol to decrease heart rate. However, the large interindividual variation makes the assumption that all older individuals would require large doses of these medications invalid. Furthermore, there is a general decrease in "homeostatic reserve," that is, the ability to withstand any physiologic perturbation, in the elderly. As such, the increased "sensitivity" to medications may be caused by this decreased ability to withstand the drug side effects.

THERAPEUTIC DRUG MONITORING

Given the changes in pharmacokinetics and pharmacodynamics, in combination with an increased prevalence of disease, **drug dosing must be individualized for the elderly. One option is to consider therapeutic drug monitoring whereby drugs are titrated to a specific plasma concentration of the drug.** Common examples include digoxin, lithium, theophylline, and various anticonvulsants. Measuring the international normalized ratio would not be in this category as it is measuring the effect of warfarin rather than the drug level itself. **One caveat: the target ranges that are quoted are often derived from younger, healthier populations and may be inappropriately high for older, frailer patients.** A common example is digoxin, where patients may be toxic despite "normal" levels. Therefore, although therapeutic drug monitoring is useful, particularly for aminoglycosides and anticonvulsants, one must be aware of the potential for side effects, even if the levels are "therapeutic." Another concern relates to changes in the concentration of binding proteins. A low albumin level may result in a low total drug level, whereas the actual unbound concentration of the drug (which generally determines the therapeutic response) may still be therapeutic, for example, phenytoin. If the same patient with a low albumin level has a "high therapeutic range" total drug level, the actual unbound concentration may be toxic for that patient.

SIDE EFFECTS IN THE ELDERLY

Side effects are more common in the elderly, particularly those older than 85 years. Older patients have nearly double the number of side effects as younger patients, and side effects account for up to 20% of hospital admissions in the elderly. However, age is not believed to be an independent risk factor for side effects. Instead, the medical conditions that are more prevalent with increasing age are much more significant. **Risk factors for side effects include** increasing number of prescription medications (especially > 4); multiple medical problems; cardiac, hepatic, or renal insufficiency; malnutrition; cognitive impairment (particularly when medication supervision is questionable); more than 2–4 new medications added to an existing regimen during hospitalization; and inappropriate prescribing. Despite these recognized risk factors, **many actual side effects go unrecognized.** Physicians and families may misinterpret side effects or other adverse events as "normal aging changes." The problem is further compounded when the side effects are then treated with more medications. An example includes using antipsychotic agents, which may cause extrapyramidal side effects, and then starting antiparkinsonian agents, assuming (incorrectly) that the patient now has Parkinson's disease. Similarly, beta-blockers can induce depression, which then triggers use of an antidepressant. A review of all side effects is beyond the scope and intent of this chapter, but some side effects are more common in the elderly (Table 7–2). An important point for the physician or caregiver to keep in mind is that when any new symptom occurs, side effects should always be considered a possibility.

COMPLIANCE IN GERIATRICS

Noncompliance with medication occurs more commonly in the elderly but is not related to age. Instead, the **factors that affect compliance occur more commonly in the elderly, thus putting this group at**

Table 7–2. Common Side Effects in the Elderly

Side Effect	Typical Medications
Acute renal failure	ACE inhibitors
	Aminoglycosides
	Cyclo-oxygenase-2 inhibitor
	NSAIDs
Constipation	Anticholinergics
	Calcium channel blockers
	Iron
	Opioids
Delirium (people with baseline dementia are especially at risk)	Anticholinergics
	Anticonvulsants
	Benzodiazepines or other sedatives
	Digoxin
	H_2 antagonists
	NSAIDs
	Steroids
Falls	Anticholinergics
	Antidepressants
	Antihypertensives*
	Antiparkinsonian medications*
	Diuretics*
	Nitrates*
	Any sedative
Gastrointestinal bleeding	NSAIDs
Orthostatic hypotension	Antihypertensives
	Antiparkinsonian medications
	Diuretics
	Nitrates
Urinary incontinence	Diuretics
Urinary retention	Anticholinergic agents (e.g., TCAs)
	Sympathomimetic agents (e.g., pseudoephedrine)

ACE = angiotensin-converting enzyme; NSAIDs = nonsteroidal anti-inflammatory drugs; TCAs = tricyclic antidepressants.

*Medications that can cause orthostatic hypotension, which can contribute to falls in the elderly.

Table 7–3. Factors Influencing Compliance

Level of Compliance	Factors Influencing Level of Compliance
No effect	Age, education, effectiveness of the drugs, ethnicity, severity of disease, sex
Increased compliance	Careful explanation by the physician or health care provider, patient's belief that the drug is effective
Decreased compliance	$\geq$ 12 medication dosages per day, complex schedule, cognitive impairment (when patient has no caregiver), functional impairment (especially decreased vision or manual dexterity), increase dosing frequency, multiple prescribers or pharmacies, number of drugs (especially if $>$ 5), use of child-resistant drug containers

higher risk (Table 7–3). In addition to the factors listed in the table, there are some other special circumstances to consider. Discharge from the hospital represents a particularly vulnerable time for noncompliance to start. Up to 20% of prescriptions are not filled at discharge, and the confusion that ensues between new and old medications can be significant. Conversely, on admission to the hospital, "**enforced compliance**" may occur. In a previously noncompliant patient, this may induce side effects, especially if the patient was practicing "intelligent noncompliance" (i.e., they were not taking the recommended dose because of side effects). **Dietary changes that occur between hospital and home may have an impact on treatment effectiveness.** This may inadvertently be assumed to be caused by medication effectiveness or compliance with resultant changes in medication or dosing when, in fact, dietary changes are primarily responsible. Examples include noncompliance to a diabetic diet or, for patients in congestive heart failure, not following a fluid and salt restriction diet. On admission to the hospital, these dietary restrictions may be enforced, leading to much more "effective" pharmacotherapy.

APPROPRIATE PRESCRIBING IN GERIATRICS

In the past, polypharmacy was described as an excessive number of medications. **However, there is no "right" number of medications for any patient.** Instead, one must consider appropriate medication use, which considers drug indications, dosing, frequency, drug interactions, safety, and expense. Most clinicians are aware of the importance of not **overtreating** patients, although overtreating still occurs with 25%–50% of elderly patients taking medications for which there is no apparent indication. There is also the important notion of **undertreating** patients, and this is less well appreciated. **Overall, it is important to provide effective therapy with appropriate dosages for diseases in the elderly with the goal of maintaining functional independence and quality of life.**

GERIATRIC SYNDROMES

Commonly encountered conditions in the elderly include dementia, delirium, sleep disturbances, pressure ulcers, urinary incontinence, and falls.

Dementia, Delirium, and Sleep Disturbances

See Ch 19 Psychiatry.

Pressure Ulcers

See Ch 4 Dermatology.

Urinary Incontinence

See Ch 22 Urology.

Falls

KY Falls are associated with significant morbidity and mortality rates in geriatrics. Although environmental hazards may sometimes precipitate a fall, **it is usually a combination of intrinsic factors within the individual that precipitates the fall.** This can occur when there is a decline in the normal homeostatic mechanisms that maintain postural stability, as well as underlying age-related declines in balance, ambulation, and cardiovascular function. Falls could be caused by an acute illness (e.g., infection, fever, dehydration, arrhythmia), an environmental stress (e.g., newly initiated medication), or an unsafe walking surface. It is unlikely, however, for an extrinsic (environmental) stress alone to completely explain the circumstances of a fall. **Risk factors for falls** in the elderly include age, female sex, past history of a fall, cognitive impairment, lower-extremity weakness, balance problems, psychotropic drug use, and arthritis.

TX One approach to falls in the elderly is to **consider gait and balance as a complex event requiring sensory input, a processing center, and a motor or effector output** (Table 7–4). Some drugs are more likely to cause

Table 7–4. Conceptual Approach to Falls in the Elderly

Sensory Input	Processing Center	Motor or Effector Output

Hearing
  Example: presbycusis
Proprioception
  Example: B_{12} deficiency
Sensation (in feet)
  Example: diabetes
  mellitus
Vestibular function
  Example: aminogly-
  coside toxicity
Vision
  Examples: cataracts,
  diabetic retinopathy,
  macular degeneration
	Brain
	  Examples: delirium,
	  dementia, Parkin-
	  sonism, stroke, tumor
	Spinal cord
	  Example: trauma
		Bones
		  Example: fractures
		Joints
		  Examples: arthritis,
		  toe deformities
		Muscles
		  Examples: myopathy
		  from steroids or
		  deconditioning
		Nerves
		  Example: neuropathy

Table 7–5. Therapeutic Approach to Falls in the Elderly

Cause	Characteristics	Intervention	Note
Hypotension	Orthostatic Postprandial	Behavior change (drug-meal separation, posture, meals, exercises) Drug reduction Pharmacologic intervention (e.g., fludrocortisone) Volume control (compression stockings, elevation of head of bed)	Fludrocortisone (Florinef): Promotes increased resorption of sodium and loss of potassium from renal distal tubules. Usual dose is 0.1–0.2 mg/day PO. Side effects include hypertension, edema, congestive heart failure, dizziness, hypokalemic alkalosis, peptic ulcer, and muscle weakness.
Leg extension weakness	Difficulty in climbing stairs Impaired ability to change from sitting position to standing Slow gait	Physiotherapy Resistance training	—
Medication toxicity	Alcohol use Anticholinergics Anticonvulsants Digoxin Hypotensives Nitrates Sedatives/hypnotics	Drug reduction Drug substitution Drug withdrawal	Reduce or eliminate, if possible, long-acting antihypertensives, benzodiazepines, neuroleptics, and nitrates
Poor balance	Poor vision Positive Romberg test*	Corrected vision Balance training Widened base of support (shoes, cane, walker)	—

*Romberg test: The patient stands with feet together and eyes closed; the physician should remain close to the patient to prevent injury from fall. Tests for a severe proprioceptive or vestibular lesion or for a midline cerebellar lesion causing truncal instability. The test is considered positive if the patient sways to one side.

falls (see Table 7–2), and their indications should be reconsidered in the event of a fall. The therapeutic approach to falls in the elderly is given in Table 7–5. (See page 115)

RX Table 7–5

DS Table 7–5

SE Table 7–5

8

Gynecology

HEATHER E. EDWARDS, KAREN GRONAU, CHRISTINE M. DERZKO

ABNORMAL UTERINE BLEEDING

Abnormal uterine bleeding is defined as changes in frequency of menses, duration of flow, or amount of blood loss.

Amenorrhea

KY **Primary amenorrhea** is caused by malfunction of the hypothalamic-pituitary-gonadal axis, the absence of ovaries (e.g., gonadal agenesis), or obstruction of the outflow tract (e.g., imperforate hymen, transverse vaginal septum). Causes of **secondary amenorrhea** include pregnancy, menopause, stress, hypothyroidism, polycystic ovarian syndrome, and hyperprolactinemia (which inhibits gonadotropin-releasing hormone secretion). Drugs that either increase prolactin (e.g., antipsychotics, tricyclic antidepressants, calcium channel blockers) or have endogenous estrogenic activity (e.g., digoxin, marijuana, oral contraceptives [OCs]) also induce amenorrhea.

TX Treatment depends on the cause.

RX Table 8–1

DS Table 8–1

SE OC side effects are listed in Table 8–2.

Table 8–1. Treatment of Amenorrhea

Cause of Amenorrhea	Treatment
Asherman syndrome	Hysteroscopy with lysis of adhesions, often followed by insertion of an intrauterine device for 3–6 weeks only
Chronic anovulation	Cyclic oral contraceptive, or Cyclic progestin Diet, exercise, weight loss, with or without metformin (Glucophage) 500 mg PO qd and increased to tid as needed.
Hyperprolactinemia	Discontinue drug medication that raises prolactin. Cabergoline (Dostinex) 0.25–1 mg PO, twice a week, or Bromocriptine (Parlodel) 2.5 mg PO qd qhs (maximum = 40 mg/day)
Hypothalamic dysfunction	Cyclic oral contraceptive, or Combined hormone replacement therapy
Premature ovarian failure	Hormone replacement therapy to treat vasomotor symptoms

Table 8–2. Treatment of Abnormal Uterine Bleeding

Type of Bleeding	Treatment	Side Effects
Acute severe bleeding (hemodynamically unstable)	Premarin 25 mg IV over 15 minutes q6hr for three doses **If bleeding cannot be controlled:** Dilation and curettage **If bleeding is not stopped:** Coagulation with hysteroscope or Uterine artery embolization	**Premarin:** Manifestations of excessive estrogenic stimulation, such as abnormal or excessive uterine bleeding or mastodynia; fluid retention. Prolonged unopposed estrogen may increase risk of endometrial hyperplasia.
Acute moderate bleeding (hemodynamically stable)	Conjugated estrogen (Premarin) 2.5 mg PO qd for days 1–25, followed by progesterone (Prometrium) 200 mg PO qd on days 16–25; or Oral contraceptive containing high-dose estrogen and synthetic progesterone (e.g., Ortho-Novum 1/50) qid for 7 days	**Oral contraceptives** can cause nausea, breast tenderness, mood changes, intermenstrual bleeding, amenorrhea, hypertension, venous thromboembolic disease, and stroke. There is an increased risk of coronary heart disease in cigarette smokers ($\geq$ 25 cigarettes/day). Oral contraceptives have been shown to increase risk of cerebral vein thrombosis in women with hereditary prothrombophilias (factor V Leiden, prothrombin gene mutation, and deficiencies in protein C, protein S, and antithrombin III).
Anovulatory bleeding (hemodynamically stable)	Medroxyprogesterone acetate (Provera) 10 mg PO qd 12–14 days each month Mirena: intrauterine device with levonorgestrel (releases 20 μg over 24 hours), or Danazol 100–200 mg qd, or Tranexamic acid (Cyklokapron) 1 g q6hr for first 4 days of menstrual cycle Combined oral contraceptives. Examples include ethinyl estradiol, norethindrone (Modicon 21); ethinyl estradiol, norethindrone (Ortho-Novum 1/35); ethinyl estradiol, norgestimate (Ortho-Cyclin 21, 28); ethinyl estradiol, norgestrel (Lo/Ovral)	**Progestins** can cause irregular bleeding. Caution with use of medroxyprogesterone acetate in patients with asthma, depression, renal or cardiac dysfunction, or thromboembolic disorders. Mirena: Rarely, risk of uterine perforation. Danazol: Can cause weight gain and amenorrhea. Cyklokapron: Can cause nausea and leg cramps. Other side effects of oral contraceptives are listed above.

Dysfunctional Uterine Bleeding

KY Dysfunctional uterine bleeding may be described as "anovulatory bleeding." Without ovulation, a progesterone-secreting corpus luteum does not form, and unopposed estrogen causes increased vascularity and proliferation of the endometrium. As areas of endometrium outgrow their vascular blood supply, they begin to bleed. **Causes of anovulatory bleeding:** In adolescents (13–18 years), anovulatory bleeding is the result of immaturity of the hypothalamic-pituitary system; in women of early and middle reproductive years (19–39 years), anovulatory bleeding may be caused by hyperthyroidism or hypothyroidism, hyperprolactinemia, hyperandrogenism (i.e., polycystic ovarian disease), or hypothalamic dysfunction resulting from psychologic stress, exercise, or weight loss; during the late reproductive years (40 years to menopause), anovulatory bleeding is often caused by declining ovarian function. Abnormal uterine bleeding in older women must be investigated to rule out pelvic pathology.

TX Any medical conditions identified as the cause of dysfunctional uterine bleeding (e.g., thyroid disease, hyperprolactinemia) should be corrected. The general treatment of anovulation is **cyclic progestins** or **OCs containing at least 30 μg of ethinyl estradiol. Progesterone-impregnated intrauterine devices** (such as Mirena) have also been reported to reduce menstrual bleeding. **Danazol** (Danocrine—*U.S.;* Cyclomen— *Can.*), a synthetic steroid with mild androgenic properties, can reduce menstrual flow by up to 80% by antagonizing the effect of estrogen on the endometrium. Tranexamic acid **(Cyklokapron)** is an antifibrinolytic agent that can reduce menstrual blood loss by up to 40%. For acute heavy bleeding, **high-dose estrogen is used initially, followed by a combined OC.**

RX Table 8–2

DS Table 8–2

SE Table 8–2

Polycystic Ovarian Syndrome

See Ch 5 Endocrinology.

HORMONAL CONTRACEPTION

Emergency Postcoital Contraception

KY **Emergency postcoital contraception (EPC) prevents ovulation, inhibits fertilization, and induces an unreceptive endometrium.** Although EPC should not be used as a substitute for contraceptive use, any woman of reproductive age who presents within 72 hours of an unprotected sexual encounter, at any time in her menstrual cycle, may be offered this contraception. Most patients (98%) will have a menstrual period within 21 days of treatment, most in < 2 weeks. There is no evidence of teratogenicity of failed EPC when the pregnancy is carried to term.

Table 8–3. Methods of Emergency Postcoital Contraception

Category	Medication	Dose/Regimen
Estrogen only	Diethylstilbestrol (Stilphostrol) [X]	25–50 PO 5 times/day
Yuzpe* regimen— "2 + 2" routine	Ethinyl estradiol and norgestrel (Ogestrel, Ovral†) [X]	2 tablets PO 1qhr for 1 day
	Yuzpe regimen + early pregnancy kit (Preven) [X]	(10 mg LNG + 100 µg EE$_2$) PO; repeat in 12 hours
Progestin only	Norgestrel (Ovrette) [X]	10 tablets LNG 0.074 mg PO; repeat in 12 hours
	Levonorgestrel (Mirena, Norplant, Plan B)	0.75-mg tablet PO; repeat in 12 hours
Copper IUD	Copper ions increase gamete toxicity (sterile intrauterine foreign body reaction)	Insertion into endometrial cavity postcoitally
Antiprogesterone RU 486/RU 38486	Mifepristone (Mifeprex) [X]	Single dose 600 mg PO

EE$_2$ = ethinyl estradiol; GI = gastrointestinal; IUD = intrauterine device; LNG = levonorgestrel.
*Yuzpe: [0.05 mg of EE$_2$ + 0.5 mg of LNG].
†Min-Ovral—four tablets q12hr for 1 day.

TX Methods often recommended for EPC are shown in Table 8–3. The Yuzpe method (also known as the "morning-after pill") has an effectiveness of approximately 75% and can be used for up to 72 hours. A similar response can be accomplished by using increased doses of OCs, such as Ovral, two tablets q12hr for 1 day, or Min-Ovral, four tablets q12hr for 1 day. A copper-containing intrauterine device can be used as EPC in women at low risk for sexually transmitted diseases who are unable to take hormonal contraception.

RX Table 8–3

DS Table 8–3

SE The major side effects are nausea and vomiting. Dimenhydrinate (Dramamine, Dymenate, Hydrate—*U.S.;* Gravol—*Can.*) 50–100 mg PO q4–6hr (not to exceed 400 mg/day) should be prescribed with high-dose OCs.

OC Pills

KY OCs alter the feedback regulation of luteinizing hormone and follicle-stimulating hormone, thereby inhibiting ovulation. These agents may also

Efficacy (%)	Side Effects	Comments
75	Nausea and vomiting, abdominal bloating; fetal teratogenicity	Use within 72 hours post-coitus. Not available in Canada.
75	Nausea and vomiting, high total dose of estrogen increases risk of thromboembolism	Use within 72 hours postcoitus. Give antiemetic to control nausea and vomiting.
75	—	Use within 72 hours postcoitus. Give with antiemetic.
90	Minimal GI effects	Use within 72 hours postcoitus. Not available in Canada.
90	—	—
99	Irritation, cramping, bleeding coitally.	Insert within 5 days postcoitally
Approximately 100	Minimal GI effects	Not available in Canada.

interfere with ovum transport, cause abnormal development of the endometrium, and thicken cervical mucus. OCs have a contraceptive efficacy of 99.9% when taken in a compliant manner. **Noncontraceptive benefits** include a lowered incidence of ectopic pregnancy; fewer benign ovarian cysts; reduced ovarian and endometrial cancer risk (which persists long after OC discontinuation); management of cyclical problems, including menorrhagia, dysmenorrhea, and menstrual migraine; and decreased tubal infection and resultant infertility (occurs after 1 year of OC use). **If pregnancy occurs, the OC should be discontinued immediately. OC use during early pregnancy is not teratogenic.** Postpartum, OCs should be deferred until lactation is well established (approximately 4 weeks postpartum), as OC use may decrease milk production, or a progesterone-only pill should be used. Steroids secreted into breast milk have no known effect on infants.

TX **Combination monophasic OCs** are most commonly used. These contain a fixed amount of estrogen and progestin for 21 days of the cycle. The estrogen is usually ethinyl estradiol (dose range, 0.02–0.05 mg), and the progestin varies depending on the preparation (dose range, 0.5–2 mg).

Biphasic OCs contain a fixed amount of estrogen (usually 0.035 mg) with two doses of progestin (0.5 mg in the first half of the cycle and 1 mg in the second half). **Triphasic OCs** have fixed (0.035 mg) or variable (0.03, 0.04, then 0.03 mg) estrogen content, with three progestin doses per cycle (from 0.05 to 1 mg). Before starting the OC, a complete history and physical examination, with blood pressure, should be taken. Patients should be counseled about smoking cessation and prevention of sexually transmitted diseases. The user failure rate is approximately 3% and is the result of compliance issues or drug interactions. Backup contraception is not required if the OC is started during the first 5 days of the cycle. One missed pill should be taken immediately. If a woman misses two pills during the first 2 weeks of her cycle, she should take two pills the day she remembers and two pills the next day. If two or more pills are missed in the third week, the pack should be discarded and another pack started immediately. Backup contraception should be used until pills have been taken for 7 days in a row.

RX Table 8–4

DS Table 8–4

SE Side effects are listed in Table 8–2. **Absolute contraindications** include risk of venous thromboembolus (previous venous thromboembolus, known protein C or S deficiency, active thrombophlebitis); risk of myocardial infarction or stroke (severe hypertension, premature atherosclerotic events, cigarette smoking after age 35 years, atypical migraines); acute or chronic obstructive liver disease (abnormal liver enzyme levels); history of estrogen-dependent tumor; undiagnosed vaginal bleeding; pregnancy; and hypertriglyceridemia. Women undergoing major surgery that is likely to be followed by a period of immobility should discontinue the OC for 4 weeks before the surgery. Drugs that can cause OC failure include antibiotics, rifampin, carbamazepine, phenytoin, and phenobarbital.

Progestin-Only Contraception

KY These include progestin-only pills (norethindrone 0.35 mg [Micronor]), intramuscular injection of depo-medroxy-progesterone acetate (Depo-Provera), progestin implants (which release levonorgestrel [Norplant]), and the MIRENA intrauterine system (a norgestrel-releasing intrauterine contraceptive device). **Progestin-only medication acts as a contraceptive by facilitating the development of hostile cervical mucus.** Inhibition of ovulation occurs in only 60% of patients taking progesterone-only pills. Efficacy is 90%–99.9%. Failure is related to compliance. The indications for progestin-only contraceptives are the same as for OCs, but they can also be used in women who cannot take OCs for a variety of reasons, including the inability to tolerate estrogen side effects, smoking after age 35 years, migraine, venous thromboembolism, and lactation. Progestin-only pills may be started immediately postpartum, but implants should be deferred until breastfeeding is well established.

TX **Progesterone-only pills should be started on day 1 of the cycle and must be taken at the same time every day.** If a pill is forgotten, backup contraception is required for 48 hours. Depot injections are given once every 3 months, and implants last for 5 years. The Mirena intrauterine system requires replacement every 5 years.

RX Table 8–4

DS Table 8–4

SE **Side effects** include weight gain, intermenstrual bleeding, amenorrhea, ovarian cysts, depression, acne, and headaches. **Contraindications** include pregnancy and undiagnosed vaginal bleeding. **Drug interactions** are probably similar to those for OCs, although this has not been extensively studied. It is likely that drugs metabolized through the hepatic cytochrome p450 system may reduce the efficacy of progestin-only contraceptives.

HORMONE REPLACEMENT THERAPY

KY Menopause occurs at an average age of 51 years. It is the permanent cessation of menses that occurs as a result of ovarian failure and is diagnosed after 12 months of amenorrhea. Loss of ovarian follicular activity results in lowered ovarian production of estrogen, progesterone, and androgens. These low steroid levels are insufficient to negatively feed back on pituitary gonadotropins, resulting in high basal levels of luteinizing hormone and follicle-stimulating hormone. Menopausal symptoms arise from the lack of estrogen and include vasomotor symptoms (hot flashes, night sweats, palpitations, headaches, light-headedness, insomnia), altered neural function (poor memory, mental confusion, irritability), and reduced pelvic tissue integrity (vaginal dryness, urinary incontinence, atrophic vaginitis). Estrogen depletion is associated with an increased risk of osteoporosis, since estrogen normally inhibits osteoclast activity and prevents bone resorption. It is also associated with increased cardiovascular disease, since the protective effects of estrogen (i.e., promotes endothelial vasodilation, lowers low-density lipoprotein cholesterol, and increases high-density lipoprotein cholesterol and triglycerides) are lost.

TX Hormone replacement therapy (HRT) restores hormone levels and signs and symptoms of menopause. It should be given on an individual basis, and the patient's history, symptoms, and risk factors should be used to determine whether the benefits outweigh the risks. Results from the Women's Health Initiative (WHI)—the first randomized primary prevention trial of postmenopausal hormones carried out in asymptomatic postmenopausal women 50 to 80 years old (mean age 63 years)—indicated that use of the combined CEE, 0.625 mg/day, plus MPA, 2.5 mg/day increased the risk of invasive breast cancer (hazard ratio [HR] 1.26), coronary heart disease (HR 1.29), stroke (HR 1.41), and pulmonary embolism (HR 2.13). In general, women who have had a hysterectomy may use estrogen therapy alone, whereas women with an intact uterus should always use a combination of estrogen and progesterone to lower the incidence of endometrial hyperplasia and cancer. The dose of estrogen in HRT is approximately one-sixth the potency of the standard estrogen dose in low-dose OC pills. Estrogen preparations are available in oral, transdermal, parenteral, and vaginal delivery systems. Oral estrogens are absorbed by the gastrointestinal tract, converted to estrone in the liver, and then excreted via the kidney and bil-

Table 8–4. Composition of Commonly Used Combination Hormonal Contraceptive Agents

Type	Generic (Brand) Name
Monophasic	Ethinyl estradiol/norethindrone acetate (LoEstrin 1.5/30, Minestrin 1/20)
	Ethinyl estradiol/norethindrone (Ortho-Novum 1/35, 0.5/35, Brevicon 1/35, 0.5/35)
	Ethinyl estradiol/levonorgestrel (MinOvral, Alesse)
	Ethinyl estradiol/norgestrel (Ovral)
	Ethinyl estradiol/ethynodiol diacetate (Demulen 30/50)
	Mestranol/norethindrone (OrthoNovum 1/50)
	Ethinyl estradiol/desogestrel (Apri, Cyclessa, Desogen, Mircette— *U.S.;* Marvelon—*Can.*)
	Ethinyl estradiol/cyproterone acetate (Diane 35*)
	Ethinyl estradiol/norgestimate (Ortho-Cyclen, Cyclen)
Biphasic	Ethinyl estradiol/norethindrone (Ortho-Novum 10/11, Synphasic)
Triphasic	Ethinyl estradiol/norethindrone (Ortho-Novum 7/7/7)
	Ethinyl estradiol/norgestimate (Tri-Cyclen)
	Ethinyl estradiol/levonorgestrel (Triphasil)
Progestin-only contraception	Norgestrel (Ovrette)
	Norethindrone acetate (Micronor)
	Depo-medroxy-progesterone acetate (Depo-Provera)
	Progestin implants (Mirena, Norplant)

*Not available in the United States.

iary tract. Transdermal estradiol avoids hepatic first-pass metabolism, resulting in sustained concentrations of estradiol. In addition to progesterone itself, **two different classes of progestins are used in HRT.** The first class is related to **progesterone** (i.e., medroxyprogesterone acetate, medrogesterone, megestrol). The second class comprises derivatives of 19-nortestosterone (norethindrone and norethindrone acetate). Progestin-only therapy can be used to control vasomotor symptoms in women with contraindications to estrogen.

Estrogen (mg)	Progesterone (mg)
LoEstrin 1.5/30: 0.02 Minestrin 1/20: 0.03	LoEstrin 1.5/30: 1 Minestrin 1/20: 1.5
0.035	Ortho-Novum 1/35, 0.5/35: 1, 0.5 Brevicon 1/35, 0.5/35: 1, 0.5
MinOvral: 0.03 Alesse: 0.02	MinOvral: 0.15 Alesse: 0.1
0.05	0.5
0.03, 0.05	2, 1
0.05	1
0.03	0.15
0.035	2
0.035	0.25
0.035	Ortho-Novum 10/11: 0.5 (10 tabs) 1 (11 tabs) Synphasic: 0.5 (12 tabs) 1 (9 tabs)
0.035	0.5, 0.75, 1 (7 tabs each)
0.035	0.18, 0.215, 0.25 (7 tabs each)
0.030 (6 tabs) 0.040 (5 tabs) 0.030 (10 tabs)	0.05 0.075 0.125
None	0.074
None	0.35
None	150 mg/mL released over 3 months
None	Mirena: Intrauterine system releases 20 μg of levonorgestrel/day for about 5 years. Norplant: 216 mg in six silastic capsules subdermally release 80 μg of levonorgestrel/day for 6–8 months, and and then a 25–30 μg/day release is maintained for about 5 years.

RX1 Available preparations of HRT are numerous, and description of each is beyond the scope of this text. Commonly used HRTs are listed in Table 8–5. Hormonal regimens generally combine an estrogen with a progestin or progesterone in either a **cyclic** or **continuous** fashion. There are **two forms of cyclic therapy. The first** uses estrogen on days 1–25 of the calendar month plus progestin on days 13–25. During the pill-free period (days 26–30), women have a menstrual period and may experience menopausal symptoms. **The second** uses estrogen every day of the month

Table 8–5. Hormone Replacement Therapy (HRT) Regimens to Use for the Indications Noted

Symptoms	HRT	Side Effects of HRT
Psychological	Conjugated estrogens (Premarin—*U.S.*; C.E.S., Congest—*Can.*) 0.625 mg PO qd	Side effects: breast tenderness, weight gain, nausea, thromboembolic disorders
Vasomotor	Premarin 0.3–0.625 mg PO qd transdermal estrogen patch/ Estradiol	Prolonged use of unopposed estrogen increases the risk of:
Cardiovascular*	Premarin 0.625 mg PO qd Climara (0.05 mg transdermal) Estraderm (0.05 mg transdermal) Raloxifene (Evista) (60 mg PO qd)	Endometrial hyperplasia and cancer Relative risk of breast cancer from 1/10 to 1.5/10 among women who have used it for > 15 years.
Osteoporosis**	Premarin 0.3–0.625 mg Estradiol (Estrace) (1.0 mg PO qd) Estropipate (Ogen) (1.25 mg PO qd) Estradiol (Climara) (0.05 mg transdermal) Estradiol (Estraderm) (0.05 mg transdermal)	Contraindications are listed in Table 8–6.
Genitourinary	Estring 2 mg estradiol in silastic ring—releases 7.5 mcg estradiol/day × 90 days) Vagifem: 25 mcg estradiol vaginal tablets: 1 tablet qhs × 7, then 1 tablet twice weekly Premarin Vaginal Cream (1 applicatorful = 4 gm; 1 gm = .625 mg Premarin cream): 1–2 gm qhs × 7, then 1–2 gm two to three times weekly	
Colorectal	Premarin 0.625 mg PO qd	

*Results from WHI indicate that the combined postmenopausal hormones CEE, 0.625 mg/d, plus MPA, 2.5 mg/d, should not be initiated or continued for the primary prevention of coronary heart disease.

**Based on the WHI results, HRT is no longer considered first line therapy for the prevention or treatment of osteoporosis. Despite the proven efficacy of HRT in reducing colorectal and endometrial cancers, as well as osteoporotic fractures, a decision to choose HRT from among the agents available to treat osteoporosis must clearly weigh for each individual patient these benefits as well as her need for symptomatic relief against the statistically significant increased risks for cardiovascular disease and breast cancer in users of continuous combined HRT (CEE .625 mg + MPA 2.5 mg).

plus progestin on days 1–14. This regimen eliminates the menopausal symptoms but still results in a menstrual bleed mid month following completion of progestin therapy. **Combined continuous HRT consists of continuous daily treatment with both an estrogen and progestin.** This method eliminates the withdrawal bleeding associated with cyclic regimens. Women using the continuous combined regimen may have irregular

Table 8–6. Contraindications to Hormone Replacement Therapy

Absolute	Relative
Estrogen-responsive breast cancer	Seizure disorders
Active or chronic liver disease	Hypertension
Unexplained vaginal bleeding	Severe hypertriglyceridemia
Recent vascular thrombosis	Endometriosis
Thrombophilia	Thrombophlebitis
	Gallbladder disease
	Migraine headaches
	Uterine leiomyomas
	History of malignant melanoma
	FHx thrombophilia
	Endometrial carcinoma
	History of other estrogen-dependent neoplasia
	History of cardiovascular disease/stroke

breakthrough bleeding during the first 3–6 months, but virtually all are amenorrheic by 12 months.

DS1 Table 8–5

SE1 **Side effects** are shown in Table 8–5. **Contraindications** to HRT are shown in Table 8–6.

or

RX2 **Serum estrogen receptor modulators (SERMs)** are increasingly prescribed instead of HRT for osteoporosis prevention and treatment, particularly in women at risk for breast cancer; however, currently available SERMS, raloxifene (Evista) and tamoxifen (Nolvadex—*U.S.;* Tamofen—*Can.*) do not relieve urogenital or vasomotor symptoms. They act as an estrogen receptor agonist, antagonist, or both, depending on the tissue.

Tamoxifen acts as an antiestrogen in the breast but has estrogenic effects on the bones, lipids, and uterus. Its estrogenic effect on the uterus limits its usefulness, as it increases the risk of endometrial hyperplasia. Tamoxifen is therefore used primarily as a chemotherapeutic agent in women with estrogen-positive breast cancer.

Raloxifene has antiestrogenic effects on the breast, endometrium, and vagina, but good estrogenic effects on the bones and lipids. It acts as an antagonist in the hypothalamus and, therefore, worsens hot flashes. Raloxifene significantly lowers the risk of invasive breast cancer in low risk for breast cancer women (MORE trial); a major study (STAR) looking at the effect of raloxifene use in high risk for breast cancer women is underway. If the results are favorable, given raloxifene's benign endometrial effects, it is likely to be the preferred treatment for asymptomatic, high risk for breast cancer women requiring hormone replacement therapy.

DS2 Tamoxifen 20 mg PO qd; Raloxifene 60 mg PO

SE2 Hot flashes. SERMS are associated with increased risk of thromboembolic disorders. Tamoxifen is associated with endometrial hyperplasia and cancer, thrombocytopenia, and leukopenia.

SEXUALLY TRANSMITTED DISEASES

Bacterial Vaginosis

KY **Caused by** *Gardnerella* infection. If untreated, it can cause pelvic inflammatory disease (PID), abnormal cervical cytology, preterm labor and delivery, premature rupture of membranes, chorioamnionitis, and postcesarean endometritis. **Symptoms** include a gray vaginal discharge that has a fishy odor and gray secretions coating the vaginal walls on examination.

TX **First-line treatment:** Oral or topical **metronidazole (Flagyl). Do not use oral therapy in the first trimester of pregnancy.**

  Second-line treatment: Oral or topical **clindamycin** (Cleocin—*U.S.*; Dalacin—*Can.*).

RX Table 8–7

DS Table 8–7

SE Table 8–7

Chlamydia

KY This is caused by infection with *Chlamydia trachomatis,* an obligate intracellular bacterium that infects the columnar epithelial cells of the cervix. If untreated, genital disease can progress to the uterus and fallopian tubes, causing PID and tubal scarring. This may cause ectopic pregnancies or infertility. **Symptoms** may include dysuria, vaginal discharge, postcoital bleeding, dyspareunia, and lower abdominal pain. Chlamydia may also remain asymptomatic. The bacterium can be spread vertically, causing conjunctivitis and pneumonia in newborns.

TX **Oral antibiotics** (Table 8–7). Treatment is the same in pregnancy. **Sexual partners should be treated, and a test of cure should be performed.**

RX Table 8–7

DS Table 8–7

SE Table 8–7

Condyloma Acuminata (Genital Warts)

KY These lesions are caused by the **human papillomavirus, nononcogenic subtypes 6 and 11.** After contact, two-thirds of people develop exophytic warts in the lower genital tract within 3 months. Most vaginal warts occur without symptoms. Rarely, women experience itching and vaginal discharge.

TX **Treatment should focus on wart removal** rather than on virus eradication. Selection of a treatment regimen should be based on site, size, and number of warts. Efficacy varies widely for various methods (32%–81% for topical preparations and 43%–93% for cryotherapy and cautery or laser ablation). Recurrence ranges from 20% to 60%.

RX Table 8–7

DS Table 8–7

SE Table 8–7

Endometritis

KY This occurs most commonly with chlamydial or gonorrheal infection. Patients present with intermenstrual bleeding, breakthrough bleeding on OCs, dyspareunia, or vague, lower abdominal pain. The diagnosis can be established by endometrial biopsy.

TX **Treatment is the same as for chlamydia or gonorrhea.**

RX Table 8–7

DS Table 8–7

SE Table 8–7

Genital Herpes

KY Caused by infection with **herpes simplex virus, types 1 and 2.** Type 2 causes 85% of primary genital herpes, and type 1 is responsible for the remaining 15%. Primary infections are characterized by severe local pain with multiple superficial ulcers and vesicles in the vulvar, perineal, and perianal areas. Clinically, patients may experience fever, malaise, headaches, myalgias, vaginal paresthesia, and burning with urination. The incubation period is 3–7 days, and lesions can persist for weeks. Recurrent infections have a shorter duration of 3–5 days, with milder local symptoms, and they rarely have systemic symptoms. Nearly 25% of recurrences are asymptomatic and manifested only by viral shedding. Diagnosis is made on clinical examination and by viral cultures of the vesicles (100% sensitive) or ulcers (30% sensitive). If a primary infection occurs during pregnancy (> 28 weeks' gestation) or if a recurrent infection occurs at parturition, the baby is at risk of developing neonatal herpes (systemic infection involving the skin, mouth, eyes, liver, and central nervous system).

TX **Acyclovir** (Zovirax—*U.S.;* Avirax—*Can.*). Although **treatment can reduce recurrences, it does not eradicate the disease** or affect viral shedding or transmission rates. For primary infection during pregnancy, prophylactic treatment with acyclovir from 36 weeks' gestation should be given.

RX Table 8–7

DS Table 8–7

SE Table 8–7

Gonorrhea

KY The infectious agent is *Neisseria gonorrhoeae,* a **gram-negative, intracellular diplococcus** that has a predilection for columnar mucosal cells. When untreated, gonorrhea may progress locally to cause PID and sterility. It also can spread to cause septic arthritis and disseminated gonococcal infection. **In newborns, vertical transmission can cause conjunctivitis (ophthalmia neonatorum) and blindness, if untreated. Symptoms** may include dysuria, vaginal discharge, postcoital bleeding, dyspareunia, and lower abdominal pain. **Signs on physical examination** include discharge, cervical motion tenderness, cervical friability, and adnexal tenderness. **There is a 60% rate of coinfection with chlamydia.**

Table 8–7. Treatment of Common Vaginal Infections

Vaginal Infection	Treatment
Bacterial vaginosis	**Topical:** • 0.75% metronidazole [B] gel, 1 applicatorful (37.5 mg) intravaginally bid for 5 days; or • 2% clindamycin cream [B], 1 applicatorful (40 g) intravaginally qhs for 7 days **Oral:** • Metronidazole 500 mg PO bid for 7 days; or • Metronidazole 2 g PO single dose; or • Clindamycin 300 mg PO bid for 7 days
Chlamydia	**Oral:** • Doxycycline [D] 100 mg PO bid for 7 days; or • Ofloxacin 300 mg PO bid for 7 days; or • Erythromycin [B] 500 mg PO qid for 7 days, or • Azithromycin [B] 1 g PO single dose
Condyloma acuminata (human papillomavirus)	**Topical:** • 10%–25% podophyllum resin [X], 1–2 times/week; or • 0.5% podofilox (Condylox) [C] bid for 3 days/week for 4 weeks; or • 80%–90% Trichloroacetic acid, once q1–2wk; or • 5% 5-fluorouracil (Efudex) [X] solution, 1–3 times/week **Surgical:** Cryotherapy, cautery, laser, or electrodesiccation
Genital herpes	**Oral:** • Acyclovir [B] 200 mg PO 5 times/day for 1 week (first outbreak) • Acyclovir 400 mg PO bid as suppressive therapy (if recurrent outbreaks > 6 per year)
Gonorrhea	**Oral:** • Ofloxacin [C], 400 mg PO single dose; or • Cefixime [B] 800 mg PO single dose; or • Ciprofloxacin [B] 500 mg PO single dose **IM:** • Ceftriaxone [B] 250 mg IM single injection
Syphilis	**Parenteral:** • Penicillin G benzathine [B], 50,000 U/kg (maximum 2.4 million U/dose) every week for 3 doses
Trichomoniasis	**Oral:** • Metronidazole 500 mg PO bid for 7 days; or • Metronidazole 2 g PO single dose • Metronidazole 2 g PO qd for 5 days (for resistant cases)

Side Effects

Stomach upset, nausea, and vomiting can be caused by both medications. Metronidazole can cause a metallic taste and a disulfiram-like reaction when co-ingested with alcohol. Rare side effects of metronidazole are convulsions and peripheral neuropathy. Clindamycin can give regional enteritis, hepatic impairment, and antibiotic-related pseudomembranous colitis.

Diarrhea, abdominal pain, nausea, vomiting
Doxycycline may cause a photosensitivity reaction and hepatic dysfunction.
Ofloxacin can give renal impairment, seizures, and headache.

Local pain, burning and irritation (6–24 hours after treatment) scarring

Gastrointestinal upset, renal failure, confusion, seizures, hypersensitivity reactions

Diarrhea, nausea, abdominal pain, rashes
Ofloxacin can give renal impairment, seizures, and headaches.

Local redness and pain if injection used.

The Jarisch-Herxheimer reaction is a well-described acute febrile reaction to treatment of syphilis that consists of fever, headache, and myalgias. Other side effects include an IgE-mediated allergic reaction (urticaria, lymphadenopathy, asthma, edema, anaphylactic shock) or the more common rash, which usually appears weeks later.

—

TX First-line treatment: Oral antibiotics (Table 8–7). **Treatment of sexual partners is mandatory, and a test of cure should be performed in all patients.** Second-line treatment: Parenteral antibiotics (Table 8–7).

RX Table 8–7

DS Table 8–7

SE Table 8–7

Pelvic Inflammatory Disease

KY PID is a spectrum of disease in which microorganisms infecting the vagina ascend, causing cervicitis or endometritis and salpingitis, with ultimate progression to pyosalpinx or tubo-ovarian abscess (TOA). Sexually transmitted disease infection (chlamydia, gonorrhea) is the most common cause, although *Haemophilus influenzae*, Group A streptococcus, and pneumococcus are also culprits. **The classic triad of signs and symptom**s is pelvic pain, cervical motion and adnexal tenderness, and fever greater than 38°C. **Clinical criteria for diagnosis** are leucorrhea or mucopurulent endocervicitis, pelvic organ tenderness, fever, and leukocytosis. Many women will be asymptomatic. Infertility, ectopic pregnancy, or chronic pelvic pain occurs in 25% of treated patients.

TX Outpatient treatment is acceptable in mild to moderate illness in a compliant patient who can tolerate oral antibiotic medications. These patients must be reevaluated in 48–72 hours, and, if not improved, hospital admission should be considered at that time. Patients should be admitted to hospital if an adnexal mass or TOA is found, if severely ill, if unable to toler-

Table 8–8. Treatment of Pelvic Inflammatory Disease

	Treatment*	Side Effects
Outpatient	**Oral:** Ofloxacin 400 mg PO bid for 14 days, plus Metronidazole 500 mg PO bid for 14 days; or Clindamycin 450 mg PO qid for 14 days	Metronidazole can cause metallic taste, stomach upset, nausea, vomiting, and a disulfiram-like reaction when co-ingested with alcohol. **Ofloxacin** can give renal impairment, seizures, and headaches. Rare side effects of **metronidazole** are convulsions and peripheral neuropathy. **Clindamycin** can give regional enteritis, hepatic impairment, and antibiotic-related pseudomembranous colitis.
Inpatient	**IV** Clindamycin 900 mg IV + gentamicin 1 mg/kg IV q8hr; or Cefoxitin 2 g IV q6hr; or Cefotetan 2 g q12hr plus Doxycycline 100 mg PO single dose	**Cephalosporins** can give an allergic reaction that includes urticaria, anaphylaxis, and rash.

*See Ch 10 Infectious Diseases for more detail on antibiotics.

ate oral medications, if immunocompromised or pregnant, or if emergency surgery is required. If an intrauterine device is in place, it should be removed after 24 hours of intravenous antibiotics. Most patients with TOA can be successfully treated medically with antibiotics. If the abscess is thick walled and multiloculated, antibiotic penetration may be suboptimal, and surgical intervention may be required.

RX Table 8–8

DS Table 8–8

SE Table 8–8

Syphilis

KY The infectious agent is an **anaerobic spirochete, *Treponema pallidum*.** The incubation period is 10–90 days, with an average of 3 weeks. The clinical course is divided into primary, secondary, and tertiary phases. **Primary syphilis** is characterized by a smooth, indurated, painless ulcer that resolves in 3–6 weeks. Hematogenous dissemination results in the **secondary stage,** which is characterized by lymphadenopathy, skin rash (on soles and palms), and vulvar condylomata lata (wartlike lesions). This lasts 2–6 weeks. The patient then enters **a latent stage** (seroreactive, but clinically asymptomatic), lasting 2–30 years. One-third of patients develop **tertiary syphilis,** which consists of progressive damage to the central nervous system, cardiovascular system, and musculoskeletal system. Clinical symptoms include tabes dorsalis, generalized paresis, aortic aneurysm, and gummata of soft tissues and bones. Diagnosis of infection is made via a positive VDRL or treponemal test.

TX Penicillin G benzathine (Bicillin, Permapen—*U.S.;* Megacillin—*Can.*) for primary and secondary syphilis. Latent syphilis should be treated similarly, but patients should receive one dose of medication per week for 3 weeks. Serum titers should be repeated at 6-month intervals after treatment and should be one-quarter of the original level.

RX Table 8–7

DS Table 8–7

SE Table 8–7

Trichomoniasis

KY Caused by the parasite ***Trichomonas vaginalis***. There is often coinfection with bacterial vaginosis. High transmission rate of $> 70\%$ per sexual encounter. Patients may be asymptomatic. **Symptoms** include vulvar pruritus and profuse foul-smelling vaginal discharge.

TX Oral **metronidazole. Sexual partner must also be treated.** If infection is resistant to metronidazole, a parasite culture and sensitivity analysis must be performed.

RX Table 8–7

DS Table 8–7

SE Table 8–7

9

Hematology

RENAUD WHITTOM

This chapter covers most of the hematologic disorders for which a pharmacologic treatment is available. Certain diseases are difficult to classify, as they are clonal but yet do not behave like cancers; paroxysmal nocturnal hemoglobinuria (PNH) is such a disease and is discussed herein.

DISORDERS OF BLOOD COAGULATION

When a blood vessel is injured, platelet aggregation occurs (primary hemostasis). The platelet plug that is formed is relatively fragile; hence, plasma proteins use the surface provided and react to produce a fibrin clot, which is solid enough to provide time for the vessel to repair itself (secondary hemostasis). Most of the coagulation factors are proenzymes that need to be activated; others are nonenzymatic cofactors. The coagulation factors are synthesized in the liver, except for von Willebrand factor, which indirectly participates in coagulation by protectively binding factor VIII. Megakaryocytes, macrophages, and endothelial cells have some synthetic capacity. Four factors (VII, IX, X, II) require vitamin K to become active. The classic coagulation cascade is shown in Figure 9–1. This cascade is controlled by other proteins, including tissue factor pathway inhibitor, antithrombin III (AT III), protein C, and protein S.

Disseminated Intravascular Coagulation (DIC)

KY The process of DIC involves both the consumption of coagulation factors and platelets to form deposition of fibrin in the microcirculation (thrombosis) and the destruction of this fibrin (fibrinolysis). It is important to remember that this fibrinolysis prevents major ischemic events.

TX **The first principle of treatment** is to eliminate the cause whenever possible. **A second principle** is to replace the consumed factors and platelets when the patient is bleeding and their levels are sufficiently low. Appropriate goals would be a prothrombin time (PT) within 2–3 seconds of normal, a fibrinogen level > 100 mg/dL, and a platelet count of 50,000/μL. **The third principle** is the judicious use of heparin. A low-dose regimen is sometimes advised when replacement therapy is not successful in controlling hemorrhage and factor levels are not rising. Low-dose heparin is also useful in cases in which thrombosis is obvious, and in rare cases such as a retained dead fetus or a giant hemangioma that is associated with bleeding. The role of other therapeutic agents in the treatment of DIC is controversial. **Antifibrinolytic agents should *never* be used without heparin.** Preliminary reports of the use of AT III concentrates are promising, especially in sepsis.

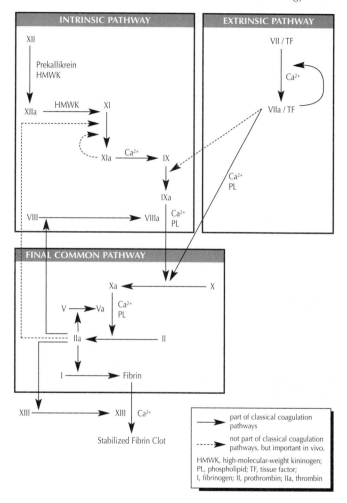

FIGURE 9–1 The coagulation cascade. HMWK = high-molecular-weight kininogen; PL = phospholipid; TF = tissue factor; I = fibrinogen; II = prothrombin; IIa = thrombin.

RX **Heparin:** See THROMBOEMBOLIC DISORDERS.

DS Approximately 500–700 U/hr

SE See THROMBOEMBOLIC DISORDERS.

Factor Deficiencies

KY Deficiencies of all these coagulation factors, except tissue factor, have been described in patients. The most well known are hemophilia A and B, which result from factor VIII and IX deficiencies, respectively. When severe enough, these deficiencies cause spontaneous bleeding, mostly in the joints but also in soft tissues. Available therapies in factor deficiencies are discussed here.

Vitamin K is a fat-soluble vitamin that is found in green vegetables, but it is also produced by intestinal bacteria. Deficiencies are found in malnourished patients (especially if they are taking antibiotics), in newborns (prevented by prophylaxis), in malabsorption (especially with cholestasis), and secondary to oral anticoagulants.

In the absence of vitamin K, the γ-carboxylation of the glutamic acids on factors II, VII, IX, and X, and also on protein C and protein S, is prevented. As a result, the level of functional proteins will fall according to their half-life.

Factor concentrates are characterized by:
- Source: Volunteer donors, commercial donors, commercial pigs, or mammalian cells that are transfected with a human factor gene. This last source is now preferred because of its absolute lack of viruses (even those that have not yet been identified).
- Preparation and virus inactivation: When prepared from human sources, techniques such as solvent/detergent inactivation or pasteurization in solution at 60°C for 10 minutes are used to eliminate human immunodeficiency virus (HIV) and virulent hepatitis strains.
- Purity: This refers to the amount of factor units per milligram of proteins in the preparation. Currently, products of intermediate (5 U/mg), high (9–22 U/mg) and very high (2,000–3,000 U/mg) purity are available.
- Half-life: The half-life and effective level are the same for all products of one factor but vary between different factors (Table 9–1).

Table 9–1. Half-life of Coagulation Factors

Factor	Half-life (hr)	Factor	Half-life (hr)
I	90–120	X	24–60
II	48–120	XI	45–80
III	Unknown	XII	40–70
V	12–24	XIII	72–200
VII	2–6	HMWK	150
VIII	10–12	Prekallikrein	48–52
IX	18–30		

HMWK = high-molecular-weight kininogen.

TX1 **Factor VIII concentrates:** There are many different types of factor VIII concentrates that are available in the United States and Canada. They are used for treatment and sometimes prophylaxis of hemophilia A, in some cases of inhibitors of factor VIII, and in the case of Haemate P in von Willebrand disease.

RX1 Factor VIII concentrates [C]: Koate HP (high-purity product), Kogenate (high-purity recombinant factor VIII recommended as first-line treatment in patients with newly diagnosed hemophilia), Hyate C (porcine factor primarily used in patients with inhibitors to factor VIII), and Humate P or Haemate P (intermediate purity prepared from commercial donors and inactivated by pasteurization). Haemate P is safer than cryoprecipitates, so that its use is recommended whenever patients with von Willebrand disease require factor treatment; the other factor VIII concentrates do not have the high-molecular-weight multimers of von Willebrand that are necessary to treat that disease.

DS1 As much as possible, factor VIII must be administered in a hemophilia center; appropriate levels are given in Table 9–2. A dose of 1 U/kg of factor VIII will elevate the plasma level by 2%.

SE1 Infectious (viral) complications have been almost eliminated, but hepatitis B vaccination is recommended. Allergic reactions are rare. Plasma-derived factors contain anti-A and anti-B hepatitis, which can cause hemolysis. Inhibitors develop in 5%–10% of patients (seen more in those with severe hemophilia), and this can complicate therapy.

TX2 **Factor IX concentrates:** Derived from commercial donors. Purity can be intermediate or very high. Viruses are inactivated by vapor, solvent/detergent, or ultrafiltration. Half-life is 18–24 hours.

RX2 Factor IX concentrates [C]: Immunine VH—*Can.* (very high purity); Mononine (purified with monoclonal antibodies and inactivated by ultrafiltration), and BeneFix (high-purity recombinant product).

DS2 Because of the larger volume of distribution compared with factor VIII, a dose of 1 U/kg of factor IX will produce a 1% elevation in plasma levels. Target levels are given in Table 9–2.

SE2 Similar to factor VIII. Inhibitors develop less commonly (2%–5%).

Table 9–2. Appropriate Therapeutic Levels of Factors VIII and IX in Patients With Hemophilia

Clinical Situation	Hemophilia A (Factor VIII)	Hemophilia B (Factor IX)
Mild bleeds (%)	20–30	20–30
Major bleeds (e.g., muscle bleeds, head trauma, obvious hemarthrosis) (%)	40–50	40–50
Life-threatening bleeds (e.g., major trauma or surgery, advanced or recurrent hemarthrosis) (%)	70–100	70–100
Dental extraction (%)	40–50	40–50

TX3 **Other factor concentrates** (not widely available).

RX3 **Factors XI, XIII, I, and VII** are all available in specific, virally inactivated concentrates of intermediate purity. Recombinant **factor VIIa** (NiaStase) is also available. Activated prothrombin complex concentrate (Autoplex T, FEIBA) is licensed but is rarely used; it can be useful in patients who have inhibitors to factor VIII or IX.

DS3 Use is restricted, and hemophilia centers and specialists have to be involved. Therapeutic levels for relevant factors, other than VIII and IX, are given in Table 9–3.

SE3 Activated prothrombin complex concentrate has the potential to induce thrombosis.

TX4 **Therapies other than factor concentrates** can improve hemostasis in appropriate situations. Desmopressin can be used in fairly mild hemophilia A (factor VIII > 5%) and von Willebrand disease. In borderline cases, it is best to test patient response before undertaking full-fledged administration. It is best avoided in von Willebrand type 2B and in the platelet type.

RX4 **Desmopressin** (DDAVP, Stimate—*U.S;* Octostim—*Can.*) [B]: A synthetic analog of vasopressin. It has the capacity to release both von Willebrand factor and factor VIII from their sites of storage. A peak in clotting factor level will be seen 30–60 minutes after administration; the increment is variable, with an average of threefold to fourfold from baseline.

DS4 Dose: 0.3 µg/kg (not to exceed 20 µg) infusion in 50–100 mL of normal saline over 30 minutes. SC administration is possible at the same dose. Intranasal therapy, at a dose of 300 µg for adults, can be used in patients with minor bleeding. DDAVP is most efficient when it is given as a single dose. Tachyphylaxis may be seen when given q12–24hr; factor level should be measured and therapy should be adjusted accordingly. The initial level of response is restored within 7–10 days from the last desmopressin exposure.

SE4 Side effects are minor, including flushing, headache, nausea, cramps reminiscent of menstrual pain, and some mild cardiovascular effects. Hyponatremia can develop with repeated administration, especially in children, and sodium levels should therefore be closely monitored.

Table 9–3. Appropriate Therapeutic Levels in Uncommon Factor Deficiencies

Factor	Target Levels
I	100 mg/dL (1 g/L)
II	20%–40% (0.2–0.4 U/mL)
V	10%–20% (0.1–0.2 U/mL)
VII	10%–20% (0.1–0.2 U/mL)
X	10%–20% (0.1–0.2 U/mL)
XI	15%–25% (0.15–0.25 U/mL)
XIII	3%–5% (0.03–0.05 U/mL)

TX5 **Antifibrinolytic agents.**

RX5 **Aprotinin** (Trasylol)[B]: A bovine protein with potent plasmin inhibitor properties. Epsilon-aminocaproic acid or EACA (Amicar) [C] and tranexamic acid or AMCA (Cyklokapron) [B] are synthetic lysine analogs that prevent clot lysis; their half-life is short, and repeated doses are required.

DS5 Typical dose: **Amicar** 75 mg/kg (up to 4 g) PO q6hr. **Cyklokapron** 25 mg/kg PO q8hr. IV preparations are available; the dose of Cyklokapron must be lowered to 10 mg/kg IV when given by this route. In patients with hemophilia: a 5-day course of Amicar or Cyklokapron can be given for the treatment of mucosal, oral, or dental bleeds. **It should not be used with urinary tract hemorrhage.** These agents are also used in patients with menorrhagia and in rare conditions such as isolated hyperfibrinolysis.

SE5 Frequently, these agents produce minor side effects, mainly gastrointestinal (GI) discomfort (EACA>AMCA); infrequently, they can cause thrombosis, myonecrosis, and hypersensitivity reactions.

TX6 **Therapy of vitamin K deficiency:** When bleeding is severe, fresh frozen plasma (FFP) must be relied on to correct it. Otherwise, SC or IV vitamin K is used.

RX6 **Phytonadione** (AquaMEPHYTON, Mephyton) [C] is the therapeutic form of vitamin K1 used. A complete, or at least major, improvement in the PT and normal hemostasis is expected to occur in approximately 24 hours; PT can improve in 8 hours but does not represent the true bleeding tendency because only factor VII has had the time to respond.

DS6 Dose: 10 mg IV/SC is appropriate for most situations and can be repeated every week if needed. A dose of 1–2 mg is sufficient when it is necessary that the effects of oral anticoagulants be reversed, without the elimination of warfarin sensitivity. IV administration is usually avoided because it is associated with hypotension.

SE6 Hypotension; related to rate of IV infusion.

TX7 In certain situation, only **FFP** or **cryoprecipitates** can be used. **FFP** contains all the coagulation factors, at levels $\geq$ 80% (in general, 1 mL of plasma = 1 unit of factor activity). **Cryoprecipitate** is the cold, insoluble precipitate that remains after FFP is thawed. One unit contains at least 80 units of factor VIII, 200 mg of fibrinogen, 40%–70% of the von Willebrand factor, and 20%–30% of the factor XIII of the parent unit.

RX7 **FFP and cryoprecipitates.**

DS7 The FFP dose of approximately 15–20 mL/kg should bring all factors to at least 30% of the normal level. The **cryoprecipitate** dose varies with the indication; in the average-sized adult, 10 bags will increase the fibrinogen level by approximately 75 mg/dL.

SE7 Detailed discussion of side effects of blood products is beyond the scope of this chapter. They are not treated for viruses, so transmission is a potential problem. Hypervolemia and allergy are also possible.

DISORDERS OF HEMATOPOIESIS

Hematopoiesis is the process by which the stem cells in the marrow give rise to progenitor cells, which can then proliferate and differentiate into the different blood cells. The capacity for self-renewal is maximal for the most primitive cell and is eventually lost when cells become specialized to produce a specific blood cell. Marrow cells also stop dividing through the last few stages of differentiation. The microenvironment of the marrow provides the supporting stroma and some of the regulatory signals that stimulate stem cell growth in vivo. This includes glycoproteins called colony-stimulating factors (CSFs) or cytokines, such as stem cell factor (Kit-ligand), interleukin-3, granulocyte-macrophage CSF (GM-CSF), granulocyte CSF (G-CSF), erythropoietin (EPO), and thrombopoietin, among others. Some of these CSFs are used in therapeutics. **The disorders of hematopoiesis are diseases of the stem cells and progenitors.** They can be neoplastic (not covered here) or result in an altered cellular function or a bone marrow failure state.

Aplastic Anemia (AA)

KY The **congenital forms** of AA are genetically transmitted and include Fanconi's anemia, familial aplastic anemia, and dyskeratosis congenita. **Acquired forms** are idiopathic approximately 50% of the time. Other cases are related to drugs (e.g., chloramphenicol), toxins (e.g., benzene), ionizing irradiation, infections (viral hepatitis), pregnancy, or thymoma (rarely) or may be a prelude to PNH or myelodysplasia. Several mechanisms are suspected, including stem cell injury (virus, toxin, etc.), an abnormal microenvironment (e.g., after radiation therapy), abnormalities of the cytokines (rare), and immunologic suppression of hematopoiesis. **Whatever the mechanism, the end result is pancytopenia,** with symptoms related to the degree of cytopenia. In severe cases, the reticulocyte count is < 1%, the neutrophil count is < 500/μL, or the platelet count is < 20,000/μL.

TX Some **general measures** apply: (1) When granulocytopenia is severe, at least minimal prophylactic measures, such as thorough hand washing and masks for those with respiratory infection, should be followed by staff and visitors. Antibiotics are used for fever. (2) If bleeding is a potential problem, IM injection should be avoided. Anovulatory agents can help with menstrual bleeding. (3) Transfusions must be used with caution, especially if bone marrow transplantation is considered. Prophylactic platelets are considered only when the platelet count is < 10,000–20,000/μL.

Nonsevere AA can often be observed. A small group of patient can benefit from the combination of EPO and G-CSF.

For severe AA, allogeneic (human leukocyte antigen–compatible donor) stem cell transplantation is the most successful curative treatment, with approximately two-thirds of the patients alive and well at 5 years. A twin donor makes transplantation possible at almost any age, but otherwise the toxicity of that treatment limits its use to patients younger than approximately 40 years or some very fit patients up to 50 years old. Unrelated donors are only used in young patients who failed immunosuppressive therapy.

In all other severe cases, immunosuppressive therapy is the treatment of choice. The combination of cyclosporine and antilymphocyte globulin or antithymocyte globulin is the current standard. Response, which is usually seen 6–12 weeks after treatment, varies according to severity of disease. Combination regimen in severe AA shows improvement in the blood count in two-thirds of the patients, but most responses are partial, with some residual abnormalities. A second course may be successful in 25% of the failures and even better in relapses. A product made from rabbit sera instead of horse sera can be used the second time around.

Occasionally, patients whose initial therapy fails can have some benefit from androgens. High-dose cyclophosphamide has induced remissions in 7 of 10 patients in a small series.

RX1 **Antilymphocyte globulin** and **antithymocyte globulin** [C]: There is little evidence of significant variation between batches or between different products. Their mode of action is unclear, although their immunosuppressive effects are well known. Anti–horse immunoglobulin can be demonstrated 1 week after exposure to a product made from horse sera, but there is no concrete evidence that it should alter protocol duration.

DS1 Table 9–4

SE1 Table 9–4. Serum sickness, a syndrome of fever, myalgia, arthralgia with a maculopapular rash, and, more rarely, GI symptoms would be seen in 75% of the patients, making corticosteroid prophylaxis necessary.

RX2 **Cyclosporine** (Gengraf, Neoral, Sandimmune) [C]: Inhibits T-helper and T-cytotoxic cells but spares T-suppressor cells. Has a vasoconstrictive effect that is probably the main cause of its nephrotoxicity combined with some renal tubular defects. Bioavailability and pharmacokinetics are quite variable. Monitoring necessary.

DS2 Table 9–4

SE2 Table 9–4

RX3 **Androgens** (Danazol, Oxymetholone) [X]: This category of drugs has been believed to increase EPO production. Erythroid and granulocytic progenitors are also stimulated.

DS3 Table 9–4

SE3 Table 9–4

RX4 **Epoetin alpha** (Epogen, Procrit—*U.S.*; Eprex—*Can.*) [C]: This glycoprotein normally secreted mainly by the kidney stimulates proliferation and maturation of erythroid progenitors. Not effective alone in AA.

DS4 Table 9–4

SE4 Table 9–4

RX5 **Filgrastim** or G-CSF (Neupogen) [C]: See LEUKOPENIA.

DS5 Table 9–4

SE5 Table 9–4

RX6 **Azathioprine** (Imuran) [D]: Cytotoxic agent. Inhibits B-cell, T-cell, and natural killer (NK) cell function.

Table 9–4. Therapeutic Agents Used in Hematopoietic Disorders

Generic (Brand) Name	Dose	Side Effects
Antilymphocyte globulin (ALG) Antithymocyte globulin (ATG)	Can vary widely between products. Given IV mixed in saline (0.9%) through central venous catheter. **10-mg test dose can be used.** ALG: 40 mg/kg/day infused up to 18 hours for 4–5 days. ATG: 15 mg/kg/day infused up to 18 hours for 8–10 days.	Anaphylaxis (to the animal proteins), fever, hypertension, hypotension, lymphopenia, neutropenia (rare), positive Coombs' test, sclerosis of peripheral veins, seizures (rare), serum sickness syndrome, thrombocytopenia
Danazol (Danocrine—*U.S.*; Cyclomen—*Can.*) [X]	200 mg PO bid-tid	Hypertension, edema, anxiety, seizure, alopecia, hirsutism, allergic reactions, amenorrhea, hyperglycemia, blood dyscrasias, jaundice, hepatic adenoma, cataracts, voice changes
Oxymetholone (Anadrol—*U.S.*; Anapolon—*Can.*) [X]	3–5 mg/kg PO qd	Gynecomastia, priapism, insomnia, decreased libido, prostatic hyperplasia (in elderly patients), anemia, hepatic necrosis, hepatocellular carcinoma
Azathioprine (Imuran) [D]	2–3 mg/kg PO qd	Fever, blood dyscrasias, hepatotoxicity, hypotension, alopecia, dyspnea, hypersensitivity reactions
Corticosteroids	For AA: methylprednisolone [C] or prednisone [B] 1 mg/kg PO qd For PNH: prednisone 15–30 mg q48 hr	Avascular necrosis, cataract, cushingoid features, gastric ulcer, glaucoma, glucose intolerance, hypertension, increased susceptibility to infections, mood changes, myopathy, osteonecrosis, osteoporosis, skin fragility

Drug	Dose	Adverse effects
Cyclophosphamide (Cytoxan, Neosar—*U.S.*; Procytox—*Can.*) [D]	For AA: high-dose treatment with 45 mg/kg IV qd for 4 days For PRCA: 2–3 mg/kg PO qd	Headache, GI intolerance, alopecia, infertility, hemorrhagic cystitis, urinary fibrosis, leukopenia, SIADH, CHF, cardiac necrosis, hemorrhagic myocarditis, anaphylactic reactions, renal tubular necrosis, pulmonary fibrosis
Cyclosporine (Gengraf, Neoral, Sandimmune) [C]	Based on ideal weight (75 kg): 1.5 mg/kg IV q12hr or 5–6 mg/kg PO q12 hr Note: Neoral and Sandimmune are not bioequivalent and **cannot** be used interchangeably.	Arterial thrombosis, central and peripheral CNS symptoms, cholestasis, gingival hyperplasia, gynecomastia, hepatotoxicity, hyperglycemia, hyperkalemia, hypersensitivity reactions, hypertrichosis, nausea and vomiting, nephrotoxicity,* pancreatitis, tremors, venous thrombosis
Epoetin alfa (Epogen, Procrit—*U.S.*; Eprex—*Can.*) [C]	50–100 U/kg SC 3 times/week usual dose 150–300 U/kg SC 3 times/week in cancer and bone marrow failure syndromes 400 U/kg SC 3 times/week found to be more efficient in AA	Hypertension, thrombosis; rarely, PRCA
Filgrastim (Neupogen) [C]	5–10 µg/kg SC qd; 400 µg/m² SC qd then titrated for neutrophil count 1000–5000/µl in AA (with epoetin alfa)	Bone pain, fever

AA = aplastic anemia; CHF = congestive heart failure; CNS = central nervous system; GI = gastrointestinal; PNH = paroxysmal nocturnal hemoglobinuria; PRCA = pure red cell aplasia; SIADH = syndrome of inappropriate secretion of antidiuretic hormone.

*Monitor creatinine levels: if level is 1.5 times the upper normal limit then decrease by 50%; 2 times the upper normal limit then decrease by 75%; and if > 2 mg/dL then stop cyclosporine.

DS6 Table 9–4

SE6 Table 9–4

RX7 **Cyclophosphamide** (Cytoxan, Neosar—*U.S.*; Procytox—*Can.*) [D]: Cytotoxic agent. Produces lymphocytopenia (B and T cell). Decreases antibody synthesis.

DS7 Table 9–4

SE7 Table 9–4

Paroxysmal Nocturnal Hemoglobinuria (PNH)

KY PNH is an acquired clonal disease of the stem cell. Hemolysis, often sporadic, is a hallmark of the disease. The red cell is susceptible to complement lysis because it has lost membrane proteins that control it. Other characteristics of the disease include occasional splenomegaly, iron deficiency from urinary losses, thrombocytopenia with occasional bleeding, thrombosis, and some renal and neurologic manifestations. A few patients may evolve toward AA, acute leukemia, or myelodysplasia.

TX **Supportive therapy is important** and includes packed red cell transfusion, which does not need to be washed, for symptomatic anemia, iron replacement, and folic acid. **Prednisone** is used to suppress hemolysis. **Androgens** sometimes help the anemia. Thrombotic episodes are managed in a standard way with the addition of prednisone to control complement activation. **Allogeneic stem cell transplantation** can be used in patients with life-threatening complications, depending on the availability of a suitable donor. **Immunosuppressive therapy** as described under Aplastic Anemia (AA) can also be used when aplasia is the main feature.

RX Table 9–4

DS Table 9–4

SE Table 9–4

Pure Red Cell Aplasia (PRCA)

KY This problem can be acute or chronic. **Acute** cases are most often caused by a viral infection, mainly Parvovirus B19, and more rarely by some drugs. An antibody-mediated mechanism has been proposed, that usually resolves within several weeks. Diamond-Blackfan syndrome is the **congenital** form of PRCA, with defect suspected to be at the stem cell or at the microenvironment level. **Acquired chronic** PRCA is immune-related about 50% of the time, with antibody demonstrated against erythroblasts. Fifteen percent of the cases are related to a thymoma. A persistent Parvovirus B 19 infection or some lymphoproliferative disorders have been associated with the disease.

TX When thymoma is present, its resection can put the patient in remission. Symptomatic anemia can be corrected by transfusion. Self-limited acute cases may not need any specific therapy. IV immunoglobulin (Ig) can be used after 2–3 weeks. Any suspected drug has to be stopped.

In **chronic acquired cases,** different types of immunosuppressive therapy have been used. These agents have to be used for up to 3 months before being considered ineffective. Prednisone is the first-line treatment of choice. If ineffective, an oral chemotherapeutic agent, most of the time cyclophosphamide and sometimes azathioprine, can be tried. Cyclosporine is considered in refractory patients, with a response rate of approximately 65%. All these agents are tapered once a response is achieved. IV Ig, antilymphocyte globulin, and antithymocyte globulin have all been used in refractory cases with some effect.

RX **IV immune globulin** (Gamimune, Gammagard) [C]: Contains antibodies against Parvovirus B 19. See Aplastic Anemia (AA) for other treatment agents.

DS 400 mg/kg IV for 1 day in acute cases, with up to 5 days of treatment in chronic refractory cases.

SE Tachycardia, hypotension, fever, headache, aseptic meningitis syndrome, myalgia, nephrotic syndrome, dyspnea, hypersensitivity reactions, and anaphylaxis.

DISORDERS OF IRON AND HEME SYNTHESIS

Iron physiology: Iron is absorbed in the duodenum and upper jejunum. Approximately 10% of elemental iron is usually absorbed, although this can be increased fourfold with iron deficiency and decreased in iron overload. Ferrous iron is better absorbed than the ferric form, and heme iron is better absorbed than inorganic forms at any pH. Gastric acid, ascorbate, and citrate positively influence absorption, and phytates and tannins (found in teas) negatively influence it. Accelerated erythropoiesis, of any cause, tends to increase iron uptake. Transferrin is the protein involved in iron transport, and ferritin is the main protein involved in iron storage. About 1 mg/day of iron is lost through the sloughing of cells from the GI tract, the genitourinary tract, and the skin. Menses can increase the loss to approximately 2 mg, and growth and pregnancy also increase iron requirements. Iron is indispensable for hemoglobin (Hb) synthesis, and it also catalyses redox reactions. Iron overload can cause the production of free radicals that can hurt the cell.

Heme synthesis: this process occurs virtually everywhere but mostly in the bone marrow and liver. The pathway is illustrated in Figure 9–2. δ-Aminolevulinic acid (ALA) synthetase is the rate-limiting enzyme in the liver and requires pyridoxine (vitamin B_6). Iron is added in the mitochondria. Excess porphyrinogens are oxidized into fluorescent byproducts called porphyrins (red). **Defects in heme synthesis can occur because of iron deficiency, anemia of chronic disease, porphyria, and sideroblastic anemia.**

Iron Deficiency

KY This is by far the most common cause of anemia (usually microcytic). A negative iron balance is most of the time caused by spoliation of blood. Menses is a common cause in premenopausal women and GI bleeding in

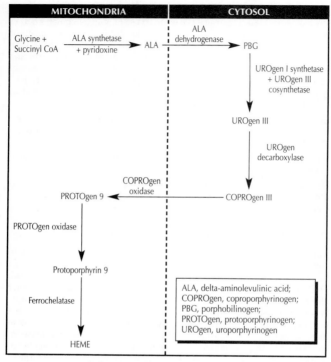

FIGURE 9-2 Heme synthesis pathway.

men and postmenopausal women. Low intake is a cause in children. Defective absorption and iron loss from other sites are rare causes.

TX The first step in the treatment of iron deficiency is correction of the cause whenever possible. Iron supplements are preferably taken by mouth. Iron should be taken on an empty stomach, unless it is not tolerated, because food and especially milk can decrease iron absorption by as much as 50%. An optimal regimen provides approximately 200 mg of elemental iron per day. Anemia should be corrected in 6–8 weeks and iron stores rebuilt in an extra 2–3 months. Parenteral iron is used only when the patient does not absorb iron or cannot tolerate a sufficient dose because of side effects; this route does not increase the speed of correction. Efficacious treatment will increase the reticulocyte count by 7–10 days and Hb by 2 g/dL at 3 weeks. Normal range (12–16 g/dL for women and 14–18 g/dL for men) is reached by approximately 6–8 weeks. A ferritin of about 50 ng/mL (50 μmol/L) is suggestive of replenished stores.

RX1 **Oral iron supplements:** Tablets usually include ferrous iron combined with an anion that can be sulfate (the cheapest), fumarate, or gluconate (more expensive but sometimes better tolerated). Enteric-coated pills are to be avoided. Sustained-release pills or gelatin capsules (gastric delivery system) can reduce commonly experienced side effects but are up to 20- to 30-fold more expensive. Some forms of medicinal iron are combined with vitamin C, which can facilitate absorption, but this can also increase side effects and cost. For maximal absorption, iron should be taken 1–2 hours before meals, at bedtime, or both.

DS1 The amount of elemental iron varies between the different available preparations. Lower dosage can be used as maintenance when needed (e.g., continuous loss). Typical dosages in iron deficiency anemia:

Ferrous sulfate (Feosol, Feratab—*U.S.;* Ferodan—*Can.*) [A]: 300 mg PO tid
Ferrous fumarate (Femiron, Feostat, Hemocyte, Ircon, Nephro-Fer—*U.S.*; Palafer—*Can.*) [A]: 300 mg PO bid
Ferrous gluconate (Fergon) [A]: 600 mg PO tid.

SE1 The upper GI side effects are significant and dose related and include nausea, epigastric pain, heartburn, vomiting, and severe abdominal cramping. The other common adverse effect is a change in bowel habitus (i.e., constipation or diarrhea); not related to dosage and can be treated symptomatically.

RX2 **Parenteral iron supplements:** Iron dextran (DexFerrum, INFeD—*U.S.*; Infufer—*Can.*) [C] can be administered IM and IV. In Canada, iron sorbitol (Jectofer—*Can.*) is provided for IM injection only; similarly to iron dextran, it is rapidly absorbed in the first few hours of administration, mainly in the blood.

DS2 The concentration of iron dextran and iron sorbitol solution is 50 mg/mL, and a single dose usually consists of two 1-mL injections into the gluteal muscles using the "Z" technique to avoid staining. A test dose of approximately 25 mg should be administered, and the patient should be observed for 20 minutes to detect any severe anaphylactic reaction. The following formula helps establish the total dose:

Hb deficit (g/L) × weight (kg) × 0.22 = iron deficit (mg);

or

Hb deficit (g/dL) × weight (lb) = iron deficit (mg)

Subsequently, 500–1,000 mg to replete iron stores can be added. As many as 20 visits may be required to provide 2 g of iron. If the undiluted solution of iron dextran is to be given IV, 2 mL is again the limit. The problem of repeated administration can be overcome by diluting up to 2 g of iron into 250–1,000 mL of normal saline and infusing it over 3–4 hours.

SE2 Iron dextran: Anaphylactic reaction can occur 0.2%–0.3% of the time, so that epinephrine should be readily available during treatment. Mild to moderate arthralgias, myalgia, urticaria, chest pain, chills, and headache. Contraindicated in rheumatoid arthritis because it can induce a crisis.

Iron sorbitol: This form is not associated with anaphylaxis or with the myalgia/arthralgia syndrome described with iron dextran.

Iron Overload

KY Increased body iron stores develop either from increased GI absorption (e.g., hemochromatosis, accelerated erythropoiesis) or from parenteral administration in chronic anemia with multiple transfusions. Hemochromatosis is an autosomal-recessive disease (mutation of HFE gene on chromosome 6); homozygotes can accumulate toxic amounts of iron in 30–40 years. Iron overload can cause dysfunction in the liver, heart, pancreas, pituitary, and thyroid. It can be associated with excessive tanning and with an arthropathy, mainly of the distal phalanges of the hands. When liver cirrhosis is present, occurrence of hepatoma can be as high as 30%–40%.

TX In hemochromatosis, it is possible to eliminate the excess iron with successive phlebotomies (ideally 1–2 times/week) until a state of iron-deficient erythropoiesis is created or according to recent guidelines a ferritin of 25–50 ng/mL. Subsequently, 1 unit of blood every 3–4 months is taken from these patients to maintain iron stores at an acceptable level. Phlebotomy is sometimes used in mild anemia associated with iron overload. When phlebotomy is not an option, chelators must be relied on. The goal of therapy is to remove approximately 0.5 mg/kg/day of iron. Because there is no ideal way to measure this, **careful monitoring of the organs that can suffer from excessive iron load is mandatory.**

RX **Deferoxamine** (Desferal, Mesylate) [C]: Binds iron by its hydroxamic acid side groups, and the complex is subsequently cleared. Administered as a 24-hour infusion or as a continuous SC administration.

DS Deferoxamine is dissolved in sterile water. Dose: 2–2.5 g/day (**PEDS:** — 25–50 mg/kg/day) SC (preferred route)/IV (requires central venous access) infusion over 12–16 hours using a 27-gauge needle attached to a syringe pump by infusion tubing. The site of infusion is rotated daily. Ascorbic acid can increase iron removal but is potentially toxic; thus, the maximum daily dose should be limited to 200–500 mg (to 100 mg at the beginning of therapy).

SE Inflammation at the site of infusion is the most common side effect. It can be minimized by inclusion of 2–3 mg of hydrocortisone in the solution. If the inflammation is too severe, infusion by a permanent venous access port can be used. Anaphylaxis has been reported, but it is rare. Mucormycosis incidence is increased and can be serious. Other rare side effects include cataracts, optic and vestibular neurotoxicity, decreased creatinine clearance, and adult respiratory distress syndrome. Failure of linear growth and metaphyseal and spinal abnormalities have been reported and thus should be monitored in children.

Porphyrias

KY Porphyrias occur as a result of a deficient enzyme activity in the heme synthesis pathway, which leads to an increase in the earlier precursors that are formed. There are many different types of porphyrias, but, for practical purposes, there are only three presentations of importance:

- The acute attacks typical of acute intermittent porphyria; characterized by abdominal pain, nausea, vomiting, constipation, and peripheral neuropathy. Associated with an increase in urine porphobilinogen and ALA. Attacks can be triggered by drugs inducing hepatic cytochrome P450.

- The chronic skin damage of porphyria cutanea tarda
- The acute photosensitivity of erythropoietic protoporphyria

TX1 **Acute attack of porphyria:** Treatment of the acute attack involves the following:

- Avoiding the offending drugs (e.g., barbiturates and sulfa drugs).
- Administration of estrogens if the attacks are related to the menstrual cycle.
- Glucose infusions in an attempt to suppress ALA-synthetase activity (associated with early precursors in the heme synthesis pathway). Approximately 300–400 g/day of dextrose is necessary (basal requirements +20% and +14% per 1°C of fever). This is administered through a central venous catheter.
- Hemin infusion: Heme provides negative feedback to ALA-synthetase. Hemin is a derivative of heme that is used for this purpose. Its administration is appropriate when the patient does not respond to glucose loading.
- Electrolyte management: Hyponatremia must be corrected *slowly* when present; this is best achieved through fluid restriction (1.5 L qd), with 75 mEq Na/L.

RX1 **Hemin** (Panhematin)

DS1 A dose of 1–4 mg/kg IV qd in two divided doses is often given, with appropriate monitoring.

SE1 Potential significant toxicity, including DIC. Local phlebitis possible.

TX2 **Chronic skin damage of porphyria:** Treatment of chronic skin damage involves the following:

- Removal of the toxin (mostly alcohol).
- Phlebotomy is used to remove excess iron; the fall in ferritin level is achieved much more rapidly than it is in hemochromatosis. Once hepatic iron is normalized, porphyria cutanea tarda is usually asymptomatic.
- Because the effects of phlebotomy are delayed, small doses of chloroquine phosphate can be used in the meantime; this drug tends to remove porphyrins stored in the liver.
- Sun protection.

RX2 Chloroquine (Aralen) [C]

DS2 250 mg PO twice a week

SE2 Nausea and diarrhea. **Retinopathy is rare but irreversible.**

TX3 **Photosensitivity of porphyria:** Treatment of photosensitivity involves (1) **sun screens** (opacity to light), and (2) **beta carotene** (can increase tolerance to light).

RX3 **Beta carotene**

DS3 200–600 mg PO qd

SE3 Yellow staining of skin (mainly palms and soles) is frequent.

Sideroblastic Anemia

KY Sideroblastic anemia can be congenital or acquired. Some of the acquired forms are reversible if the causative agents are removed; these agents include alcohol, antituberculosis agents, chloramphenicol, and copper deficiency.

TX The acquired myelodysplastic form rarely responds to pyridoxine, and treatment usually relies on transfusional support and iron chelation. EPO is rarely useful. In the hereditary form, the defect seems to involve ALA-synthetase. Because pyridoxal phosphate is a cofactor in this reaction, it follows that pharmacologic doses of pyridoxine can overcome the defect. Folic acid can be added if megaloblastic changes are seen.

RX **Pyridoxine** (vitamin B$_6$) (Aminoxin, Nestrex—*U.S.*; Carthamex, Hexa-Betalin—*Can.*) [A/C in high doses]

DS 50–200 mg PO qd

SE Elevated doses are associated with nonspecific side effects that are not considered serious, including nausea, headache, and paresthesia.

HEMOGLOBINOPATHIES

Hb is composed of a heme moiety, which contains one ferrous iron atom and a globin tetramer. Hb A contains two α-globin and two β-globin chains (α_2, β_2), Hb A$_2$ contains two α-globin and two δ-globin chains, and Hb F contains two α-globin and two γ-globin chains.

Normal adult Hb is composed of 96%–98% Hb A, 1.5%–3% Hb A$_2$ and 0.5%–1% Hb F. Hemoglobinopathies can be very complex; only the most common will be discussed.

Methemoglobinemia

KY In this condition, Hb M, an Hb that contains iron in the ferric state instead of the ferrous state, is the culprit. Hb M can be either congenital (a mutation in a globin chain or an enzyme deficiency) or acquired (oxidizing agents such as nitrate). Methemoglobin binds oxygen tightly, causing hypoxia of the tissues. It has a brownish blue color.

TX **Ascorbic acid** is used to treat the congenital form of methemoglobinemia. **Methylene blue** can also be used orally, but it causes blue urine. **Riboflavin** is another choice. **Acquired methemoglobinemia can be fatal when Hb M increases more than 50%**; it requires treatment with IV methylene blue, which acts via the nicotinamide adenine dinucleotide phosphate reductase system. Because this system requires glucose-6-phosphate dehydrogenase (G-6-PD) activity, it is ineffective in patients with G-6-PD deficiency, who may then need exchange transfusions.

RX1 **Ascorbic acid** (vitamin C) [A/C in high doses]

DS1 300–600 mg PO qd

SE1 Hyperoxaluria and kidney stones

or

RX2 **Methylene blue** (Urolene Blue) [C]

DS2 60 mg PO tid–qid; or 1 mg/kg IV in 1% saline solution, infused in approximately 15 minutes.

SE2 Blue-green urine, stools, or both and skin staining.

or

RX3 **Riboflavin** (Riobin) [A/C in high doses]

DS3 20 mg PO qd

SE3 Discoloration of urine (yellow-orange)

Sickle Cell Anemia and Related Syndromes

KY Certain Hbs have a tendency to polymerize inside erythrocytes. The most important of these Hbs are Hb S and Hb C. Both of these result from amino acid substitutions on position 6 of the β chain, which is usually occupied by glutamate. In Hb S, valine is the anomaly; in Hb C, it is lysine.

The amount of abnormal Hb per cell is critical to the development of the syndrome. People with just one abnormal gene live a normal life, except in extreme situations such as hypoxia or dehydration (or both). People with two abnormal genes are symptomatic. It can be two Hb S genes, two Hb C genes, a combination of the two, or one gene in combination with a β-thalassemia gene. Although there are some clinical differences depending on the combination, treatment guidelines are similar.

The abnormal Hbs polymerize at a lower pO_2 such that the cells tend to be of normal morphology in the arteries and of abnormal morphology in the veins. When cells become irreversibly sickled (or Hb C crystals become permanent), they can cause (1) extravascular hemolysis (splenic infarct eventually results in the loss of spleen function, but the reticuloendothelial system continues to destroy the cells) and (2) tissue damage from obstruction of the microcirculation.

TX **Treatment is mainly supportive:** Painful vaso-occlusive crisis requires adequate hydration, treatment of the precipitating factors (infections or inflammation), adequate analgesics, and, occasionally, exchange transfusions. **Maintenance therapy** includes vaccination ideally against *Streptococcus pneumoniae* (23 types), *Haemophilus influenzae* type b, and *Neisseria meningitidis* in endemic areas (see Ch 18 Pediatrics); supplementation with folic acid; and, rarely, a regular transfusion program. The antineoplastic agent hydroxyurea has the capacity to increase Hb F (inhibits polymerization of deoxyhemoglobin S) to a level of 15%–20% or more, and severely affected patients can benefit (e.g., more than three severe crisis per year).

RX **Hydroxyurea** (Hydrea) [D]

DS The average dose: 20 mg/kg PO qd, titrated to reach Hb F improvement and to keep neutrophil count > 2,000/μL.

SE Minimal when supervised by dedicated facilities. Myelosuppression is dose limiting.

Thalassemia Syndromes

KY Thalassemia syndromes are quantitative defects in globin chains. α-Thalassemia is a deficit of α-globin production that is caused by gene deletion. The severity is correlated with the number of genes that are deleted (from one to all four). β-Thalassemia is a deficit of β-globin production that is caused by gene mutation rather than deletion. There are two β genes; in β-thalassemia, one or both contain mutations. Thalassemia syndromes and their most common genotypes and manifestations are listed in Table 9–5.

RX Table 9–5

DS Table 9–5

SE Table 9–5

HEMOLYTIC ANEMIA

Normal red blood cells (RBCs) survive in the circulation for approximately 120 days. They have to pass through tissue capillaries and slitlike orifices in the spleen. The flexibility of RBCs depends on the maintenance of a biconcave shape, a healthy membrane, and adequate fluid content. In hemolysis, RBCs have a shortened life span. When hemolysis is mainly extravascular the spleen is the primary site of destruction of the RBCs, with the liver and bone marrow as alternative sites. In intravascular hemolysis, the membrane of RBCs is attacked within the blood vessels. Hemolysis can also be divided into intracorpuscular and extracorpuscular.

Acquired Hemolytic Anemia

KY Acquired hemolytic anemia is **extracorpuscular** most of the time. **Immune hemolytic anemias** are recognized by the presence of Igs or complement fractions (C3) on the surface of the RBCs (positive Coombs' test). **Alloimmune anemia** occurs when the body responds appropriately to a foreign antigen, such as an incompatible transfusion.

When autoantibodies are produced, the anemia is described as being **autoimmune.** It can be **warm reactive or cold reactive.** In **warm-reactive anemia,** the antibody is an IgG, which reacts maximally at 37°C toward a part of Rh antigens. Warm-reactive anemias can be idiopathic, associated with lymphoproliferative disorders (e.g., chronic lymphocytic leukemia, lymphoma) and connective tissue diseases (e.g., systemic lupus erythematosus), or associated with drugs.

In **cold-reactive anemia,** IgM is usually responsible and is more reactive at low temperatures. When temporarily bound to the RBC, it fixes complement, which will either activate and destroy the cells by creating holes in the membrane (intravascular hemolysis) or leave C3 on the surface of the cells (removed mainly in the liver). Cold-reactive anemias can be

Table 9–5. Thalassemia Syndromes and Their Most Common Genotypes, Manifestations, and Treatments

Syndrome	Genotype*	Manifestation**	Transfusion	Folic Acid	Other Treatment(s)
α2-Thalassemia	α-/αα	None or microcytosis	No	No	No
α1-Thalassemia	α-/α- or αα/- -	Microcytosis Anemia +/-	No	No	No
Hb H disease	α-/- -	Microcytosis Anemia ++ Hemolysis ++ Ineffective erythropoiesis +	Yes (occasionally)	1 mg PO qd	Avoidance of oxidant drugs Splenectomy
Hb Bart	- -/- -	Hydrops fetalis (lethal)			
β-Thalassemia minor	β/βo or β+	Microcytosis Mild anemia	No	No	No
β-Thalassemia intermedia	β+/β+ (many other possibilities)	Microcytosis Anemia ++ Hemolysis +/- Ineffective erythropoiesis ++	Yes (occasionally)	1 mg PO qd	Splenectomy Iron chelation
β-Thalassemia major	βo/βo	Microcytosis Anemia ++ Hemolysis + Ineffective erythropoiesis ++	Yes Keep hemoglobin ≥ 10 g/dL	1 mg PO qd	Early iron chelation Bone marrow transplantation Splenectomy

*α = normal alpha (α) gene; - = deletion; β = normal beta (β) gene; βo = no β chain produced; β+ = decrease production of β chain.
** +/- = mild to normal; + = mild to moderate; ++ = moderate to severe.

idiopathic or can be associated with lymphomas and infections (e.g., Epstein-Barr virus, mycoplasma).

Paroxysmal cold hemoglobinuria (PCH) is a special type of cold-reactive anemia in which IgG is directed at the blood group antigen P. PCH is sometimes seen after viral infections.

Transfusion hemolytic reactions are alloimmune (the antigen is foreign), and acute types are caused by IgM and are almost always the result of ABO incompatibility. The delayed-type is caused by IgGs against blood groups such as Rh, Kidd, Kell, and Duffy. The delayed type is not as severe as the acute type and is often subclinical.

Mechanical hemolysis is seen when blood flows rapidly through an area of turbulence (e.g., a leaking prosthetic valve, aortic stenosis, malignant hypertension, tumors, giant hemangioma, and intravascular coagulation). Some infections are associated with hemolysis and include *Clostridium perfringens*, plasmodium, bartonellosis, and HIV (autoimmune type). Spur cell anemia and PNH are examples of acquired defects of the red cell membranes.

℞ **General measures:** see Hereditary Hemolytic Anemia. Remove or treat the cause whenever possible (e.g., drugs).

Acute transfusion hemolytic reactions can be life-threatening and require vigorous hydration and use of diuretics.

Therapy for immune-type hemolysis is more elaborate. **Corticosteroids** (e.g., prednisone) are used as first-line therapy in warm-reactive type. When prednisone is withdrawn, many patients do not remain in remission. Some patients are stable with acceptable toxicity at a dose of approximately 10 mg/day. Steroids are not effective in cold-reactive type and yield disappointing results in PCH.

Splenectomy removes the major site of RBC destruction in warm-reactive autoimmune anemia. Up to 75% of patients will have an appropriate response to splenectomy, but relapse may occur. Some patients require a lower dose of steroids after splenectomy. It is recommended that patients be **immunized** with polyvalent pneumococcal, *Haemophilus influenzae* b, and quadrivalent meningococcal polysaccharide vaccines, at least before surgery. Antibiotic prophylaxis is controversial. **When symptoms of a bacterial infection develop, the patient must either consult a physician immediately or, if a delay is inevitable, start penicillin or erythromycin empirically.** As with corticosteroids, splenectomy yields disappointing results in cold-reactive type or PCH.

Immunosuppressive agents and **cytotoxic therapy** are the next steps in warm-reactive type and the first pharmacotherapeutic steps in the cold-reactive type if avoidance of the cold is not sufficient. **Azathioprine** or **cyclophosphamide** is used. **Cyclosporine** has been used in resistant disease. With cold-reactive type, **chlorambucil** is preferable. **Danazol**, a modified androgen, is used by some before immunosuppressive therapy.

℞ Table 9–6

DS Table 9–6

SE Table 9–6

Table 9-6. Drugs Useful in Hemolytic Anemias

Generic (Brand) Name	Dose (PO)	Side Effects	Note
Azathioprine (Imuran) [C]	50–200 mg qd	See Table 9-4	Monitor blood counts. Delayed effectiveness (3–4 weeks).
Chlorambucil (Leukeran) [D]	2–4 mg qd	GI upset, elevated liver enzymes, leukemogenic, myelosuppression, rash	First choice for cold-type immune hemolysis. Monitor blood counts. Allow 3–4 weeks' trial.
Cyclophosphamide (Cytoxan, Neosar—*U.S.*; Procytox—*Can.*) [D]	50–150 mg in a single morning dose	See Table 9-4	Monitor blood counts. Delayed effectiveness (3–4 weeks). Recommend good hydration PO and voiding before bedtime.
Cyclosporine (Gengraf, Neoral, Sandimmune) [C]	See Table 9-4	See Table 9-4	See Table 9-4
Danazol (Danocrine—*U.S.*; Cyclomen—*Can.*) [X]	200–800 mg qd	Table 9-4	Liver function tests must be monitored. Gradually increase the dose as required.
Folic acid (Folvite—*U.S.*; Flodine—*Can.*) [A/C in high doses]	1 mg qd	Nonspecific and rare, including flushing, malaise, rash, and allergic reactions.	Do not use alone if associated pernicious anemia.
Iron supplements	See Iron Deficiency	See Iron Deficiency	Use with caution in PNH (reticulocytes are hemolysis prone).
Prednisone (Deltasone) [B]	1–1.5 mg/kg	See Table 9-4	Wait 3 weeks before failure is considered. Taper down slowly (subtract 10 mg from daily dose per once week) hemoglobin levels become stable. Alternate-day therapy possible at $\leq$ 30 mg/day.

GI = gastrointestinal; PNH = paroxysmal nocturnal hemoglobinuria.

Hereditary Hemolytic Anemia

KY Hereditary hemolytic anemia is of the **intracorpuscular** type. It can be caused by a membrane defect, the most frequent being hereditary spherocytosis (HS) and the second most frequent being elliptocytosis. HS is caused by a deficiency of spectrin with or without ankyrin (primarily defective in 40%–70% of cases), which are cytoskeletal proteins. The RBC loses part of its membrane, which decreases its surface-volume ratio and makes it less flexible. These cells become trapped in the spleen, which leads to extravascular hemolysis, splenomegaly, pigment gallbladder stones, and, occasionally, jaundice.

The RBC requires anaerobic glycolysis to produce energy and to maintain Hb in a reduced state. Defective enzymes in the glycolytic pathway can cause hemolytic anemia; pyruvate kinase (PK) deficiency, which is autosomal recessive, is one of these rare deficiencies. The anemia is severe and is accompanied by hepatosplenomegaly. A more common enzyme deficiency is G-6-PD deficiency, which is x-linked recessive. In this disorder, hemolysis can be episodic and of varied severity.

TX Folic acid should be given to any patient with chronic hemolysis. In G-6-PD deficiency, any oxidant drug or compound should be avoided. Iron can be lost through the urine in intravascular hemolysis, and supplements should be provided when stores are depleted. Splenectomy is most useful when the spleen is the main site of RBC destruction. It is very useful in symptomatic spherocytosis, less useful in PK deficiency, and occasionally useful in hemoglobinopathies. If possible, surgery should wait until a child reaches 5 years of age.

RX Table 9–6

DS Table 9–6

SE Table 9–6

IMMUNODEFICIENCY STATES RELATED TO LYMPHOCYTES

Lymphopoiesis and lymphocyte functions are very complex, beyond the scope of this book. The following description is very succinct and simplified. Humans produce three types of lymphocytes: B cells, T cells, and NK cells. B cells differentiate into plasma cells and produce antibodies (humoral immunity). T cells ($\geq$ 85% of blood lymphocytes) are divided into help-inducer (CD4+) and cytotoxic-suppressor (CD8+) subsets. With the NK cells, they constitute the cellular immunity. Igs are composed of two heavy chains (γ, α, μ, δ, or ϵ) and two light chains (κ or λ), producing IgG, IgA, IgM, IgD, and IgE. IgG is important in therapeutics and has a half-life of approximately 21 days.

Conditions Associated With Immunodeficiency

KY See Table 9–7

TX In the treatment of immunodeficiency states, **immunoglobulin prepa-**

Table 9–7. Conditions Associated With Immunodeficiency

B-Cell Deficiencies
Common variable immunodeficiency*
Malignancies of lymphocytic origin*
Newborns
Specific immunoglobulin deficiencies†
X-linked agammaglobulinemia*
X-linked lymphoproliferative disease*

T-Cell Deficiencies‡
Congenital thymic aplasia
Human immunodeficiency virus infection
Human T-cell leukemia virus type 1
Wiskott-Aldrich syndrome*

B-Cell and T-Cell Deficiencies
Ataxia-telangiectasia
Leukocyte adhesion deficiency
Severe combined immunodeficiency disorder (SCID)*

* Immunoglobulin can be beneficial.

†Immunoglobulin can be beneficial when a significant IgG subclass is involved.

‡An efficient humoral response cannot be mounted in cases of severe T-cell deficiency.

rations remain the principal treatments. Other treatments include antibiotics (to control secondary infections), bone marrow transplantation (in severe disorders, i.e., SCID, Wiskott-Aldrich), splenectomy (occasionally used in Wiskott-Aldrich to control thrombocytopenia), and fetal thymic transplantations (thymic aplasia). For management of HIV, refer to Ch 10 Infectious Diseases.

Immune globulins or immunoglobulins (Igs) are available in IV preparations and contain almost only IgG, with less than 2% of IgA and IgM. The antibody profile reflects the serologic responses to endemic pathogens and immunization states of the donor population.

IV Ig can block the activity of harmful antibodies by interfering with the receptor of effector cells or by combining with the antibody in the blood or on the surface of lymphocytes (which decreases antibody synthesis).

RX IV immune globulin (Gamimune N)

DS Dosage depends on the indication.

Primary immunodeficiencies: doses were classically 100–200 mg/kg, but this was increased to a range of 200–800 mg/kg q3–5wk; the goal is to keep the trough level of Igs > 400–500 mg/dL. Many different companies produce IV Ig. The concentration of Gamimune is 50 or 100 mg/mL. Because most side effects are related to the rate of administration, infusion should be started slowly (approximately 0.01–0.02 mL/kg/min) and the rate increased every 15 minutes until a rate of 0.08 mL/kg/min is attained.

SE Side effects occur in ≤ 5% of patients. They include minor systemic reactions, such as headaches, fever and chills, nausea and vomiting, and light-headedness; changes in blood pressure; tachycardia; hypersensitivity; and, rarely, anaphylactic reactions, mainly in IgA-deficient individuals.

Aseptic meningitis might occur several days after infusion, but it is rare. Slowing the rate of infusion can reduce most of these effects. Note that HIV and hepatitis B are not transmitted by Ig infusions. Anecdotal reports of hepatitis C were linked to certain products that are now no longer used. Nevertheless, Igs are blood products and should be used wisely.

LEUKOPENIA

It is beyond the scope of this book to discuss all of the possible causes of leukopenia. It is, however, useful to know the physiology of granulopoiesis and the mechanisms of neutropenia, which is the most important of the leukopenias.

Granulocytes are found in three major compartments—bone marrow, blood, and tissues. Granulopoiesis occurs in the medullary compartment, starting with the myeloid stem cells. During the first three stages of maturation (i.e., myeloblast, promyelocyte, and myelocyte), the cell is still capable of division. In the more advanced stages (i.e., metamyelocyte, band, and polymorphonuclear), the cell no longer has the ability to divide.

The second compartment is the blood, where about 50% of the granulocytes are marginated (next to the endothelium) and 50% are circulating. Normal neutrophil counts are 1,800–7,000/µL in adults. Neutrophil granulocytes survive only 6–10 hours in the blood, where most of them appear as polymorphonuclear neutrophils, with ≤ 5% bands.

Granulocytes are attracted to the tissue compartment by chemotactic factors released from areas of inflammation. They squeeze between endothelial cells (a phenomenon called diapedesis) to reach their destination. They finally fulfill their role of phagocytosis and are destroyed.

The production of granulocytes is stimulated by growth factors (i.e., cytokines), which are produced mostly by T cells, endothelial cells, and mesenchymal cells. The most important growth-stimulating factors for neutrophils are IL-3, GM-CSF, and G-CSF, the latter being more specific.

Neutropenia

KY Neutropenia is defined by a neutrophil count < 1,800–2,000/µL; it is considered to be severe when the neutrophil count is < 500/µL. In the latter condition, mucosal ulcers, pharyngitis, spiking fever and chills, skin infections, septicemia from different sources, and shock are seen. Neutropenia can result from defective proliferation (e.g., postchemotherapy), defective maturation (e.g., pernicious anemia), shortened survival (e.g., autoimmune diseases), or excessive margination or hypersplenism. Another way to classify neutropenia is to separate isolated neutropenia from the neutropenia associated with other cytopenias. Isolated neutropenia can then be divided into toxic (drug-related), infection-related, immune-related, and idiopathic (including congenital) neutropenia.

TX **Treatment options vary depending on the cause of the neutropenia** (see classification in the previous paragraph). In the case of drug-related neutropenia, the cessation of all relevant medications is required. In cases of severe neutropenia, the presence of fever should be sought, and, if present, the appropriate cultures (i.e., blood, urine, +/- throat, sputum, stool) and a chest x-ray of the lungs should be obtained. Broad-spectrum antibiotics should be administered. Treat the cause whenever possible (see Ch 14 Oncology).

G-CSF or filgrastim (Neupogen) and GM-CSF or sargramostim (Leukine, Prokine) can be useful pharmacologic treatments; GM-CSF is rarely used and will not be discussed further. **G-CSF** is used to treat certain congenital and cyclic neutropenias and to alleviate the neutropenia caused by zidovudine (Retrovir) [C] in acquired immunodeficiency syndrome. It reduces the duration of severe neutropenia that is caused by conventional or high-dose chemotherapy in cancer. The American Society of Clinical Oncology has published guidelines for its appropriate use. Maximum stimulation of hematopoiesis occurs when the exposure is constant.

RX **Filgrastim or G-CSF** (Neupogen) [C]: Promotes the maturation of granulocyte/macrophage progenitors to neutrophils, stimulates the neutrophils to leave the marrow and enhances their function, and causes demargination.

DS Recommended dosage: 5 μg/kg SC qd. The duration of treatment depends on the indication. When G-CSF is used in nonneoplastic disorders, it can be continued for much longer, if not for life. With neoplastic disorders, it is usually given for 10–14 days after chemotherapy (with blood count monitoring). A short-lived drop in neutrophil count can be expected after initiation of G-CSF treatment, but it is not considered to be clinically significant. Therapy is usually terminated when neutrophils reach 10,000/μL.

SE Bone pain; elevated liver enzymes, uric acid, and lactate dehydrogenase (LDH) (all of which are reversible); and, rarely, mild dysuria.

MEGALOBLASTIC ANEMIAS

Megaloblastosis describes the morphology of cells that show delayed nuclear maturation, with respect to cytoplasmic maturation. The reason for this delay lies in abnormal DNA synthesis. The most frequent and treatable causes of megaloblastic anemia are deficiencies of vitamin B_{12} (cobalamin), folic acid, or both. Other causes include some antineoplastic agents, rare inborn errors of pyrimidine or folate metabolism, and myelodysplastic syndromes. Treatment is usually ineffective in the latter two.

Cobalamin (Vitamin B_{12}) Deficiency

KY Vitamin B_{12} is found in food that contains animal proteins (e.g., meat, fish, eggs, milk) and can also be synthesized by bacteria in the GI tract. A standard diet will provide > 5 μg/day, largely exceeding the daily requirements of 1 μg/day. Normal absorption depends on intrinsic factor, produced by the stomach, and a healthy distal ileum. Vitamin B_{12} blood levels are normally approximately 200–610 pg/mL; liver storage capacity is approximately 2–5 mg, or enough to last at least 2–5 years.

Cobalamin is an enzyme linked to folic acid metabolism. A deficiency causes intracellular folate deficiency.

Cobalamin deficiency can result from reduced intake, malabsorption (i.e., lack of intrinsic factor, decreased absorption surface, blind-loop syndrome, parasitic infection), and, rarely, impaired cellular utilization. Cobalamin deficiency can cause folic acid deficiency, defective myelin synthesis, and neurotoxicity.

TX **Transfusion** is more often indicated in cobalamin-deficient patients than it is in folate-deficient patients. Because these are chronic anemias, patients must be transfused very slowly (1 U/day is appropriate) and with appropriate diuretics. In pernicious anemia (atrophic gastritis with lack of intrinsic factor) and in any other irreversible cause of B_{12} malabsorption, the treatment is to administer B_{12} supplements. Response is usually dramatic, with an increase of the reticulocyte count by the first week and resolution by about the sixth week. If these criteria are not met, the diagnosis should be reevaluated.

RX **Cyanocobalamin (vitamin B_{12})** supplements [A/C in high doses]

DS Administered IM or by deep SC injection. Regimens are quite variable: Some experts administer a very low dose (5–10 µg) of the drug for the first day or two to avoid the drop in K^+ that is caused by the rapidly ensuing erythrocyte maturation. Then, 100 µg/day can be administered for 7–10 days, followed by 100 µg/month.

Other experts suggest doses of 1,000 µg because even if 80%–85% of the of the dose is lost in the urine, the net absorption of B_{12} is quite large. When neurologic damage is present, it is suggested that weekly injections be continued until maximum recovery is achieved, which can take up to 6 months. **Life-long therapy is required.** Oral supplements in very large doses are efficient but more dependent on compliance; a dose is 1,000–2,000 µg PO qd.

SE In elderly patients with heart problems, K^+ supplementation should be considered (i.e., possible hypokalemia with arrhythmia). Other side effects are nonspecific.

Folate Deficiency

KY Folic acid (pteroylglutamic acid) and dietary folates are polyglutamates; they must be reduced to the monoglutamate form in the small bowel before they can be absorbed by the intestinal microvilli (primarily in the proximal jejunum). The main dietary source of folic acid is green vegetables. **An adult requires about 100 µg of folate per day,** which is more than adequately supplied by a normal diet (up to 5 times that amount). **Pregnancy increases the requirements by up to 10-fold, so that folate supplementation is indicated.**

Serum levels of 1.75–11 ng/mL are considered normal, but these values can vary widely depending on the laboratory. Up to 5 mg of folate can be stored in the body, equivalent to a 3- to 4-month supply.

Different forms of folic acid are used as coenzymes in metabolic systems, including DNA synthesis.

Folate deficiency can be caused by nutritional deficiencies, malabsorption (abnormal intestine, as in celiac disease, or from anticonvulsant drugs), increased requirements found in pregnancy or states of increased cell turnover, or impaired cellular folate use (alcohol or folate antagonists).

TX **Oral supplements** can correct the problem even with malabsorption. Response is similar to that described for cobalamin deficiency.

RX **Folic acid** (Folvite—*U.S.;* Flodine—*Can.*) [A/C in high doses]: Main supplement used orally. In specific situations, **folinic acid** (Leucovorin) can be used orally or IV and has the ability to bypass the blockade of dihydrofolate reductase that is caused by the chemotherapeutic agent methotrexate.

DS Folic acid 1 mg PO qd.

SE Well tolerated. Neurologic problems associated with vitamin B_{12} deficiency can deteriorate on folate alone so when in doubt, start folate and vitamin B_{12} together.

PLATELET DISORDERS

Platelets are produced in the marrow by the megakaryocyte, a cell that is much larger than other hematopoietic precursors. When its cytoplasm matures, it actually separates into fragments that become platelets, leaving the nucleus behind. Thrombopoietin, a recently identified cytokine, is the major stimulus of thrombopoiesis.

One-third of the platelets are sequestered in the spleen; the remainder circulate in the blood. Platelet survival is approximately 7–10 days, for senescence and a minor effect from ongoing hemostasis consumes about 15% of the daily pool. Normal counts range from 150,000–400,000/μL.

When a vessel is injured, platelets adhere to the subendothelial surface through platelet receptors; the most important ligands include collagen and von Willebrand factor. The platelets then have to aggregate; this aggregation progresses in two waves, stimulated by adhesion, adenine dinucleotide phosphate, thrombin, or adrenaline. Primary aggregation (the first wave) is reversible, but the second wave, which results from prostacyclin metabolism and thromboxane A_2 release, is irreversible.

The platelet is also involved in coagulation: (1) it provides the very important phospholipid surface that is required by coagulation factors and (2) it contains some of the coagulation factors.

Platelet function can be crudely assessed by bleeding time or, more precisely, by studying platelet response to certain agonists.

Disorders of Platelet Function

KY Functional defects can be congenital or acquired. **Congenital disorders** can involve many platelet structures that would be too long to describe. **They cannot be corrected on a long-term basis.** Desmopressin can correct mild cases, and some patients with severe symptoms can improve with the use of antifibrinolytic drugs. **Acquired disorders of platelet function include** uremia, myeloproliferative diseases, monoclonal gammopathies (e.g., myeloma, Waldenström macroglobulinemia), drugs (e.g., antiplatelet agents, heparin, fibrinolytic agents), chronic liver disease, cardiopulmonary bypass, and some antiplatelet antibodies.

TX The treatment of acquired disorders of platelet function is directed at the cause whenever possible (e.g., dialysis in uremia). Maintenance of an adequate Hb level (approximately 9 g/dL) is also helpful. Desmopressin may provide some beneficial effects in uremia and in cardiopulmonary bypass, some mild defects in myeloproliferative disorders and monoclonal gammopathies, and may also prove to be beneficial after acetylsalicylic acid (ASA) treatment. Conjugated estrogens seem to help in uremia.

RX1 **Desmopressin** (DDAVP, Stimate—*U.S.*; Octostim—*Can.*) [B]

DS1 See Disorders of Blood Coagulation

SE1 See Disorders of Blood Coagulation

RX2 **Antifibrinolytic drugs:** See Disorders of Blood Coagulation

DS2 See Disorders of Blood Coagulation

SE2 See Disorders of Blood Coagulation

Disorders of Platelet Number

KY **Increased platelet number (thrombocytosis)** can be either primary or secondary (reactive). **Primary thrombocytosis** is caused by myeloproliferative and rare myelodysplastic disorders. **Secondary thrombocytosis** results from some common conditions such as iron deficiency, inflammatory disorders, hemorrhage or hemolytic anemia, nonhematopoietic malignancies, or splenectomy. Most of the time, the count is < 600,000/μL. If it is above this number, treatment of the underlying cause can be useful; ASA is of no proven benefit.

Thrombocytopenia can be **mild** (100,000–150,000/μL), **moderate** (50,000–100,000/μL), or **severe** (< 50,000/μL). Provided that the platelets are functioning appropriately, no symptoms are seen when the count is > 50,000/μL. At 20,000–50,000/μL, bleeding can be prolonged after an injury, and at < 20,000/μL, spontaneous bleeding can be seen. Classification of thrombocytopenia is shown in Table 9–8.

TX1 **Therapy of thrombotic thrombocytopenic purpura/hemolytic uremic syndrome: Plasma exchange (plasmapheresis) is the cornerstone of therapy.** In idiopathic cases, exchange should be started as soon as possible. In pregnancy-related cases, it is used especially when delivery is not possible, although in some cases, it must be initiated postpartum. It is useful in some cancer-associated and drug-induced states.

RX1 Plasma exchange (plasmapheresis)

DS1 Plasma exchange of 40–80 mL/kg qd through a double-lumen central venous catheter should be continued until neurologic symptoms are resolved and normal platelet count and LDH levels are obtained for a few days. At this point, the interval is gradually increased over 1–2 weeks, then

Table 9–8. Classification and Management of Thrombocytopenia

Class of Thrombocytopenia	Mechanism or Associated Diseases	Note on Treatment
Pseudothrombocytopenia	Platelet clumping on blood smears No clinical manifestation	No treatment
Hypersplenism	Increase splenic pool up to 90% of platelets. Rarely < 30,000/μL	No bleeding on its own. Splenectomy is of no benefit unless an additional platelet-lowering mechanism is at play.
Decreased production Congenital Acquired	Very rare AA AMT Infiltration of marrow (by cancer, leukemia, dysplasia) Drugs (e.g., thiazide diuretics, DES) Toxic substances (e.g., alcohol) Chemotherapy	Supportive treatment Specific treatment for many of the associated diseases Otherwise: Antifibrinolytic drugs (see Disorders of Blood Coagulation) Danazol or cyclosporine is sometimes useful in AMT Removal of the cause
Radiation therapy	Severe B$_{12}$, folate, or iron deficiency PNH Renal failure (mild) Viral infection	Supportive treatment
Dilutional	Massive hemorrhage treated with fluid replacement	Supportive treatment

(continued)

Table 9–8. Classification and Management of Thrombocytopenia (Continued)

Class of Thrombocytopenia	Mechanism or Associated Diseases	Note on Treatment
Accelerated platelet destruction: Nonimmunologic TTP or HUS	Most cases are idiopathic. Secondary causes can be epidemic (*Escherichia coli, Shigella*), pregnancy-related, carcinoma-related, drug-related.	See Disorders of Platelet Number for treatment.
Pregnancy related	Preeclampsia Incidental (most common)	See Ch 13 Obstetrics
Infection related	Mostly bacterial	Supportive treatment
Macroangiopathy or microangiopathy	Other than TTP/HUS, includes: DIC Dysfunctional cardiac valves Giant cavernous hemangioma Large aortic aneurysms	Supportive treatment See Disorders of Blood Coagulation and DIC.
Accelerated platelet destruction: Immunologic Autoimmune (ITP)	Primary HIV related Secondary (SLE, rare solid tumors, lympho-proliferative disorders)	Therapy for all immune-related thrombocytopenia (see Table 9–9)

Drug induced	Antibiotics (e.g., sulfa drugs, many others) HIT Quinine-related drugs Valproic acid	See Thromboembolic Disorders for HIT (SE2a)
Infection induced	Epstein-Barr virus	Supportive treatment
Neonatal isoimmune Posttransfusion purpura	Exposures to fetal blood or transfusion; antibodies to a platelet antigen (mostly HPA-1a) can cross the placenta; platelet drop delayed by 1 week after transfusion.	Discussed in text, Therapy of Immune Thrombocytopenia See Table 9–9
Alloimmune	Destruction of transfused platelets. Often HLA related.	

AA = aplastic anemia; AMT = amegacaryocytic thrombocytopenia; DIC = disseminated intravascular coagulation; DES = diethylstilbestrol; HIT = heparin-induced thrombocytopenia; HIV = human immunodeficiency virus; HLA = human leukocyte antigen; HUS = hemolytic uremic syndrome; ITP, immune thrombocytopenic purpura; PNH = paroxysmal nocturnal hemoglobinuria; SLE = systemic lupus erythematosus; TTP = thrombocytopenic thrombotic purpura.

therapy is discontinued, although some specialists carry on with one or two pheresis for 1 month. The replacement fluid should be either plasma or cryosupernatant plasma because it is thought that the therapy works by either removing a harmful plasma component or replacing a putative deficiency.

SE1 Changes in fluid volume, hypotension, and symptoms of hypocalcemia.

TX2 **Therapy of immune thrombocytopenia:** Treatment should be **individualized.** In most situations, a platelet count as low as 30,000/µL may be tolerated. Therapy aims at inhibiting removal of platelets by the spleen and decreasing the amount of antiplatelet antibodies. **Corticosteroids** are usually the first line of treatment.

IV Igs are often used in severe or refractory cases. IV anti-D globulins can also be used. In cases that are refractory to these first options, or in which it is impossible to lower the steroids to a reasonable chronic dose (maximum 10 mg/day), **splenectomy** is the treatment of choice; this removes the most important site of destruction. **Plasmapheresis** with immunoabsorption over a staphylococcal A column can also be considered.

Therapy in HIV-related cases follows similar guidelines: Steroids, provided that they can be sufficiently tapered, and splenectomy have both been shown to be safe. Therapy directed at the virus can also increase the platelet count.

The only major difference in secondary immune thrombocytopenic purpura is the added use of therapy directed at the cause (e.g., chemotherapy of lymphoproliferative disorders).

Posttransfusion purpura and **neonatal isoimmune thrombocytopenia** are self-limited but **can be very dangerous, and treatment of moderate to severe cases is mandatory.** Steroids are used, and IV Ig can prove to be beneficial. Plasmapheresis is another useful treatment modality. Platelet concentrates that are negative for the antigen are the only appropriate treatment for major bleeding.

RX2 Table 9–9

DS2 Table 9–9

SE2 Table 9–9

THROMBOEMBOLIC DISORDERS

Individual diseases caused by thromboembolic disorders are discussed in their respective specialty chapters. Here, the focus is on the treatment of thromboembolic disease, with emphasis on anticoagulant agents.

KY The pathophysiology of venous thrombosis includes stasis, endothelial injury, and hypercoagulability. Disease entities associated with this pathology include deep venous thrombosis and pulmonary embolus, and both are discussed in Ch 20 Pulmonology. The **pathophysiology of arterial thrombosis** is slightly different. Here, a dysfunctional endothelium (from atherosclerosis, hypertension, etc.) is important. The rheologic abnormalities are different because thrombosis often starts at bifurcations and expands via turbulent flow and high shear forces. Finally, platelets are more important than in venous thrombosis; in arterial thrombosis, the clot is platelet rich. Disease entities associated with this include unstable angina and myocardial infarction (discussed in Ch 3 Cardiology) and stroke (discussed in Ch 12 Neurology).

TX1 **Antiplatelet drugs**

RX1 See Ch 3 Cardiology.

DS1 Doses differ depending on the disease entity being treated: See Ch 3 Cardiology for doses of antiplatelet agents used to treat chronic ischemic heart disease and Ch 12 Neurology for doses used to treat acute stroke syndromes.

SE1 See Ch 3 Cardiology.

TX2 **Anticoagulant drugs**

RX2a **Heparin:** Standard heparin (Calciparine—*U.S.*; Calcilean—*Can.*) [B] and low-molecular-weight heparin (LMWH), enoxaparin (Lovenox) [B], dalteparin (Fragmin) [B], and tinzaparin (Innohep) [B] are among the most commonly used anticoagulants. Heparin works by potentiating AT III, the natural inhibitor of thrombin, factor Xa, and factors IXa, XIa and XIIa. Standard heparin primarily inhibits thrombin because the length of the molecules enables them to bind both thrombin and AT III ("template effect"), which is necessary to provide thrombin inhibition. The LMWH acts primarily on factor Xa, which can be inhibited without the template effect.

The commercial LMWH preparations have an average molecular weight of 4,000–6,500 d, compared with 15,000 daltons for standard heparin. Their anti-Xa/antithrombin activity is 2:1–4:1.

Heparin must be administered either IV or SC. The effects are instantaneous. **Standard heparin** has a low and variable bioavailability (approximately 30%) because of protein binding and a variable half-life (0.5–6 hour) that becomes longer when the dose in increased. It also has an affinity for platelets. **LMWH** does not have the same affinity, has 90% bioavailability, and has a longer, more stable half-life (approximately 3 hours).

Activated partial thromboplastin time (aPTT) can be used to monitor standard heparin's therapeutic effect. The therapeutic range of heparin is 0.3–0.6 IU of anti-Xa activity per 1 mL. The corresponding range of aPTT in a hospital could be used as the therapeutic target (Table 9–10).

LMWH's better bioavailability makes monitoring unnecessary, but if desired (e.g., with renal failure or rather small or large patients), only anti-Xa activity can be used.

DS2a **Standard heparin:** many variations of the protocol for treatment have been published. The principles are as follows:

IV:

- Bolus of 5,000–10,000 U (approximately 70–80 U/kg).
- Heparin 15–18 U/kg/hr IV infusion

Table 9–9. Treatment of Immune Thrombocytopenia

Treatment	Generic (Brand) Name
Corticosteroids	Prednisone (Deltasone) [B]
	Methylprednisolone (SoluMedrol) [C]
	Dexamethasone (Decadron) [C]
Immunoglobulin	Intravenous immune globulin (Gamimune, Gammagard) [C]
Anti-D globulin	Intravenous Rho (D) immune globulin (WinRho SDF) [C]
Androgen	Danazol (Danocrine—*U.S*; Cyclomen—*Can.*) [X]
Antibiotic (mechanism of action unclear)	Dapsone (Avlosulfon—*Can.*) [C]
Antineoplastic agents with immunosuppressive activity	Cyclophosphamide (Cytoxan, Neosar—*U.S.*; Procytox—*Can.*) [D]
	Vincristine (Oncovin, Vincasar) [D]
	Azathioprine (Imuran) [D]
Immunosuppressive agent	Cyclosporine (Neoral, Sandimmune) [C]

- aPTT is measured before and 4–6 hours after the beginning of treatment.
- Adjustments are made according to the aPTT results (see Table 9–10).
- Where the IV dose exceeds 35,000 U/day without a therapeutic aPTT, the anti-factor Xa level can be measured.
- When anticoagulation is required for several weeks or months, warfarin should be started on the first or second day. Heparin can then be discontinued when warfarin has achieved therapeutic levels for 2 days. In severe iliofemoral thrombosis, treatment is heparin for 10 days.

Dose	Side Effects
Starting dose: 1–2 mg/kg PO qd; taper down over 1–2 months when normal count is achieved. (*Peds*—1–4 mg/kg PO qd tapered down over 1–2 [rarely 3] weeks)	See Table 9–4 Dose for chronic use should be limited to a maximum of about 10 mg/kg qd to limit side effects. Note: Methylprednisolone is used for life-threatening bleeding.
1 g IV qd for 3 days	
40 mg PO qd on days 1–4, 7–12, and 17–20 of a 28-day menstrual cycle.	
400 mg/kg IV qd for 5 days or 1 g/kg IV qd for 2 days	See Conditions Associated with Immunodeficiency. Note: Tendency is to use it in very severe cases (platelets < 5–10,000/µL).
50–75 µg/kg IV	Hemolysis usually not significant. Note: 70% response in nonsplenec-tomized Rh-positive patients.
400–600 mg PO qd	Elevated transaminases, mild mas-culinizing effects
50–125 mg PO qd	Hemolysis and methemoglobinemia, hepatitis
2–4 mg/kg PO qd for 6 months, or 750–1,500 mg/m^2 IV q3–4wk	See Table 9–4
2 mg IV weekly for 4 weeks See Ch 14 Oncology	
1–3 mg/kg PO qd for 9–12 months See Table 9–4	
6–12 mg/kg/day in divided doses See Table 9–4	

- Complete blood count should be checked every 3 days (see below).

SC:

Starting dose: 17,500 U q12hr with adjustments made according to aPTT performed 6 hours postdose. (5,000–10,000 U IV bolus can be added at the start of treatment.)

Therapeutic doses of LMWH:

Enoxaparin 1 mg/kg SC q12hr or
Dalteparin 200 U/kg SC qd or
Tinzaparin 175 U/kg SC qd

Table 9–10. **Dosing Instructions According to aPTT Results for a Therapeutic Range of 55–95 Seconds, With 25,000 U of Heparin in 500 mL of D-5-W (50 U/mL)***

aPTT (seconds)	Repeat Bolus (U)	Stop Infusion (minutes)	Change Rate		Next aPTT
			U/hr	mL/hr	
< 40	5,000	0	+200	+4	6 hours
40–54	0	0	+100	+2	6 hours
55–95	0	0	0	0	Morning
96–105	0	0	−100	−2	Morning
106–120	0	30	−100	−2	6 hours
> 120	0	60	−200	−4	6 hours

aPTT = activated partial thromboplastin time; D-5-W = 5% dextrose in water.
*When anticoagulation is required for several weeks or months, warfarin should be started on the second day. Heparin can be discontinued when warfarin has achieved therapeutic levels for 2 days.

SE2a **Serious bleeding** is an obvious side effect. This risk is approximately 14% with repeated IV bolus (no longer used), 5%–6% with continuous heparin, and approximately 4% with SC heparin. ASA can increase the risk, but this risk is acceptable provided that a short course of heparin is given. **Management of bleeding is discussed in** Table 9–11.

Nonimmune, mild thrombocytopenia (> 100,000/μL) can occur early and is of no consequence. **Immune-type heparin-induced thrombocytopenia** occurs within 3–15 days of the first dose, unless the patient has been previously exposed to the antigen. The incidence is 2%–5% with porcine heparin, and it can lead to thrombosis (not bleeding) in 30%–75% of these patients at therapeutic levels. The incidence of thrombocytopenia decreases to 0.3% at smaller prophylactic doses. LMWH is also associated, but with lower incidence, to this type of thrombocytopenia (one-tenth the incidence).

If the platelet count decreases by 40%–50% (for no apparent reason) while the patient is taking heparin, then heparin should be stopped and danaparoid, hirudin, or argatroban should be started at therapeutic doses even without thrombosis The platelet count should return to normal in approximately 4 days. Initiation of warfarin is possible, preferably once the platelet count has reached 100,000/uL.

Osteoporosis can be seen with long-term SC administration (i.e., > 4–6 months); this can be associated with fractures. **Other rare side effects** include hypersensitivity, alopecia, skin necrosis, and hypoaldosteronism.

Contraindications to heparin are numerous and can be divided into absolute and relative (Table 9–12).

RX2b **Warfarin** (Coumadin) [B]: Interferes with vitamin K metabolism. This vitamin must be in its reduced form to act as a cofactor in the post-translational carboxylation of glutamate residues on factors II, VII, IX, and X; protein C; and protein S. Half-life is about 35 hours, and the effect lasts

Table 9–11. Management of Anticoagulant Therapy–Related Bleeding*

Anticoagulant Therapy–Related Bleeding	Management
Heparin	Mild severity of bleeding:
	Local measures and discontinuation of heparin only if necessary.
	Protamine sulfate usually not used (1% risk of anaphylaxis if previously exposed).
	Serious severity of bleeding:
	Protamine sulfate IV may be used as a neutralizer; 1 mg combines with 100 U of heparin. The dose is calculated according to an estimated half-life of heparin of 60 minutes, and it may be necessary to repeat the dose because protamine's half-life is shorter than 60 minutes.
Warfarin	Various situations can occur:
	INR too high, < 5, no bleeding: Lower or omit a dose.
	INR from 5–9, no bleeding: Omit a few doses until INR decreases to therapeutic levels. Vitamin K 0.5–1 mg SC may be administered, repeated at 24 hours if still too high. Oral vitamin K 2.5 mg is another option.
	INR from 9–20, no bleeding: Administer vitamin K 3–5 mg SC. Omit warfarin until INR decreases to therapeutic levels.
	INR > 20 or serious bleeding: Administer vitamin K 10 mg SC and consider plasma transfusion. Omit warfarin until INR decreases to therapeutic levels.
	Life-threatening bleeding or with serious overdose (suicide attempt, etc.): Administer fresh frozen plasma and vitamin K 10 mg SC, repeated as needed.

INR = international normalized ratio.

*Bleeding related to anticoagulation therapy is managed according to the severity of the bleeding and to the agent that is being used.

for 2–3 days. Stored vitamin K will change the sensitivity to the drug from extreme sensitivity to relative resistance, especially after a large dose of vitamin K.

PT is used to follow warfarin treatment. It is sensitive to low levels of factors VII, X, and II; it is most affected by factor VII. The results are now expressed in the international normalized ratio (INR) to standardize variability among the different reagents that are used.

DS2b A **starting dose of 5 mg** is now recommended for most patients, unless the patient has a condition that is suggestive of increased sensitivity to its effect (e.g., malnourishment, liver disease, congestive heart failure), a high risk of bleeding, or a high risk of early thrombosis (e.g., defect in protein C pathway), in which case a **dose of 2.5–5 mg** can be used instead. Doses are then prescribed according to desired INR (weak intensity,

Table 9–12. Contraindications to Heparin

Absolute
Severe active hemorrhage
Cerebral hemorrhage
Malignant hypertension
Recent surgery to the brain, eye, or spinal cord
Severe hemostatic defect
Major side effects to heparin in the past (heparin-induced thrombocytopenia is not
   an absolute contraindication once the antibody has disappeared)
Subacute endocarditis
Severe hemorrhagic retinopathy

Relative
Peptic ulcer or irritation of the stomach with less than severe hemorrhage
Recent stroke
Recent surgery or trauma (within 14 days)
Severe hypertension
Mild to moderate hemostatic defect
Liver or kidney failure
Diabetic retinopathy
> 75 years of age

1.3–1.9; standard, 2.5 [range, 2–3]; strong, 3 [range, 2.5–3.5]; some special
settings, 3–4.5). It takes 4–5 days for the INR to be reliable since it is
mostly affected by lowered factor VII in the first few days. Average dose
would be **4–5 mg/day.**

SE2b The annual risk of major bleeding is estimated to be 3%; minor
bleeding is at least twice as frequent. This can be minimized by keeping
INR in the lower part of the standard range. **Management of bleeding
is discussed in** Table 9–11. Other side effects are skin necrosis (most
common with protein C deficiency), skin rash, a rare alopecia, and,
rarely, blue toes. **The problems associated with pregnancy are typical
embryopathy (nose hypoplasia and skeletal defects) that occurs at
6–12 weeks' gestation, central nervous system defects (occur anytime
during pregnancy), and bleeding (more prevalent at birth).**

Absolute contraindications to warfarin are the same as those
described for heparin, plus the first trimester and the last month of
pregnancy, newborns, and high-risk suicide patients. Relative contraindications to warfarin are mainly related to unreliable follow-ups.

A large number of drugs can interact with warfarin, and this
should always be checked. Decreased anticoagulant effects occur with concomitant use of barbiturates, carbamazepine, phenytoin, rifampin, oral contraceptive pills, vitamin K, and spironolactone. Enhanced anticoagulant
effects occur with concomitant use of salicylates, certain antibiotics, acetaminophen, and propranolol. Increased bleeding tendency is reported with
concomitant use of certain antibiotics, salicylates, antimetabolites, quinidine, quinine, corticosteroids, and potassium products. These lists are not

exhaustive. Diet (vitamin K–rich food) and alcohol can also interact with warfarin.

RX2c **Hirudin:** A potent antithrombin drug that is found in leech saliva; the recombinant molecule lepirudin (Refludan) [B] is now available.

DS2c Bolus of 0.1–0.4 mg/kg IV, then 0.06–0.15 mg/kg/hr IV infusion. Monitor with aPTT. Dosage has to be adjusted in cases of renal impairment.

SE2c Bleeding, hemorrhage, DIC, fever, and allergic reactions.

RX2d **Ancrod** (Viprinex): Discontinued due to lack of material. Ancrod was a rapid-acting defibrinogenerating enzyme derived from Malayan pit viper venom (*Agkistrodon rhodostoma*). It reduced fibrinogen levels by removing fibrinopeptide A, which created an inefficient fibrin that could be removed by the reticuloendothelial system. It was indicated for short-term anticoagulation, when heparin was contraindicated.

DS2d Will not be discussed since this drug is no longer available.

SE2d Will not be discussed since this drug is no longer available.

RX2e **Danaparoid** (Organan) [B]: A mixture of heparan sulfate, dermatan sulfate, and chondroitin sulfate that inhibits factor Xa in a way similar to heparin. Effect is immediate. Cross-reactivity with heparin seems to be less than 10%.

DS2e **Loading dose:** 2,250 U IV bolus, followed by 400 U/hr infusion over 4 hours, and then 300 U/hr infusion over 4 hours. **Maintenance dose:** 150–200 U/hr. Danaparoid has a long half-life, about 25 hours, so it can be discontinued earlier than heparin when combined with warfarin. Anti-Xa levels can be used for monitoring. **Prophylactic dose:** 750 U SC q12hr.

SE2e Hemorrhage, abdominal discomfort, edema, urinary retention, urinary tract infections, anemia, and allergic reactions.

RX2f **Argatroban** [B]: A highly selective thrombin inhibitor that reversibly binds to active (both free and clot-associated) thrombin. It inhibits fibrin formation and the activation of factors V, VIII, and XIII; protein C; and platelet aggregation. It is a safer agent to use compared with hirudin in patients with renal impairment.

DS2f No bolus. Start with a dose of 2 µg/kg/min continuous IV infusion (0.5 µg/kg/min if hepatic dysfunction). Target steady-state aPTT is 1.5–3 times baseline (maximum, 100 seconds). Measure aPTT 2 hours after the initial dose or modification. Do not exceed 10 µg/kg/min.

SE2f Hemorrhage, hypotension, arrhythmias, fever, abdominal discomfort, and infection.

TX3 **Thrombolytic therapy:** Drugs in this category target plasminogen, which contains an enzymatically active site. Plasminogen is transformed to plasmin when a cut is made at its enzymatic site, rendering it active, and it is then that fibrinolysis can occur. All of the activators cleave the same bond, Arg560-Val561.

RX3 **Thrombolytic agents.** See Ch 3 Cardiology.

DS3 **Doses differ depending on the disease entity being treated:** See Ch 3 Cardiology for the doses used in the treatment of acute coronary syndromes and Ch 12 Neurology for acute stroke syndromes.

SE3 See Ch 3 Cardiology. Contraindications to the administration of a thrombolytic agent are listed in Ch 3 Cardiology.

10

Infectious Diseases

WAYNE L. GOLD

PRINCIPLES OF ANTIMICROBIAL THERAPY

When selecting an antimicrobial regimen for the management of an infectious disease, several factors must be taken into consideration. If the identity of the infecting organism is known, specific therapy may be administered. In many circumstances, however, the causative pathogen is not known. Therefore, initial antimicrobial therapy must be empiric and is targeted against the pathogens that are most likely to cause the clinical condition. In these circumstances, information regarding local antimicrobial resistance and the patient's recent exposure to antibiotic agents must be incorporated into the decision-making process. Recent antibiotic exposure is a risk factor for infection with drug-resistant pathogens.

Host factors, including the presence of immunodeficiency states, neutropenia, renal insufficiency, liver disease, site of infection, and previous adverse drug reactions, must also be taken into consideration. **Potential drug interactions** must be anticipated, as dose adjustment of the antimicrobial agent may be necessary.

The ability of the patient to metabolize and excrete antimicrobial agents must be considered when choosing an antibiotic agent or combination. Renal excretion is the most important route of elimination for most antibiotic agents. Drugs that are highly excreted by the kidney must be administered with caution in patients with impaired renal function. Failure to alter the dose or dosing interval of these agents may result in drug toxicity. Creatinine clearance calculations are outlined in Ch 7 Geriatrics.

The **site of infection** is another important factor that must be considered when choosing an antimicrobial agent. The ability of an antibiotic to penetrate the site of infection will determine the choice of antimicrobial agent as well as the dose and route by which the drug will be administered. Concentrations of antibiotics must be in excess of the minimum inhibitory concentration of the infecting organism. Failure to achieve appropriate drug concentrations may result in treatment failures. This is particularly important in the management of bacterial meningitis in which the peak concentration–minimum inhibitory concentration ratio should be ≥ 10.

Finally, in certain clinical conditions, **combinations of antimicrobial agents** may be required. Indications for combination antimicrobial therapy might include the treatment of polymicrobial infections and the treatment of infections in the neutropenic host. Combinations of antimicrobial agents may also be indicated when the combination of agents provides **synergistic killing activity** against the infecting pathogen.

Table 10–1 lists commonly used classes of antimicrobials, their mechanisms of action, side effects, and mechanisms of antimicrobial resistance. Table 10–2 lists their spectrum of activity.

(Text continues on page 184)

Table 10-1. Summary of Commonly Used Antimicrobial Drug Classes

Class	Generic (Brand) Name	Mechanism of Action, Route(s) of Elimination, Dose Adjustments	Side Effects	Mechanism(s) of Resistance
Aminoglycosides	Amikacin (Amikin) [C] Gentamicin (Garamycin—U.S.; Cidomycin—Can.) [C] Streptomycin [D] Tobramycin (Nebcin, Tobrex) [C]	**Bactericidal.** Inhibit protein synthesis by binding to the 30S subunit of the bacterial ribosome. Aminoglycosides are not absorbed after oral administration; they must be administered parenterally. Dose adjustments are necessary in the presence of renal insufficiency.	Nephrotoxicity, ototoxicity Neuromuscular blockade may occur when large doses are rapidly infused, especially in patients with myasthenia gravis.	Production of aminoglycoside inactivating enzymes. Inability of the aminoglycoside to penetrate to the target site of action. Alteration of the binding site in the 30S ribosomal subunit.
Cephalosporins*	**First generation:** Cefazolin (Ancef, Kefzol) [B] **Second generation:** Cephalexin (Keflex) [B] Cefamandole (Mandol) [B] Cefotetan (Cefotan) [B] Cefoxitin (Mefoxin) [B] Cefuroxime (Ceftin, Kefurox, Zinacef) [B]	**Bactericidal.** Inhibit bacterial cell wall synthesis in a similar manner as the penicillins. Excreted almost exclusively by the kidney, except for cefoperazone and ceftriaxone, which have significant biliary excretion. Dosage adjustments are necessary in the presence of renal insufficiency.	Drug-induced hemolytic anemia; GI upset; hypersensitivity reactions, including fever and rash; thrombocytopenia	Production of beta-lactamases. Alteration of the target penicillin-binding proteins. Decreased ability of the cephalosporins to reach their target site of action.

Cephalosporins*	**Third generation, *without* antipseudomonal activity:** Cefixime (Suprax) [B] Cefotaxime (Claforan) [B] Ceftriaxone (Rocephin) [B] **Third generation, *with* antipseudomonal activity:** Ceftazidime (Ceptaz, Fortaz, Tazicef, Tazidime) [B]		
Fluoroquinolones	Ciprofloxacin (Ciloxan, Cipro) [C] Gatifloxacin (Tequin) [C] Levofloxacin (Levaquin) [C] Moxifloxacin (Avelox) [C] Norfloxacin (Chibroxin, Noroxin) [C] Ofloxacin (Floxin) [C]	**Bactericidal.** Inhibit bacterial DNA synthesis by binding to bacterial topoisomerases (DNA gyrase and topoisomerase IV); DNA gyrase is an essential bacterial enzyme that is needed for superhelical twisting of bacterial DNA. The concomitant oral administration of calcium- or magnesium-containing compounds may reduce the bio-availability of fluoroquinolones. Dosage adjustment is required in the presence of renal insufficiency, except for moxifloxacin.	Dizziness, GI intolerance, headache, photosensitivity, QTc prolongation, Torsade de pointes	Stepwise increasing resistance occurs as a result of sequential mutations in the target topoisomerases.

(continued)

177

Table 10-1. Summary of Commonly Used Antimicrobial Drug Classes (Continued)

Class	Generic (Brand) Name	Mechanism of Action, Route(s) of Elimination, Dose Adjustments	Side Effects	Mechanism(s) of Resistance
Lincosamides	Clindamycin (Cleocin—U.S.; Dalacin C—Can.) [B]	**Bacteriostatic.** Binds to the 50S ribosomal subunit, resulting in the inhibition of bacterial protein synthesis. Penetrates well into most tissues and body spaces. Metabolized by the liver and excreted in bile and urine. Dose adjustments not required in the presence of renal insufficiency.	Hypersensitivity reactions, including fever and rash; diarrhea in up to 20% of patients; *Clostridium difficile*-associated diarrhea or pseudomembranous colitis.	Alteration of the 50S ribosomal subunit protein confers resistance to clindamycin and cross-resistance to macrolide agents.
Macrolides	Azithromycin (Zithromax) [B] Clarithromycin (Biaxin) [C] Erythromycin [B]	**Bacteriostatic.** The site of action is the 50S ribosomal subunit. Macrolides inhibit protein synthesis at the step of chain elongation. Erythromycin and azithromycin: Excreted in bile. Dosage adjustment is not required in the presence of renal insufficiency. Clarithromycin: Metabolized in the liver and excreted in the bile and urine. Dosage adjustments must be made in the presence of severe renal insufficiency.	Cholestasis Important **drug interactions** include elevation of serum theophylline and digoxin concentrations. GI upset, QTc prolongation, Torsade de pointes	Efflux mechanisms, which pump the drug out of the bacterial cell. Alterations of the 50S ribosomal protein, which is the target site of action; less common mechanisms of resistance include enzymatic inactivation and decreased ability of the drug to permeate the bacterial cell wall in gram-negative bacteria.

Nitroimidazoles	Metronidazole (Flagyl) [B/X in first trimester]	Bactericidal. After entry of the drug into the bacterial cell, metronidazole undergoes reductive activation. The reduced intermediate product interacts with bacterial DNA, resulting in its bactericidal activity. Metronidazole is well absorbed in the GI tract after oral administration and diffuses well into all body sites, including CSF. It is metabolized in the liver and excreted in the urine. Dosage adjustment is not necessary in renal failure.	Disulfiram reactions if ingested with alcohol, metallic taste (may occur after ingestion), peripheral neuropathy	Despite extensive use, acquired resistance to metronidazole among anaerobic bacteria is rare. Possible mechanisms of resistance include decreased uptake into the bacterial cell and reduced rates of reductive activation.
Penicillins	**Natural penicillins** Penicillin V potassium (Suspen, Truxillin, Veetids) [B] Penicillin G [B] **Aminopenicillins** Amoxicillin (Amoxil) [B] Amoxicillin and clavulanate potassium (Augmentin—U.S.; Clavulin—Can.) [B] Ampicillin (Marcillin, Polycillin, Principen—U.S.; Ampicin—Can.) [B]	Bactericidal. Inhibit bacterial cell wall synthesis by binding to PBPs in the bacterial cell wall. PBPs are responsible for the cross-linkage of peptidoglycans in the bacterial cell wall. Failure of cross-linkage results in osmotic lysis of bacteria. Penicillins are variably absorbed after oral ingestion. These agents penetrate into most body spaces, including CSF, and are rapidly excreted by the kidney. The dosage must be altered in the presence of renal insufficiency.	GI upset; hemolytic anemia; hypersensitivity reactions, including fever, skin rash, serum sickness, and anaphylaxis; seizures; thrombocytopenia	Production of beta-lactamases, which are enzymes that hydrolyze the beta-lactam ring (examples include penicillin resistance in *Staphylococcus aureus* and ampicillin resistance in *Escherichia coli*). Alteration of bacterial PBPs (examples include methicillin-resistant *S. aureus* and penicillin resistance in *Streptococcus pneumoniae*). Inability of the antibiotic to penetrate to the target site of action.

(continued)

179

Table 10–1. Summary of Commonly Used Antimicrobial Drug Classes *(Continued)*

Class	Generic (Brand) Name	Mechanism of Action, Route(s) of Elimination, Dose Adjustments	Side Effects	Mechanism(s) of Resistance
Penicillins (cont.)	**Antipseudomonal penicillins** Carbenicillin (Geocillin, Geopen) [B] Piperacillin (Pipracil) [B] Piperacillin-tazobactam† Ticarcillin (Ticar) [B] Ticarcillin-clavulanic acid‡ **Antistaphylococcal penicillins** Cloxacillin (Cloxapen) [B] Oxacillin (Bactocill) [B]			
Sulfonamides and trimethoprim	Trimethoprim and sulfamethoxazole (Bactrim, Septra, Sulfatrim) [C/D at term]	Sulfonamides (**bacteriostatic**): Antimicrobial agents that are similar in structure to PABA. Sulfonamides competitively inhibit binding of PABA to hydropteroate synthetase, an enzyme that is required for folic acid synthesis. Metabolized by the liver and excreted in the urine. Dosage adjustments are required in severe renal insufficiency.	Aseptic meningitis, bone marrow suppression, drug-induced hepatitis, fever, rash	Sulfonamide resistance is mediated by the changes in the structure of hydropteroate synthetase or by overproduction of PABA. Trimethoprim resistance is mediated by structural alteration of bacterial dihydrofolate reductase.

Trimethoprim (bacteriostatic): A dihydrofolate reductase inhibitor. Trimethoprim is excreted in the urine. Dosage adjustment is required in severe renal insufficiency.

| Vancomycin (Lyphocin, Vancocin, Vancoled) [C] | **Bactericidal.** A glycopeptide antibiotic agent that inhibits bacterial cell wall synthesis. For systemic activity, vancomycin must be given IV. It has poor CSF penetration in the presence of a normal blood-brain barrier. Vancomycin is almost exclusively eliminated by the kidney via glomerular filtration. Dose adjustment must be made in the presence of renal insufficiency | Bitter taste, GI upset, fever, chills, eosinophilia, vasculitis, thrombocytopenia, ototoxicity, renal failure, hypotension, allergic reactions

Phlebitis at the infusion site

Rapid infusion may result in histamine release, leading to flushing and pruritus of the face, neck, and thorax (red person's syndrome).

Vancomycin-induced neutropenia may occur. | Vancomycin resistance can occur in enterococcal species; *S. aureus* isolates with reduced susceptibility to vancomycin have been reported to cause clinical infections. |

CSF = cerebrospinal fluid; GI = gastrointestinal; PABA = para-aminobenzoic acid; PBP = penicillin-binding protein.

*Cephalosporins lack activity against enterococci and *Listeria monocytogenes*.

†Addition of tazobactam provides coverage against beta-lactamase–producing organisms.

‡Addition of clavulanic acid provides coverage against beta-lactamase–producing organisms.

Table 10–2. Spectrum of Activity of Commonly Used Antimicrobial Agents

Antimicrobial Agent	Antimicrobial Spectrum of Activity/ Clinical Indications for Use
Aminoglycosides	Gram-negative bacilli (documented or presumed infections); tobramycin should be used for pseudomonal infections Empiric treatment of the patient with febrile neutropenia Enterococcal infections in combination with penicillin or ampicillin Mycobacterial infections—streptomycin, amikacin
Cephalosporins First generation*	Staphylococcal species (not MRSA or MRSE) Streptococcal species (not recommended for the treatment of infections that are likely to be caused by *Streptococcus pneumoniae*) Indicated for the treatment of skin and soft-tissue infections *Escherichia coli* *Klebsiella pneumoniae* *Proteus mirabilis*
Second generation*	Indicated for the treatment of community-acquired pneumonia Staphylococcal species (not MRSA or MRSE) Streptococcal species (some isolates of *S. pneumoniae* may be resistant) *Haemophilus influenzae* *Moraxella catarrhalis* Some members of the Enterobacteriaceae family of gram-negative organisms
Third generation, *without* antipseudomonal activity*	Indicated for the treatment of community-acquired and nosocomial pneumonia and bacterial meningitis Aerobic gram-negative bacilli (not *Pseudomonas aeruginosa*) *H. influenzae* *M. catarrhalis* *Neisseria meningitidis* Streptococcal species (some isolates of *S. pneumoniae* may be resistant) Modest *Staphylococcus aureus* activity
Third generation, *with* antipseudomonal activity*	Aerobic gram-negative bacilli, including *P. aeruginosa* *H. influenzae* *M. catarrhalis* *N. meningitidis*

**Table 10–2. Spectrum of Activity of Commonly Used
Antimicrobial Agents** *(Continued)*

Antimicrobial Agent	Antimicrobial Spectrum of Activity/ Clinical Indications for Use
Clindamycin	Staphylococcal species Streptococcal species, including group A streptococci Anaerobic bacteria, including *Bacteroides fragilis*: indicated for the treatment of anaerobic infections, including pelvic and abdominal infections, infections of the oral cavity alone or in combination with other antimicrobial agents *Pneumocystis carinii* in combination with primaquine *Toxoplasma gondii* in combination with pyrimethamine
Fluoroquinolones Ciprofloxacin	Indicated for the treatment of urinary tract infections except moxifloxacin Gram-negative bacilli, including *P. aeruginosa* Poor staphylococcal, streptococcal activity *Mycoplasma pneumoniae* *Chlamydia pneumoniae* *Legionella pneumophila* *Chlamydia trachomatis* *Neisseria gonorrhoeae* *Mycobacterium tuberculosis* Atypical mycobacteria
Gatifloxacin Levofloxacin Moxifloxacin	Gram-negative bacilli, excluding *P. aeruginosa* Increased gram-positive activity compared with ciprofloxacin *M. pneumoniae* *C. pneumoniae* *L. pneumophila* *C. trachomatis* *N. gonorrhoeae* *M. tuberculosis* Indicated for the treatment of respiratory tract infections Atypical mycobacteria
Macrolides	Staphylococcal species Streptococcal species, including group A streptococci, *S. pneumoniae* *H. influenzae* (clarithromycin, azithromycin) *M. pneumoniae* *C. pneumoniae* *L. pneumophila* *C. trachomatis* Indicated for the treatment of respiratory tract infections Clarithromycin and azithromycin are used in the treatment of atypical mycobacterial infections, including *Mycobacterium avium* complex, *Mycobacterium chelonae* *(continued)*

Table 10–2. Spectrum of Activity of Commonly Used Antimicrobial Agents *(Continued)*

Antimicrobial Agent	Antimicrobial Spectrum of Activity/ Clinical Indications for Use
Penicillins	
Natural penicillins	Aerobic gram-positive cocci
	Group A streptococci
	Group B streptococci
	Viridans group streptococci
	S. pneumoniae: some isolates may be resistant
	Majority of *Staphylococcus* species are resistant
	Anaerobes (not *B. fragilis*)
	Treponema pallidum
Aminopenicillins	See Natural penicillins
	Enterococcal species (serious infections should be treated in combination with an aminoglycoside)
	E. coli
	P. mirabilis
Antipseudomonal penicillins	Streptococcal species
	Gram-negative bacilli, including *P. aeruginosa*
	Anaerobes
Antistaphylococcal penicillins	Aerobic gram-positive cocci, including methicillin-sensitive *S. aureus* and methicillin-sensitive *S. epidermidis*
Trimethoprim and sulfamethoxazole	Staphylococcal species, including some isolates of MRSA and MRSE
	Enteric gram-negative organisms: indicated for the treatment of urinary tract infections
	H. influenzae
	M. catarrhalis
	P. carinii
	T. gondii
Vancomycin	Staphylococcal species, including MRSA and MRSE
	Enterococcal species (not vancomycin-resistant enterococci)
	Clostridium difficile

MRSA = methicillin-resistant *Staphylococcus aureus*; MRSE = methicillin-resistant *Staphylococcus epidermidis*.

*As you move from first-generation cephalosporins to third-generation cephalosporins, there is a reduction in gram-positive activity and an increase in gram-negative activity. Only third-generation cephalosporins have reliable cerebrospinal fluid penetration.

ACUTE BACTERIAL MENINGITIS

KY **Acute bacterial meningitis is a life-threatening infection of the central nervous system.** Acute meningitis is a clinical syndrome characterized by fever, neck stiffness, and altered level of consciousness. The most common causes of adult bacterial meningitis are *Streptococcus pneumoniae*, *Neisseria meningitidis*, and *Listeria monocytogenes*. Meningitis caused by *L. monocytogenes* most frequently occurs in immunocompromised patients and during pregnancy. For cases of bacterial meningitis caused by *S. pneumoniae* and *N. meningitidis*, pathogenesis involves colonization of the nasopharynx by the infecting organism followed by local invasion of the nasopharyngeal mucosa, resulting in bacteremia and secondary hematogenous seeding of the meninges. Bacterial replication in the subarachnoid space results in an acute inflammatory response in the cerebrospinal fluid (CSF). The inflammatory response results in increased permeability of the blood-brain barrier, which in turn causes cerebral edema and increased intracranial pressure. Complications of acute bacterial meningitis include cranial nerve palsies, focal neurologic deficits, and seizures.

The diagnosis of bacterial meningitis relies on examination of CSF by lumbar puncture. Typical CSF findings in acute bacterial meningitis include elevation of the opening CSF pressure, neutrophilic pleocytosis, elevation of CSF protein concentration, and a decrease in CSF glucose concentration.

TX The most common microbial etiologies and the recommended empiric antibiotic regimens for the treatment of patients with acute bacterial meningitis differ among age groups (Table 10–3). Patients should remain in respiratory isolation until they have received at least 24 hours of effective antimicrobial therapy.

For cases of bacterial meningitis caused by *N. meningitidis*, rifampin must be given to the index patient and close contacts to eradicate pharyngeal carriage of *N. meningitidis*. For cases of meningitis caused by *Haemophilus influenzae,* rifampin must also be given to the index patient and all household contacts, irrespective of age, if there is at least one unvaccinated household contact younger than 4 years.

RX Table 10–3

DS Table 10–3

SE Table 10–1

HUMAN IMMUNODEFICIENCY VIRUS (HIV) INFECTION

KY Advances in the understanding of HIV-1 disease pathogenesis, the development of molecular techniques to measure levels of HIV-1 RNA in plasma (viral load measurement), and the development and introduction of highly active antiretroviral treatment (HAART) combinations into clinical practice have significantly reduced the morbidity and mortality associated with chronic HIV-1 infection.

Recommendations for the initiation of antiretroviral therapy must incorporate clinical, virologic, and immunologic assessments of the patient. The health status of the patient (symptomatic or asymptomatic HIV infection), plasma HIV-1 RNA level, CD4 cell count, and commitment of the patient to comply with a complex, long-term treatment regimen must be considered.

HAART is defined as a simultaneous combination of three or more antiretroviral agents that includes either a protease inhibitor or non-nucleoside analogue reverse transcriptase inhibitor as part of the multidrug regimen.

Table 10–3. Empiric Treatment of Bacterial Meningitis

Age of Patient	Pathogens	Therapy (IV)

0–4 weeks	*Escherichia coli*
	Group B streptococci
	Listeria monocytogenes
		Ampicillin 150–200 mg/kg/day in four to six divided doses
		plus
		Third-generation cephalosporin
		  Cefotaxime 200 mg/kg/day in four divided doses
		  Ceftriaxone 100 mg/kg/day in two divided doses

4 weeks to 23 months	*Streptococcus pneumoniae*
	Neisseria meningitidis
	Group B streptococci
	Haemophilus influenzae
	E. coli
		Ampicillin 150–200 mg/kg/day in four to six divided doses
		plus
		Third-generation cephalosporin
		  Cefotaxime 200 mg/kg/day in four divided doses
		  Ceftriaxone 80–100 mg/kg/day in two divided doses

2–18 years	*N. meningitidis*
	S. pneumoniae
	H. influenzae
		Vancomycin* 40–60 mg/kg/day in four divided doses
		plus
		Third-generation cephalosporin
		  Cefotaxime 200 mg/kg/day in four divided doses
		  Ceftriaxone 80–100 mg/kg/day in two divided doses

19–50 years	*S. pneumoniae*
	N. meningitidis
	H. influenzae
		Vancomycin* 1 g IV q12hr
		plus
		Third-generation cephalosporin
		  Cefotaxime 2 g IV q6hr
		  Ceftriaxone 2 g IV q12hr

> 50 years	*S. pneumoniae*
	N. meningitidis
	L. monocytogenes
	H. influenzae
		Ampicillin† 2 g IV q4hr
		plus
		Vancomycin 1 g IV q12hr
		plus
		Third-generation cephalosporin
		  Cefotaxime 2 g IV q6hr
		  Ceftriaxone 2 g IV q12hr

*Empiric coverage for penicillin- and cephalosporin-resistant strains of *S. pneumoniae*.

†Empiric coverage for *L. monocytogenes*.

TX **Initiation of antiretroviral therapy** (Table 10–4) is recommended for all patients with symptomatic HIV infection; plasma HIV-1 RNA level > 30,000 copies/mL, irrespective of CD4 cell count; and CD4 cell count < 350/mm³, irrespective of plasma HIV-1 RNA level. Treatment is also recommended for all patients with a plasma HIV-1 RNA level of 5,000–30,000 copies/mL with a CD4 cell count of 350–500/mm³. Treat-

Table 10–4. Possible Initial Antiretroviral Treatment Regimens*

2 NRTIs + protease inhibitor
2 NTRIs + NNRTI
2 NRTIs + 2 protease inhibitors
3 NRTIs
NRTI + NNRTI + protease inhibitor

*NRTI = nucleoside reverse transcriptase inhibitor; NNRTI, non-nucleoside reverse transcriptase inhibitor. Refer to Table 10–5 for members of each class of antiretroviral agents.

ment may be considered for HIV-1 infected individuals with plasma HIV-1 RNA levels of 5,000–30,000 copies/mL with a CD4 cell count > 500/mm³and (2) plasma HIV-1 RNA level < 5,000 copies/mL with a CD4 cell count of 350–500/mm³. **The risks and benefits of antiretroviral therapy should be discussed** with all patients having both a plasma HIV-1 RNA level < 5,000 copies/mL and a CD4 cell count > 500/mm³. Balancing the potential benefits of early antiretroviral therapy against potential drug side effects, the need for long-term compliance to a complex treatment regimen, and the possible emergence of drug resistance must be considered. If antiretroviral therapy is deferred, ongoing monitoring of the patient's virologic (plasma HIV-1 RNA level) and immunologic (CD4 cell count) status must be conducted.

Measurements of both CD4 cell counts and plasma HIV-1 RNA levels should be obtained to assess response to therapy. HIV-1 RNA assays have a lower limit of detection of 50 copies/mL. Suppression of plasma HIV-1 RNA levels to below the lower limit of detection of the assay is a goal of therapy. A 1.0- to 2.0-log decline in plasma HIV-1 RNA levels should be expected by 4–8 weeks after the introduction of therapy. Lack of compliance to the antiretroviral regimen is a major cause of early treatment failure. Failure to achieve viral suppression (50 copies/mL) by week 24 of therapy should prompt consideration of a change in the entire drug regimen. Other indications of drug failure include a blunted CD4 cell count response and clinical progression of HIV-1 infection, including the development of new opportunistic infections, while receiving HAART.

RX Table 10–4 and Table 10–5

DS Table 10–5

SE Table 10–5

HIV INFECTION AND PROPHYLAXIS AGAINST OPPORTUNISTIC INFECTIONS

KY Opportunistic infections have been a major cause of morbidity and mortality in patients living with chronic HIV infection (see *Pneumocystis carinii* pneumonia [PCP]). Before the introduction of HAART, improved recognition and characterization of opportunistic infections led to the development of strategies to prevent these infections that resulted in improved patient outcomes. Primary prevention of opportunistic infections may involve avoidance of exposure to opportunistic pathogens or antimi-

Table 10-5. Antiretroviral Agents, Dosages, and Side Effects

Generic (Brand) Name	Dose	Side Effects
Nucleoside reverse transcriptase inhibitors		
Zidovudine (AZT) (Retrovir) [C]	200 mg PO tid 300 mg PO bid	Anemia, headache, myopathy, nausea, neutropenia, vomiting
Didanosine (ddI) (Videx) [B]	200 mg PO bid (> 60 kg) 125 mg PO bid (< 60 kg)	Diarrhea, nausea, pancreatitis, peripheral neuropathy, vomiting
Zalcitabine (ddC) (Hivid) [C]	0.75 mg PO tid	Peripheral neuropathy, rash, stomatitis
Stavudine (d4T) (Zerit) [C]	40 mg PO bid (> 60 kg) 30 mg PO bid (< 60 kg)	Peripheral neuropathy
Lamivudine (3TC) (Epivir) [C]	150 mg PO bid	Anemia in combination with AZT
Abacavir (Ziagen) [C]	300 mg PO bid	Hypersensitivity In cases of suspected toxicity, the drug should be stopped. Rechallenge can be associated with life-threatening toxicity and mortality.
Non-nucleoside reverse transcriptase inhibitors		
Nevirapine (Viramune) [C]	200 mg PO daily for first 14 days 200 mg PO bid after day 14	Rash, transaminase elevation, hepatitis
Delavirdine (Rescriptor) [C]	400 mg PO tid	Rash, transaminase elevation, hepatitis
Efavirenz (Sustiva) [C]	600 mg PO daily	Rash, transaminase elevation, hepatitis Central nervous system disturbances: mood and sleep disturbances may occur in ~25% of patients during the first 4 weeks of therapy, generally transient

Protease inhibitors*		
Saquinavir (hard- and soft-gel formulations) (Fortovase, Invirase) [B]	Hard-gel formulation: 600 mg PO tid; Soft-gel formulation: 1,200 mg PO tid	GI intolerance (diarrhea, nausea, vomiting), headache, rash, transaminase elevation, hepatitis
Indinavir (Crixivan) [C]	800 mg PO q8hr	Dry skin, GI intolerance (diarrhea, nausea, vomiting), hyperbilirubinemia, ingrown toenails (paronychia), nephrolithiasis, crystal nephropathy—patients should ingest > 2 L of water per day, transaminase elevation
Ritonavir (Norvir) [B]	600 mg PO bid (dose escalation is recommended when initiating therapy)	GI intolerance, hyperbilirubinemia, paresthesias, taste disturbances, transaminase elevation (including fatal hepatotoxicity)
Nelfinavir (Viracept) [B]	750 mg PO tid; 1,250 mg PO bid	Diarrhea
Amprenavir (Agenerase) [C]	1,200 mg PO bid	Rash, diarrhea, headache; Potential for hypersensitivity reactions in patients with sulfonamide allergies.
Lopinavir and ritonavir (Kaletra) [C]	Lopinavir 400 mg PO bid and ritonavir 100 mg PO bid	GI intolerance

GI = gastrointestinal.

*Use of protease inhibitors is associated with changes in body fat distribution, including peripheral fat loss and central fat accumulation (lipodystrophy). Metabolic disturbances, including hypercholesterolemia, hypertriglyceridemia, insulin resistance, and, rarely, hyperglycemia are often associated with lipodystrophy. Dosages listed are for single protease inhibitor antiretroviral therapy. When ritonavir is used in combination with other protease inhibitors, changes must be made to the dosages and dosing intervals of these agents.

crobial chemoprophylaxis to prevent a first episode of infection. Avoidance of exposure is possible for only a few infections, as most opportunistic infections result from the reactivation of latent infections that have been acquired remotely (e.g., herpes zoster, cytomegalovirus [CMV], toxoplasmosis) or from infection with pathogens that are ubiquitous in the environment (e.g., *Mycobacterium avium* complex [MAC]).

The CD4+ cell count remains the best predictor of the short-term risk of developing an opportunistic infection and should be used alone or in combination with the results of serologic tests for toxoplasma (IgG) and CMV (IgG) to decide on the most appropriate timing for the initiation of primary prophylactic regimens. At the time of the initial assessment, screening should also be conducted for hepatitis B virus (hepatitis B surface antigen, anti-HBc, and anti-HBs) infection, hepatitis C virus infection, latent syphilis infection (Venereal Disease Research Laboratory or rapid plasma reagin tests), and latent tuberculosis infection (tuberculin skin test).

TX If the patient is nonimmune to hepatitis B virus infection, **vaccination against hepatitis B virus** should be given. If pneumococcal vaccination has not been received in the past 5 years, **vaccination against *S. pneumoniae*** should also be administered; it is most effective when the CD4 cell count is $>200/mm^3$. **Influenza vaccination** should be administered annually. Vaccinations and schedules are discussed in Ch 18 Pediatrics. Therapy for latent syphilis infection (benzathine penicillin G 2.4 MU IM weekly for 3 weeks) should be provided once active disease has been excluded.

The routine administration of prophylactic drug regimens has clearly been shown to improve the quality of life and to reduce the incidence of several HIV-associated opportunistic infections. These regimens, including the indications for initiating these therapies, are listed in Table 10–6.

It has been demonstrated to be safe to discontinue primary PCP prophylaxis in patients receiving HAART whose CD4 cell count is $> 200/mm^3$ for ≥ 3 months; primary and secondary PCP prophylaxis in patients receiving HAART whose CD4 cell count is $> 200/mm^3$ for ≥ 3 months and whose plasma HIV-1 RNA level is $\leq 5,000$ copies/mL for ≥ 3 months; and primary prophylaxis against MAC in patients receiving HAART with a stable CD4 cell count $> 100/mm^3$. For other opportunistic infections, including CMV retinitis, there are ongoing studies evaluating the safety of discontinuing secondary prophylaxis in patients receiving HAART who have demonstrated sustained immunologic improvement.

RX Table 10–6

DS Table 10–6

SE Table 10–6

INFECTIVE ENDOCARDITIS PROPHYLAXIS

KY Infective endocarditis refers to an infection of the endocardial surface of the heart, including the heart valves. Cardiac conditions that predispose to the development of infective endocarditis include prosthetic cardiac

Table 10-6. Primary Prophylaxis Regimens Against Opportunistic Infections in HIV*

Pathogen	Indication	Generic Name and Dose		Side Effects
		First Line	Second Line	
Cytomegalovirus (CMV)	CMV antibody (+) and CD4+ < 50/mm^3	Ganciclovir 1,000 mg PO tid	—	Fever, diarrhea, leukopenia, anemia, rash, confusion, neuropathy, sepsis
Mycobacterium avium complex (MAC)	CD4+ < 50/mm^3	Clarithromycin 500 mg PO bid or Azithromycin 1,200 mg PO weekly	Rifabutin 300 mg PO qd; or rifabutin 300 mg PO qd + azithromycin 1,200 mg PO weekly	See Table 10-1 Rifabutin (Mycobutin) can cause discolored urine, neutropenia, leukopenia, anemia, thrombocytopenia, anemia, and elevated liver enzymes; should be used with caution in patients with liver impairment.
Pneumocystis carinii pneumonia (PCP)	History of PCP, CD4+ < 200/mm^3, or oropharyngeal candidiasis (thrush)	TMP/SMX DS PO qd	Dapsone 100 mg PO qd; or aerosolized pentamidine 300 mg by Respirgard II nebulizer q4wk; atovaquone 1,500 mg PO qd	See Table 10-9

(continued)

Table 10–6. Primary Prophylaxis Regimens Against Opportunistic Infections in HIV* (Continued)

Pathogen	Indication	Generic Name and Dose		Side Effects
		First Line	Second Line	
Mycobacterium tuberculosis (TB)	Tuberculin skin test (purified protein derivative) induration ≥ 5 mm, previous untreated positive skin test, or contact with active TB case	INH 300 mg PO qd for 9 months + pyridoxine 50 mg PO qd for 9 months; directly observed therapy with INH 900 mg PO twice-weekly + pyridoxine 100 mg PO twice-weekly for 9 months	Rifampin 600 mg PO qd for 4 months for contacts of INH-resistant, rifampin-susceptible TB	See Table 10–10
Toxoplasmosis gondii	IgG antibody (+) and CD4+ < 100/mm^3	TMP/SMX DS PO qd	Dapsone 50 mg PO qd + Pyrimethamine 50 mg PO weekly + Leucovorin 25 mg PO weekly	See Table 10–9

DS = double strength; HIV = human immunodeficiency virus; INH = isoniazid; TMP/SMX DS = trimethoprim 160 mg and sulfamethoxazole 800 mg.

valves, previous bacterial endocarditis, congenital cardiac disease, rheumatic valvular heart disease, hypertrophic cardiomyopathy, mitral valve prolapse with mitral regurgitation, and myxomatous degeneration of the mitral valve. In patients with these cardiac lesions, turbulent blood flow results in deposition of platelet-fibrin thrombi on the endocardial surface. Interruption of normal mucosal membranes during dental, gastrointestinal, or genitourinary procedures may result in transient bacteremia with secondary seeding of the thrombi.

TX Recommendations for the prevention of endocarditis in patients with predisposing cardiac lesions who are undergoing invasive procedures involving the oropharynx, gastrointestinal tract, and genitourinary tract are listed in Table 10–7.

RX Table 10–7

DS Table 10–7

SE Table 10–1

RESPIRATORY TRACT INFECTIONS

Pneumonia in children is discussed in Ch 18 Pediatrics.

Table 10–7. Recommendations for Infective Endocarditis Prophylaxis

Procedures	Prophylaxis
Esophageal procedures (dilatation, sclerotherapy) Dental procedures Oral procedures Upper respiratory tract procedures	Amoxicillin* 2 g PO 1 hour before starting the procedure (no follow-up dose recommended) or ampicillin in 2 g IV if patient is unable to take oral medications

Gastrointestinal procedures (excluding esophageal procedures)
    Biliary tract surgery
    ERCP with biliary obstruction
    Surgical procedures involving the intestinal mucosa
Genitourinary tract procedures
Prophylaxis is not recommended for endoscopy without gastro-intestinal procedures.
	High-risk patients†: ampicillin‡ 2 g IV within 30 minutes of starting the procedure + gentamicin 1.5 mg/kg IV within 30 minutes of starting the procedure; followed by ampicillin 1 g IV or amoxicillin 1 g PO 6 hours after the initial antibiotic administration
	Moderate-risk patients: ampicillin‡ 2 g IV within 30 minutes of starting the procedure **or** amoxicillin‡ 2 g PO 1 hour before starting the procedure

ERCP = endoscopic retrograde cholangiopancreatography.

*For penicillin-allergic patients: clindamycin 600 mg PO or clarithromycin 500 mg PO or azithromycin 500 mg PO or cephalexin 2 g 1 hour before the procedure. If the patient is unable to take oral medications: clindamycin 600 mg IV or cefazolin 1 g IV within 30 minutes before starting the procedure.

†Patients with prosthetic heart valves, previous infective endocarditis, complex cyanotic congenital heart disease, surgically constructed systemic pulmonary shunts or conduits.

‡For penicillin-allergic patients, vancomycin IV is recommended.

Community-Acquired Pneumonia

KY Community-acquired pneumonia is a common and potentially lethal infectious disease. It is the sixth leading cause of mortality in North America. Symptoms of community-acquired pneumonia may include fever, cough, sputum production, chest pain, and dyspnea.

S. pneumoniae is the most common bacterial cause of community-acquired pneumonia. Other common bacterial causes of community-acquired pneumonia include *H. influenzae*; *Staphylococcus aureus;* and gram-negative aerobic bacilli, including *Escherichia coli* and *Klebsiella pneumoniae.* Less commonly encountered bacterial agents include *Streptococcus pyogenes* (group A beta-hemolytic streptococci) and anaerobic bacteria. Anaerobic bacteria are the predominant pathogens in patients with aspiration pneumonia, lung abscess, and empyema. *Mycoplasma pneumoniae*, *Chlamydia pneumoniae,* and *Legionella pneumophila* have been increasingly recognized as important pathogens requiring antibiotic coverage in empirical treatment regimens. *M. pneumoniae* is a common cause of community-acquired pneumonia in young adults. *L. pneumophila* most frequently causes pneumonia in elderly individuals with underlying comorbid medical conditions, including chronic obstructive pulmonary disease, congestive heart failure, and alcoholism. The diagnosis of pneumonia caused by these agents is generally made by serologic testing. Urinary antigen testing may be used for the diagnosis of infections caused by *L. pneumophila.*

RX Table 10–8

DS See Table 10–8. Decisions regarding hospitalization for the patient with community-acquired pneumonia should be based on clinical, radiologic, and laboratory assessments. Patients with advanced age and underlying comorbid medical conditions are at greatest risk for a fatal outcome. Patients < 50 years old without comorbid medical conditions are most suitable for outpatient management. In these patients, predicted mortality is ≤ 1%.

SE See Table 10–1.

Pneumocystis carinii Pneumonia (PCP) Complicating HIV Infection

KY PCP is the most common pulmonary infection in patients with chronic HIV infection. Most patients with chronic HIV infection who are diagnosed as having PCP have a CD4 cell count < 200/mm^3. The most frequent symptom at presentation is a chronic nonproductive cough. Fever is often present, but it is usually of shorter duration than the cough. The most common physical finding is tachypnea. The diagnosis of PCP is made by examination of bronchoalveolar lavage (BAL) specimens. Examination of induced sputum specimens may also provide a diagnosis. In patients who are not receiving PCP prophylactic therapy, examination of a BAL specimen

Table 10–8. Antimicrobial Treatment of Community-Acquired Pneumonia

Generic (Brand) Name	Dose	Pathogens
Outpatients Without Comorbid Conditions		
Macrolides		*Streptococcus pneumoniae*
Erythromycin [B]	500 mg PO qid	*Mycoplasma pneumoniae*
Clarithromycin (Biaxin) [C]	500 mg PO bid	*Chlamydia pneumoniae*
Azithromycin	Initial dose 500 mg	*Legionella pneumophila*
(Zithromax) [B]	PO then 250 mg	
	PO qd × 4 days	
or		
Fluoroquinolones		
Levofloxacin (Levaquin) [C]	500 mg PO qd	
Gatifloxacin (Tequin) [C]	400 mg PO qd	
Moxifloxacin (Avelox) [C]	400 mg PO qd	
or		
Doxycycline (Adoxa, Doryx,	100 mg PO bid	
Monodox, Periostat,		
Vibramycin—*U.S.*;		
Doxycin, Doxytec—		
Can.) [D]		
Outpatients With Modifying Factors: COPD		
(No Recent Antibiotic or Steroid Use Within Past 3 Months)		
Macrolides		*S. pneumoniae*
Clarithromycin	500 mg PO bid	*Haemophilus influenzae*
Azithromycin	Initial dose 500 mg	*Moraxella catarrhalis*
	PO then 250 mg	*C. pneumoniae*
	× 4 days	*L. pneumophila*
or		
Doxycycline	100 mg PO bid	
or		
Fluoroquinolones		
Levofloxacin	500 mg PO qd	
Gatifloxacin	400 mg PO qd	
Moxifloxacin	400 mg PO qd	
Outpatients With Modifying Factors: COPD		
(Recent Antibiotic or Steroid Use Within Past 3 Months)		
Fluoroquinolones		*S. pneumoniae*
Levofloxacin	500 mg PO qd	*H. influenzae*
Gatifloxacin	400 mg PO qd	*M. catarrhalis*
Moxifloxacin	400 mg PO qd	*L. pneumophila*
or		*C. pneumoniae*
Second-generation cephalosporin		
Cefuroxime axetil (Ceftin)	500 mg PO bid	
Cefprozil (Cefzil)	500 mg PO bid	

(continued)

Table 10–8. Antimicrobial Treatment of Community-Acquired Pneumonia (Continued)

Generic (Brand) Name	Dose	Pathogens
plus		
Macrolide		
Erythromycin	500 mg PO qid	
Clarithromycin	500 mg PO bid	
Azithromycin	Initial dose 500 mg PO then 250 mg PO qd × 4 days	
Hospitalized Patients		
Second-generation cephalosporin		
Cefuroxime	750 mg IV q8hr	Gram-negative bacilli
or		*H. influenzae*
Ceftriaxone	1 g IV q24hr	*S. pneumoniae*
Cefotaxime	1–2 g IV q8–12hr	*Staphylococcus aureus*
plus		*L. pneumophila*
Macrolide		*C. pneumoniae*
Erythromycin	500 mg IV/PO qid	
Clarithromycin	500 mg IV/PO bid	
Azithromycin	Initial dose 500 mg IV, then 250 mg IV qd × 4 days	
or		
Fluoroquinolone		
Levofloxacin	500 mg IV/PO qd	
Gatifloxacin	400 mg IV/PO qd	
Moxifloxacin	400 mg PO qd	

COPD = chronic obstructive pulmonary disease.

should yield the diagnosis in up to 90% of cases. In patients receiving aerosolized pentamidine for PCP prophylaxis, the diagnostic yield of a bronchoalveolar lavage (BAL) is reduced to ≤ 60%.

TX **The choice of therapy depends on the severity of the infection and the documentation of previous adverse drug reactions.** Table 10–9 lists treatment options. Adjunctive corticosteroids may be considered for patients with severe PCP (pO$_2$ < 70 mm Hg and/or [A-a]O$_2$ >35 mm Hg) and for maximal benefit should be administered within the first 24–48 hours of treatment.

RX Table 10–9

DS Table 10–9

SE Table 10–9

Tuberculosis

KY **Tuberculosis is an infection caused by *Mycobacterium tuberculosis*.** Infection with this organism often affects the lungs, but any organ can be infected. Humans are the only reservoir for *M. tuberculosis*. Person-to-person transmission occurs through the inhalation of droplet nuclei that are gener-

Table 10–9. Treatment Options for *Pneumocystis carinii*
Pneumonia (PCP)

Generic (Brand) Name	Recommended Dose (for 21 days)	Side Effects
Atovaquone (Mepron) [C]	750 mg PO tid	Rash, nausea, diarrhea
Clindamycin + primaquine [C]	Clindamycin 300 mg PO qid or 600 mg IV q8hr × 21 days **plus** Primaquine 15–30 mg PO qd × 21 days	Clindamycin: GI intolerance, including diarrhea and antibiotic associated colitis; hypersensitivity reactions
Primaquine: hemolytic anemia in G-6-PD–deficient individuals, methemoglobinemia
Pentamidine (Pentacarinat) [C]	4 mg/kg/day IV	Cytopenias, hyperkalemia, hypocalcemia, hypoglycemia, hypotension (after rapid infusion), pancreatitis, QTc prolongation, secondary insulin-dependent diabetes mellitus
TMP/SMX (Bactrim, Septra) [C/D at term]	20 mg TMP /kg PO/IV daily in four divided doses × 21 days	Aseptic meningitis; cytopenias; hepatotoxicity; hypersensitivity reactions, including skin rash and fever; nephrotoxicity
TMP and dapsone (Avlosulfon—Can.)	20 mg/kg TMP PO in four divided doses + dapsone 100 mg PO qd	Hemolysis in G-6-PD–deficient individuals; hypersensitivity reactions, including fever and skin rash

G-6-PD = glucose-6-phosphate dehydrogenase; GI = gastrointestinal; TMP/SMX = trimethoprim and sulfamethoxazole.

ated by infected individuals who are coughing. Inhalation of droplet nuclei results in the deposition of mycobacteria in the distal airways and alveoli, where the acid-fast bacilli multiply. Both lymphatic and hematogenous dissemination to extrapulmonary sites can occur. The development of hypersensitivity (tuberculin skin test reactivity) occurs approximately 3–8 weeks after infection. Symptoms of pulmonary tuberculosis include fever, cough, sputum production, night sweats, weight loss, and fatigue. The diagnosis of pulmonary tuberculosis relies on maintaining an index of suspicion in at-risk individuals and obtaining appropriate specimens for acid-fast staining and culture.

TX The principles of modern antituberculous therapy include administration of multiple drugs for a sufficient period of time. The selection of antituberculous therapy must be based on drug susceptibility testing. Drugs must be taken regularly. First-line agents include isoniazid (INH), rifampin, pyrazinamide, ethambutol, and streptomycin. Initial selection of an antituberculous treatment regimen will depend on local resistance patterns. In North America, the initial antituberculous regimen should include INH, rifampin, pyrazinamide, and ethambutol. Short-course antituberculous therapy (≤ 9 months' duration) is only possible if the isolate is susceptible to both INH and rifampin.

Table 10–10. Antituberculous Combination Therapy

Generic (Brand) Name	Dose	Duration (months)	Side Effects
Ethambutol (Myambutol—*U.S.*; Etibi—*Can.*) [B]	15 mg/kg/day PO in single or divided doses	*	GI upset, headache, hyperuricemia, optic neuritis, peripheral neuropathy
Isoniazid (Nydrazid) [C]	300 mg PO qd	6†	GI intolerance, hepatitis, peripheral neuropathy, rash
Pyrazinamide (Tebrazid—*Can.*) [C]	15–25 mg/kg/day PO‡ in single or divide doses	2†	Fever, GI intolerance, hepatitis, hyperuricemia, gout, rash
Rifampin (Rifadin, Rimactane) [C]	600 mg PO qd	6†	Fever, hepatitis, rash, thrombocytopenia

GI = gastrointestinal.

*Should be included as a component of four-drug empiric therapy until results of susceptibility testing are available.

†For fully sensitive isolates of *M. tuberculosis*

‡Not to exceed 2 g/day

RX Table 10–10
DS Table 10–10
SE Table 10–10

SEPTIC ARTHRITIS

See Ch 21 Rheumatology.

SOFT TISSUE INFECTIONS

Cellulitis and Erysipelas

KY **Cellulitis** is an acute spreading infection of the skin and subcutaneous tissues. Common infecting organisms include *S. pyogenes* (beta-hemolytic group A streptococci) and *S. aureus*. Skin wounds may predispose to the development of cellulitis. Signs of infection include warmth, swelling, tenderness, and erythema of the affected area. **Erysipelas** is a superficial cellulitis of the skin with prominent lymphatic involvement. Lymphangitic streaking and tender regional lymphadenitis may be present. It is commonly caused by group A streptococci. The lower extremities are the most common sites of erysipelas. Other sites of involvement include the face and the upper extremities. In women with breast cancer who have undergone axillary lymph node dissection, lymphedema of the upper extremity may be a predisposing factor.

🆃🆇 Empiric therapy for cellulitis and erysipelas should include cover-age of group A streptococci and *S. aureus*. Previously healthy patients without hypotension or necrotizing fasciitis may be considered for outpatient treatment. Response to therapy is indicated by defervescence and local regression of the signs of soft-tissue inflammation. Residual edema may result.

🆁🆇 Table 10–11

🅳🆂 Table 10–11

🆂🅴 Table 10–1

Table 10–11. Empiric Antimicrobial Therapy for Soft-Tissue Infections

Generic (Brand) Name	Dose
Erysipelas (Group A streptococci, *Staphylococcus aureus*)	
Cefazolin (Ancef, Kefzol) [B]	1 g IV q8hr
Cephalexin (Keflex) [B]	500 mg PO qid
Clindamycin (Cleocin—*U.S.*; Dalacin-C—*Can.*) [B]	600 mg IV q8hr; or 300 mg PO qid
Erythromycin [B]	500 mg IV q6hr; or 500 mg PO qid
Non–Limb-Threatening Diabetic Foot Infections (Group A Streptococci, *S. aureus*)	
Cefazolin	1 g IV q8hr
Cephalexin	500 mg PO qid
Clindamycin	600 mg IV q8hr; or 300 mg PO qid
Amoxicillin and clavulanate potassium (Augmentin—*U.S.*; Clavulin—*Can.*) [B]	500/125 mg PO tid; or 875/125 mg PO bid
Limb-Threatening Diabetic Foot Infections (Anaerobes, coliforms, Group A streptococci, Group B streptococci, *S. aureus*)	
Cefotetan (Cefotan) [B]	1 g IV q12hr
Piperacillin and tazobactam sodium (Zosyn—*U.S.*; Tacozin—*Can.*) [B]	3.75 g IV q6hr or 4.5 g IV q8hr
Clindamycin	600 mg IV q8hr
+	
Ciprofloxacin (Ciloxan, Cipro) [C]	500 mg PO/IV q12hr
Necrotizing Fasciitis*	
Ampicillin (Marcillin, Polycillin, Principen) [B]	2 g IV q6hr
+	
Clindamycin	600 mg IV q8hr
+	
Gentamicin (Gentacidin—*U.S.*; Cidomycin—*Can.*) [C]	5 mg IV q24hr, with dose adjustment for renal insufficiency

*Urgent surgical consultation is required. Intravenous immunoglobulin 2 g/kg has been demon-strated to reduce mortality rates in cases caused by group A streptococci associated with strepto-coccal toxic shock syndrome.

Diabetic Foot Infections

KY Acute and chronic foot infections may occur in the patient with diabetes mellitus. Peripheral sensory neuropathy and ischemia secondary to macrovascular and microvascular disease are key factors in the pathogenesis of diabetic foot infections. Foot infections may begin after minor trauma. Signs of soft-tissue infection include skin ulceration, erythema, and wound discharge. Contiguous osteomyelitis may be present. Non–limb-threatening, superficial infections of the diabetic foot are often caused by gram-positive organisms, including *S. aureus* and streptococcal species. Deeper, limb-threatening infections are frequently polymicrobial infections caused by gram-positive cocci, coliform organisms, and anaerobic bacteria. Culture of deep-tissue aspirates provides the most reliable microbiologic data. Reaching bone by advancing a surgical probe or culture swab has a high specificity and positive predictive value for the diagnosis of osteomyelitis. Sensitivity of this procedure may be low. Other diagnostic tests include plain radiographs, bone and gallium scans, and magnetic resonance imaging scans of the affected area.

TX The antibiotic treatment of diabetic foot infections is frequently empiric. It is described in Table 10–11. **Combinations of antimicrobial agents may be needed.** Surgical débridement may also be required. Assessment of the arterial supply to the foot should be performed to identify patients who would benefit from revascularization procedures.

RX Table 10–11

DS Table 10–11

SE Table 10–1

Erysipelas

See **Cellulitis and Erysipelas.**

Necrotizing Fasciitis

KY Necrotizing fasciitis is a deep infection of the subcutaneous tissues. It requires immediate recognition and treatment. Causes include group A streptococci or mixed infections involving anaerobic organisms in combination with one or more aerobic gram-negative bacilli. Symptoms of necrotizing fasciitis include fever and pain, swelling, and erythema at the site of infection. At its onset, reports of pain may be out of proportion to the signs of soft-tissue inflammation. Signs suggestive of necrotizing fasciitis include rapid progression of the infection with development of hemorrhagic bullae and areas of cutaneous necrosis.

TX Treatment includes a combination of **surgical débridement and the administration of antimicrobial therapy.** Delay in treatment could be fatal. Intravenous immunoglobulin administration has been shown to reduce mortality in cases of necrotizing fasciitis associated with streptococcal toxic shock syndrome.

RX Table 10–11
DS Table 10–11
SE Table 10–1

URINARY TRACT INFECTIONS (UTIs)

UTIs are discussed in Ch 22 Urology. Pediatric UTIs are discussed in Ch 18 Pediatrics. Management of UTIs in pregnancy are discussed in Ch 13 Obstetrics.

11

Nephrology

MARTIN SCHREIBER

ACUTE RENAL FAILURE (ARF)

KY ARF is diagnosed when there is evidence of a reduction in glomerular filtration rate (GFR) to a significant degree (e.g., > 50% reduction) over a period of days to a few weeks. Classification of causes of ARF is divided into prerenal (e.g., bilateral renal artery stenosis, failure of renal autoregulation, renal hypoperfusion), renal (e.g., proliferative glomerulonephritis [GN], acute tubular necrosis [ATN]), and postrenal (e.g., obstruction) causes. The major complications of ARF relate to the failure of renal excretion of nitrogenous waste products, which leads to the uremic syndrome, and the failure of normal renal regulation of fluid-electrolyte and acid-base balance.

TX **Conservative management includes all measures that can be used short of providing dialysis.** Any reversible contributing factors, especially volume depletion and obstruction to urinary flow, should be corrected. Nephrotoxic drugs, including nonsteroidal anti-inflammatory drugs (NSAIDs), should be discontinued. The dosage of drugs excreted via the kidneys should be adjusted. Complications, including hyperkalemia, fluid overload, and metabolic acidosis, need to be treated, and adequate nutrition must be maintained. Dialysis is indicated for severe uremic manifestations (pericarditis, encephalopathy) and in refractory fluid-electrolyte complications (hyperkalemia, fluid overload with pulmonary edema, metabolic acidosis).

RX See the Edematous Disorders, Hyperkalemia, and Metabolic Acidosis sections.

DS Table 11–1, Table 11–6

SE Table 11–1, Table 11–6

CHRONIC RENAL FAILURE (CRF)

KY CRF is said to be present when **a significant reduction in GFR persists for longer than a few weeks.** The **major causes** are diabetic nephropathy, chronic GN, hypertension, renovascular disease (ischemic nephropathy), and tubulointerstitial kidney disease. CRF tends to be progressive, even if the initial inciting factor is eliminated because of hyperfiltration by remaining nephrons. Additional factors that may contribute to the progression of CRF include hyperlipidemia, calcium-phosphate precipitation in the renal parenchyma (caused by associated hyperphosphatemia), metabolic acidosis, and activation of cytokines (including angiotensin II).

The same complications that affect ARF can also affect CRF. Additional complications can develop in the setting of CRF that may require management (some are listed in Table 11–1).

Table 11–1. Specific Therapy Available for Some Complications of CRF

Complication	Description	Treatment Options	Medication and Dose	Side Effects and Cautions
Anemia	Mainly a consequence of insufficient renal production of erythropoietin. In addition, the uremic milieu impairs marrow function and causes shortened red blood cell survival, and there may be associated iron deficiency from occult GI losses.	Adequate iron stores, achieved via either oral or IV iron replacement.	Ferrous fumarate (Femiron, Feostat, Hemocyte, Ircon, Nephro-Fer—U.S.; Palafer—Can.) [A]; 60–100 mg PO bid Ferrous sulfate (Feosol, Ferotab—U.S.; Ferodan—Can.) [A] 300 mg PO bid	GI upset, dark stool, constipation
		SC recombinant human erythropoietin. The goal of therapy is a hemoglobin level of 11–12 g/dL, corresponding to a hematocrit of 30%–33%	Erythropoietin 100 U/kg/week SC given in two divided doses (maximum dose is 30,000 U/week)	Worsening hypertension, headaches, seizures, clotting of dialysis access grafts
Metabolic bone disease	A combination of hypocalcemia, hyperphosphatemia, and 1,25-dihydroxy-vitamin D deficiency that occurs in the setting of CRF, known as secondary hyperparathyroidism. High levels of PTH cause a bone lesion (osteitis fibrosa cystica) and pruritus, may contribute to cardiomyopathy, and may be one of the major uremic toxins.	Control of hyperphosphatemia is achieved via dietary phosphate restriction and the use of calcium-containing phosphate binders.	Calcium carbonate [C] 250–500 mg PO tid with meals The goal is a phosphate level of < 1.8 mEq/L	Headache, hypophosphatemia, hypercalcemia, GI upset
		Vitamin D administration	Calcitriol (1,25 [OH] 2-vitamin D) (Calcijex, Rocaltrol) [C] initial dose of 0.25 μg PO 3 times/week, and titrating upward to a maximum of 2 μg/day.	Hypercalcemia

(continued)

Table 11–1. Specific Therapy Available for Some Complications of CRF (Continued)

Complication	Description	Treatment Options	Medication and Dose	Side Effects and Cautions
Metabolic acidosis	This can lead to skeletal muscle catabolism and also possibly worsened metabolic bone disease and therefore should be treated.	The goal is to maintain a plasma bicarbonate level of at least 20 mmol/L and this is generally achieved using sodium bicarbonate $NaHCO_3$ tablets.	$NaHCO_3$ initial dose of 600 mg PO tid	Monitor for evidence of extracellular fluid volume overload because of the sodium given along with the bicarbonate.
Nausea, vomiting, poor appetite		These symptoms may be improved by the use of gastric prokinetic agents.	Domperidone (Motilium) 10 mg PO with each meal	Does not cross the blood-brain barrier, therefore does not cause any neurologic side effects. Not available in the United States.
Nocturnal leg cramps		These can be alleviated using quinine.	Quinine [X] 200–300 mg PO at bedtime	Headache, GI upset, hypersensitivity reactions Use with **caution** in patients with cardiac arrhythmias and myasthenia gravis.
Pruritus		Major available modalities include antihistamines and phototherapy using UVB radiation.	Hydroxyzine (Atarax, Hyzine, Restall, Vistacot, Vistaril—*U.S.*; Multipax—*Can.*) [C] 10–25 mg PO bid prn	Headache, seizure, blurred vision, bronchial secretions

CRF = chronic renal failure; GI = gastrointestinal; PTH = parathyroid hormone.

TX There is specific therapy available for some of the complications of CRF (Table 11–1). Measures that slow the progression of CRF include control of hypertension, use of angiotensin-converting enzyme (ACE) inhibitors, dietary protein restriction, and control of hyperlipidemia, hyperphosphatemia, and metabolic acidosis (Table 11–2).

RX Table 11–1 and Table 11–2

DS Table 11–1 and Table 11–2

SE Table 11–1 and Table 11–2

Table 11- 2. Measures that Slow the Progression of CRF

Strategy	Treatment Options	Side Effects and Cautions
Control hypertension	The goal BP in patients with CRF is 130/80 mm Hg, and 125/75 mm Hg if there is associated proteinuria of 1g/day or more. See Table 11–16.	See Table 11–16
Use of ACE inhibitors	The physician should attempt to use ACE inhibitors in treating patients with CRF and hypertension, particularly in the setting of proteinuria. See Table 11–16.	Hyperkalemia as a result of an ACE inhibitor–induced fall in aldosterone levels. ARF resulting from a fall in efferent arteriole resistance caused by the fall in angiotensin II levels. This is most likely to occur when there is associated ECF volume depletion, CHF, or cirrhosis or with concurrent use of NSAIDs.
Dietary protein restriction	The efficacy of this measure is controversial. Certainly, high-protein diets should be avoided, and it may be reasonable to advise a modest dietary protein restriction of 0.8–1.0 g/kg/day, plus providing in the diet roughly the same amount of protein lost in daily urinary excretion.	Excessive protein restriction may cause malnutrition.
Control of hyperlipidemia	This may contribute to progressive CRF. Lipid-lowering agents are discussed in Ch 3 Cardiology.	See Ch 3 Cardiology.

ACE = angiotensin-converting enzyme; ARF = acute renal failure; BP = blood pressure; CHF = congestive heart failure; CRF = chronic renal failure; ECF = extracellular fluid; NSAID = nonsteroidal anti-inflammatory drug.

DIABETIC NEPHROPATHY

KY Both type 1 and type 2 diabetes mellitus (DM) are frequently associated with renal disease. Chronic hyperglycemia causes diffuse microvascular disease. In the kidney, the principal target is the glomerulus. This is compounded by intraglomerular hypertension, at least partly resulting from afferent arteriolar dilatation caused by hyperglycemia. Eventually, fibrosis (referred to as glomerulosclerosis) develops. This glomerular disease leads to proteinuria (particularly albuminuria), hypertension, and progressive CRF.

TX This depends on the stage of disease, classified according to the magnitude of proteinuria.

RX Table 11–3

DS Table 11–3

SE Table 11–3

Table 11–3. Management Options in Diabetic Nephropathy

Magnitude of Proteinuria	Treatment	Side Effects and Cautions
Normoalbuminuria Excretion of < 30 mg/day of albumin	Tight glycemic control.	Hypoglycemia
Microalbuminuria Excretion of 30–300 mg/day of albumin	Tight glycemic control and ACE inhibitors (even in patients without hypertension). In type 2 DM, angiotensin II receptor antagonists are as effective. See Table 11–16.	See Table 11–16.
Macroalbuminuria Excretion of > 300 mg/day of albumin	ACE inhibitors (and angiotensin II receptor antagonists in type 2 DM) and additional antihypertensive agents as required to achieve BP < 130/80 mm Hg (see Table 11–16). Dietary protein restriction to a modest degree (0.8 g/kg/day) is probably appropriate.	See Table 11–16.

ACE = angiotensin-converting enzyme; BP = blood pressure; DM = diabetes mellitus.

DISORDERS OF POTASSIUM CONCENTRATION

Hyperkalemia

KY The major causes of hyperkalemia are classified into increased intake, shift from cells to extracellular fluid (ECF) (e.g., digoxin toxicity, insulin deficit, tumor lysis syndrome, rhabdomyolysis, tissue ischemia), and impaired renal excretion (potassium-sparing diuretics, ACE inhibitors, heparin, renal failure, renal tubulointerstitial disease, adrenal insufficiency). The main manifestations of hyperkalemia are cardiac and include various electrocardiographic abnormalities, the most important of which are the increase in height of the T wave with a peaked appearance, the loss of the P wave, broadening of the QRS complex, and then a sine wave appearance. Cardiac dysrhythmias can be seen, including bradycardia, heart block, ventricular fibrillation, and asystole.

TX Strategies for treating hyperkalemia are listed in Table 11–4.

RX Table 11–4

DS Table 11–4

SE Table 11–4

Hypokalemia

KY The major causes of hypokalemia are classified into low intake, shift into cells (e.g., anabolism, high levels of beta-adrenergic stimulus, insulin, sodium bicarbonate [NaHCO$_3$]), excess loss via the gastrointestinal tract (i.e., diarrhea, vomiting), and excess loss via urine (diuresis, hyperaldosteronism, hypomagnesemia). The major manifestations of hypokalemia include:

- **Cardiac dysrhythmias,** including ventricular premature beats and ventricular tachycardia (more likely to occur in patients taking digoxin, those with underlying heart disease, and those who have concomitant hypomagnesemia)
- **Skeletal muscle weakness** (leading occasionally to rhabdomyolysis)
- **Precipitation of hepatic encephalopathy** (caused by enhanced renal ammoniagenesis)

TX Requires **correction of the underlying cause, replacement** of potassium deficit, and **cardiac monitoring** if the potassium level is below 2.5–3.0 mEq/L. The magnitude of the potassium deficit may be very difficult to estimate, since most of the potassium deficit is intracellular, and it is hard to predict what proportion of the potassium deficit is in fact from cells. Thus, serial monitoring of the plasma potassium level is needed as potassium is being replaced.

RX Table 11–5

DS Table 11–5

SE Table 11–5

Table 11–4. Strategies for the Treatment of Hyperkalemia*

Strategy	Treatments	Side Effects and Cautions
Protect the heart	Calcium gluconate 10 mL of 10% solution; may repeat once	Avoid rapid IV administration. Use with caution in patients taking digoxin. Hypercalcemia can occur in patients with renal failure. Rarely, vasodilation, hypotension, bradycardia, and cardiac arrhythmias can occur.
Shift potassium into cells	Insulin (regular) 10–20 U IV, with 50 mL of 50% dextrose IV, followed by infusion of insulin (regular) 1 U/hr with 50 mL of 50% dextrose IV	Monitor for hypoglycemia q1h
	Salbutamol (Ventolin) 5–20 mg nebulized	Cardiac arrhythmias
	Sodium bicarbonate 100–200 mEq/L; more effective if coexisting metabolic acidosis	Contraindicated in extracellular fluid volume overload.
Enhance potassium elimination	Via gastrointestinal tract: Sodium polystyrene sulfonate (kayexalate) resin 30 g PO with 50 mL of 70% sorbitol as laxative; or 50–100 g of resin as enema with tap water	Constipation Do not give sorbitol rectally. Do not administer resins to patients who have had abdominal surgery or who have ileus or bowel obstruction or who have been using opioids (risk of intestinal necrosis)
	Via urine: Furosemide 40–200 mg IV; may need to replace intravascular volume with normal saline Via hemodialysis	See Table 11–9

*Potassium level < 6.5 mEq/L, no electrocardiographic (ECG) changes: treat underlying cause, stop IV/PO potassium, and treat with resin or furosemide; potassium level 6.5–7.0 mEq/L or ECG changes: add insulin and calcium gluconate; potassium level > 7.0 mEq/L or ECG changes: consider adding IV sodium bicarbonate and inhaled albuterol, or hemodialysis.

DISORDERS OF SODIUM CONCENTRATION

Hypernatremia

KY Chronic hypernatremia implies that there is **a problem with intake of water** caused by the inability to communicate the need for water (infants, elderly demented patients), the inability to access water (bedridden patients), or the inability to swallow. In addition, there is usually a site of excess water loss via skin (fever), urine (diuresis, diabetes insipidus), or the gastrointestinal tract (vomiting, diarrhea). **Hypernatremia, especially**

Table 11–5. Management of Hypokalemia

Treatment	Dose	Side Effects and Cautions
Oral route: KCl tablets used whenever possible; usually sufficient in cases in which the potassium level is > 2.8 mEq/L	Start at 40 mEq and re-assess over next 12–24 hours. (Slow-release tablets contain 8 or 20 mEq of KCl per tablet; liquid preparations usually contain 20 mEq per 15 mL.)	Bradycardia, hyperkalemia, muscle weakness, dyspnea. Rarely, alkalosis, arrhythmias, heart block, and hypotension.
IV route:* Used when the patient cannot take PO; in severe hypokalemia (potassium < 2.8 mEq/L), especially if taking digoxin; and in cases in which there are large, ongoing losses	Potassium must be given diluted in saline (not dextrose) solutions to avoid release of endogenous insulin. The concentration in a peripheral vein should be no more than 40 mEq/L (higher concentrations cause irritation). The amount of potassium given should not exceed 40 mEq/hr.	Use with **caution** in patients with cardiac disease or renal impairment. Local tissue necrosis with extravasation.
Potassium-sparing diuretics: Used to limit the magnitude of diuretic-induced potassium losses	Amiloride, spironolactone, triamterene (see Table 11–9).	See Table 11–9

KCl = potassium chloride.

*IV administration of KCl **must** be diluted in saline; **direct IV administration will cause death.**

when acute, leads to significant shrinkage and therefore dysfunction of brain cells and may lead to intracerebral hemorrhage.

TX Treatment requires frequent **monitoring** of plasma sodium and other electrolyte levels, **restoration** of circulating volume, **replacement** of free water deficit, replacement of ongoing fluid losses, and **correction of the underlying condition** if possible. When present, diabetes insipidus should be treated (see Ch 5 Endocrinology).

RX Table 11–6

DS Table 11–6

SE Table 11–6

Hyponatremia

KY Hyponatremia occurs when there is **an excess of water in relation to sodium in the ECF.** This develops when the rate of intake of water in the

Table 11-6. Management of Hypernatremia

Treatment Goals	Choice of Fluid	Side Effects and Cautions
Restoration of circulating volume	Hypernatremia is often associated with significant ECF volume depletion. Restoration of volume is generally accomplished with administration of 0.9% NaCl.	Normal saline (0.9% NaCl) has no free water.	Fluid overload. (This may occur with any of the fluids noted here, especially if the ECF volume is not low before starting treatment.)
Replacement of the free water deficit	This can be calculated for each patient. The deficit should be restored gradually, aiming for a rate of correction of no more than 0.5 mEq/L/hr.	Half-normal saline (0.45% NaCl) has 500 mL of free water per liter of solution. 3.3% dextrose and 0.3% NaCl (two-thirds and one-third) have 667 mL of free water per liter.	Rates of correction faster than 0.5 mEq/L/hr may lead to cerebral edema.
Replacement of ongoing fluid losses	Patients with hypernatremia may continue to lose copious amounts of fluid via the gastrointestinal or urinary tracts, even while they are being treated. These losses must be anticipated and, if possible, measured, and then an appropriate replacement fluid chosen. The concentration of sodium in the replacement fluid should be approximately equal to that in the fluid being lost. Potassium should also be replaced.	5% dextrose is entirely free water.	Hypokalemia may occur because of administration of dextrose, which causes the release of insulin.

ECF = extracellular fluid; NaCl = sodium chloride.

*Water deficit (L) = Body weight (kg) × 0.6 × (P[Na]/140 − 1). Calculate the rate of correction by noting the difference between the current P[Na] and the normal value of 140, and aiming to correct to normal in twice the number of hours.

absence of sodium (so-called free water) exceeds the rate of excretion of free water. This can happen in:

- Psychogenic polydipsia, seen mainly in patients with schizophrenia who ingest huge amounts of water that exceed the capacity of even normal kidneys to excrete free water
- Advanced renal failure with significant intake of free water
- The presence of antidiuretic hormone when it is not expected.

Most cases are due to the release of antidiuretic hormone (ADH) despite hyponatremia. Causes of ADH release include: (1) volume depletion. This may be either true volume depletion [due to excessive losses of fluid via urine (diuretics, glucose-induced osmotic diuresis, deficiency of aldosterone), gastrointestinal tract (bleeding, vomiting, or diarrhea), skin (fever, burns), or into tissues such as during pancreatitis] or "effective" circulating volume depletion (due to congestive heart failure or cirrhosis); (2) The syndrome of inappropriate secretion of ADH. This happens due to many pulmonary and central nervous system disorders, ectopic production by certain cancers (especially small cell cancer of the lung), many medications (cyclophosphamide, carbamazepine, vincristine, antipsychotics, SSRI antidepressants, bromocriptine, morphine), and many situations associated with "stress" (pain, nausea, postoperatively); (3) Deficiencies of thyroid hormone or cortisol.

The complications of hyponatremia are listed in Table 11–7.

TX **All patients with hyponatremia should have their intake of water restricted;** a reasonable initial prescription in an adult is the intake of no more than 1 L/day of fluid, but more extreme degrees of water restriction may be necessary. Also, **the underlying cause of the hyponatremia should be specifically treated,** if possible.

RX Table 11–8

DS Table 11–8

SE Table 11–7 and Table 11–8

EDEMATOUS DISORDERS

KY Under normal conditions, kidneys excrete the daily intake of sodium and water. In contrast, in edematous states, **a proportion of this ingested sodium and water is retained. The major edematous disorders are congestive heart failure (CHF), cirrhotic liver disease, nephrotic syndrome, and renal failure.** The consequences of renal retention of sodium and water is that this excess ECF then manifests as edema, the location of which depends on the causative disorder; CHF causes pulmonary edema and peripheral edema; cirrhosis causes ascites; and nephrotic syndrome causes diffuse edema but is less likely to cause pulmonary edema.

TX1 **Edema:** In addition **to treatment of the underlying disease,** management of edema involves the use of **diuretics** and **dietary restriction of salt and water.** Diuretics are drugs that act at various sites in the renal tubule to inhibit the reabsorption of sodium (Table 11–9).

Table 11–7. Complications of Hyponatremia

Complications caused by hyponatremia	If the hyponatremia develops rapidly (in < 48 hours), there is a significant risk of cerebral edema, as water moves from the hypotonic ECF to the intracellular fluid of brain cells. This can lead to cerebral dysfunction, with the risk of seizures and depressed level of consciousness. Symptomatic hyponatremia is most commonly seen in the perioperative setting when patients are given hypotonic IV fluid; with psychogenic polydipsia; or with elderly women treated with thiazide diuretics.
Complications caused by overly rapid correction of hyponatremia	When hyponatremia is present for > 24–48 hours, brain cells adapt by exporting intracellular particles, which then favors the exit of water from these cells and the return of brain cell size toward normal. If there is in addition the rapid correction of hyponatremia toward normal, then there is the risk of excessive dehydration of the brain cells, leading to a syndrome referred to as osmotic demyelination. This can cause central pontine myelinolysis (quadriplegia, cranial nerve palsies) and demyelination in other parts of the brain as well. Patients most at risk for this are those with (1) treatment that included excessive amounts of hypertonic saline; (2) psychogenic polydipsia and hyponatremia who are deprived of water; (3) hyponatremia and ECF volume depletion whose volume depletion is rapidly corrected, leading to a sudden fall in ADH levels and subsequent free water diuresis; (4) hypokalemia; (5) cirrhosis; (6) malnutrition.

ADH = antidiuretic hormone; ECF = extracellular fluid.

RX1 **Diuretics:** Table 11–9

DS1 Table 11–9

SE1 Table 11–9

TX2 **Refractory edema:** This exists when edema does not respond to treatment with a single diuretic agent, in the presence of controlled dietary sodium intake. Therapeutic options include increasing the dose of the first diuretic used, or adding a second diuretic that acts as a different nephron segment.

RX2 **Commonly used combinations** include furosemide (acts on the loop of Henle) and metolazone (acts on the distal tubule); furosemide and spironolactone (acts on the cortical collecting duct); and hydrochlorothiazide (acts on the distal tubule) and spironolactone.

DS2 Table 11–9

SE2 Hypokalemia is a common complication of therapy with both loop-acting and thiazide diuretics. The severity of hypokalemia can be reduced by the concurrent administration of a diuretic that acts on the collecting

Table 11–8. Management of Hyponatremia

Clinical Presentation	Treatment	Side Effects and Cautions*
Acute symptomatic hyponatremia This is hyponatremia developing in < 24–48 hours with the presence of seizures or a depressed level of consciousness.	This condition must be promptly treated using hypertonic (3%) saline at a rate of 1–2 mL/kg/hr until symptoms resolve or a sodium concentration of 130 mmol/L is reached.	The sodium load given here may cause pulmonary edema, so one may need to use a diuretic (furosemide) to deal with the sodium excess (see Table 11–9).
Asymptomatic acute hyponatremia There is significant risk that a patient with severe acute hyponatremia (plasma sodium level falling from normal to < 120–125 mEq/L in < 24 hours) who does not have symptoms may suddenly develop severe neurologic complications.	This rare condition should be promptly treated as described for acute symptomatic hyponatremia.	Same as for acute symptomatic hyponatremia.
Asymptomatic chronic hyponatremia Water restriction and treatment of the underlying cause are the major modalities of treatment.	If the hyponatremia is refractory, the following strategies can be used: 0.9% NaCl given together with furosemide; or Demeclocycline 300–600 mg PO bid; or Oral urea 30–60 g PO daily.	The danger is likely greater from overly rapid correction, so one should avoid hypertonic saline. Limit correction to ≤ 8 mEq/L per day.
Chronic symptomatic hyponatremia This is the most challenging situation because there is a risk both to not treating (cerebral edema) and to overtreating (osmotic demyelination).	3% NaCl 1–2 mL/kg/hr until the plasma sodium is raised by 5–7 mEq/L over the first 3–4 hours. Subsequently, slow the rate of correction so that the total 24-hour correction is < 8–10 mEq/L.	Osmotic demyelination with overtreatment of hyponatremia.

NaCl = sodium chloride.
*See Table 11–7 (complications caused by overly rapid correction of hyponatremia).

Table 11–9. Diuretics

Generic (Brand) Name	Dose (PO)	Mechanism of Action	Side Effects
Amiloride (Midamor) [B]	5–20 mg qd	Potassium-sparing diuretic: Inhibits the active transport of potassium/sodium exchange in the distal tubule, cortical collecting tubule, and collecting duct.	Hyperkalemia
Furosemide (Lasix) [C]	20 mg qd–200 mg bid	Loop diuretic: Inhibits the reabsorption of sodium and chloride in the ascending loop of Henle and distal renal tubule.	Excessive volume depletion, hypokalemia, hypomagnesemia, metabolic alkalosis, precipitation of gout, hearing loss with very high doses
Hydrochlorothiazide (Aquazide, Esidrix, Ezide, Hydrocot, HydroDIURIL, Microzide, Oretic—*U.S.*; Hydrazide, Urozide—*Can.*) [B/D]	12.5–100 mg qd	Thiazide diuretic: Inhibits sodium reabsorption in the distal tubules.	Same as for furosemide (except for hearing loss), hypercalcemia
Metolazone (Mykrox, Zaroxolyn) [B/D]	2.5–10 mg qd		
Spironolactone (Aldactone) [D]	25–400 mg qd	Potassium-sparing diuretic: Direct aldosterone antagonist in the distal renal tubules.	Gynecomastia, hyperkalemia
Triamterene (Dyrenium) [B/D]	50–100 mg qd	Same as for amiloride.	Hyperkalemia

duct (e.g., amiloride, triamterene, or spironolactone), since this later class reduces renal potassium losses.

GLOMERULONEPHRITIS (GN)

KY A classification of GN is provided in Table 11–10. There are **three major syndromes associated with GN:**

- **Nephrotic syndrome:** This is the result of heavy proteinuria, which leads to hypoalbuminemia, edema, and hypercholesterolemia from a hepatic response to hypoalbuminemia. There is also a hypercoagulable state in patients with nephrotic syndrome, leading to both renal vein thrombosis and deep venous thrombosis of the leg veins.
- **Nephritic syndrome:** This is seen with proliferative GN, which has associated marked glomerular inflammation, causing hematuria, hypertension, and edema.
- **Progressive CRF:** All glomerular diseases, except minimal change disease, may lead to glomerulosclerosis and progressive CRF.

TX1 **Nonspecific management of glomerular disease:** The major components of therapy include **control of hypertension, control of fluid overload,** and **treatment of associated hyperlipidemia.**

RX1a The goal of therapy is a blood pressure (BP) of < 125–130 mm Hg systolic and < 75–80 mm Hg diastolic; aim at the lower levels if there is associated proteinuria of more than 1 g/day. **ACE inhibitors are the drugs**

Table 11–10. Major Categories of Glomerulonephritis (GN)

	Nonproliferative	Proliferative
Primary	Minimal change disease FSGS Membranous nephropathy	IgA nephropathy Idiopathic crescentic GN Membranoproliferative GN
Secondary	Secondary forms of each of the primary forms noted above, including: • Minimal change disease caused by lymphoma and NSAIDs • FSGS caused by heroin and HIV infection • Membranous nephropathy caused by systemic lupus erythematosus, solid tumors, drugs (penicillamine and gold), and infections (hepatitis B, syphilis, malaria) Amyloidosis	Associated with immune complex deposition: • Postinfectious GN • Systemic lupus erythematosus • Cryoglobulinemia (often caused by hepatitis C) Associated with vasculitis (and antibody to antineutrophil cytoplasmic antigen): • Wegener's granulomatosis • Microscopic polyangiitis Associated with antibody to glomerular basement membrane: • Goodpasture's syndrome

FSGS = focal segmental glomerulosclerosis; HIV = human immunodeficiency virus; NSAID = nonsteroidal anti-inflammatory drug.

of choice for management of hypertension in the setting of glomerular disease.

DS1a See Table 11–16

SE1a See Table 11–16

plus

RX1b **Diuretics:** Table 11–9

DS1b Table 11–9

SE1b Table 11–9

plus

RX1c Lipid-lowering agents: See Ch 3 Cardiology.

DS1c See Ch 3 Cardiology.

SE1c See Ch 3 Cardiology.

TX2 **Specific management of inflammatory renal disease:** Certain glomerular disorders respond to **immunosuppressive therapy.** The major ones that do and the major agents used for them are listed in Table 11–11. In general, **glucocorticoids** are used, and in many instances, **cytotoxic agents** are added. In addition, **if a specific etiologic factor can be identified, then it should also be treated;** for instance, discontinuation of a causative drug or treatment of infection.

RX2 Table 11–11 and Table 11–12

DS2 Table 11–11 and Table 11–12

SE2 Table 11–11 and Table 11–12

HYPERTENSION OR HIGH BP

KY The most practical value for normal BP is < 140 mm Hg systolic and < 90 mm Hg diastolic.

Primary versus secondary hypertension: Secondary hypertension is defined as hypertension with an identifiable cause (e.g., renal artery stenosis, pheochromocytoma, hyperthyroidism, drugs). **Primary hypertension** has also been labeled essential hypertension and is characterized by increased systemic vascular resistance. The basis for it involves a complex interaction between genetic and environmental factors, including diet, activity level, and stress.

Resistant hypertension is present when patients being treated for hypertension fail to achieve their goal BP despite the use of three different antihypertensive medications, one of which is a diuretic.

Isolated systolic hypertension is diagnosed when the diastolic BP is < 90 mm Hg and the systolic BP is > 140 mm Hg (American definition) or > 160 mm Hg (Canadian and British definitions). This is most commonly relevant in the elderly population.

Accelerated-malignant hypertension is severe hypertension associated with certain end-organ manifestations. The basis for these is a critical elevation in BP that leads to acute microvascular injury.

Table 11–11. Glomerulonephritic Illnesses Most Likely to Respond to Immunosuppressive Therapy

Disease	Therapeutic Regimen(s)
Amyloidosis	Treatment of underlying condition
Antiglomerular basement membrane disease	Same as for vasculitis, plus plasma exchange
Glomerulonephritis caused by hepatitis B or hepatitis C	Treatment of underlying hepatitis with interferon
Idiopathic focal segmental glomerulosclerosis	Same as for minimal change; lower rate of response
	Cyclosporine
Idiopathic membranous neuropathy	Controversial
	Some support for prednisone and cyclophosphamide
Idiopathic minimal change disease	Prednisone 1 mg/kg PO qd until remission, then taper
	Cyclophosphamide for relapsing or steroid-dependent disease
IgA nephropathy	Some evidence for dietary fish oil supplementation and for corticosteroids in the setting of proteinuria > 1 g/day
Systemic lupus erythematosus	Prednisone as mainstay for diffuse proliferative and severe focal proliferative disease (systemic lupus erythematosus with membranous nephropathy is controversial)
	Prednisone often combined with cyclophosphamide in monthly IV infusions
Vasculitis	Prednisone and cyclophosphamide, often changed to azathioprine after 3–6 months

Hypertensive crises are situations in which the BP is quite high (generally, diastolic BP > 120 mm Hg, although occasionally a crisis may be present with diastolic BP as low as 100 mm Hg), and rapid reduction of BP is necessary to avoid serious end-organ consequences for the patient.

Hypertensive emergency is a situation in which there needs to be a significant reduction of BP within 1 hour. The clinical features and management of hypertensive emergencies are discussed in Table 11–13 and Table 11–14.

Hypertensive urgency is a situation in which the end-organ manifestations that constitute emergencies are not present but the BP is still elevated to a severe degree. These conditions are generally asymptomatic. The BP should be significantly reduced within 24–48 hours. The major situations that constitute hypertensive urgencies are (1) asymptomatic hypertension with diastolic BP > 120 mm Hg, (2) preoperative or postoperative hypertension with diastolic BP > 110 mm Hg, and (3) accelerated malignant hypertension if the only end-organ manifestation is a change seen on funduscopy (see Table 11–15).

TX1 **Chronic hypertension:** Investigations appropriate for all patients with suspected or diagnosed hypertension include urinalysis, plasma crea-

Table 11–12. Immunosuppressive Drugs Used in Nephrology

Generic (Brand) Name	Dose	Side Effects and Cautions
Azathioprine (Imuran) [D]	1–2 mg/kg/day	Anemia, leukopenia, thrombocytopenia, hepatitis, infection, pancreatitis **Caution:** Concomitant allopurinol administration will increase azathioprine levels and thus can cause toxicity.
Cyclophosphamide (Cytoxan, Neosar—*U.S.*; Procytox—*Can.*) [D]	1–3 mg/kg/day	Anemia, leukopenia, thrombocytopenia, hemorrhagic cystitis, bladder cancer, lymphoma, infection
Cyclosporine (Neoral, Sandimmune) [C]	5 mg/kg/day	Hypertension, renal insufficiency, seizures, gum hypertrophy, infection
Prednisone (Deltasone—*U.S.*; Winpred—*Can.*) [B]	1 mg/kg/day, with taper	Edema, hypertension, fat accumulation in face, neck (cushingoid appearance), muscle weakness, osteoporosis, avascular necrosis of long bones, diabetes mellitus, hypertension, psychosis, infection, cataracts, glaucoma

tinine, plasma potassium, fasting glucose, fasting cholesterol and triglyceride levels, and electrocardiogram. Factors influencing the decision to prescribe antihypertensive therapy are described in Figure 11-1. **There are many medications from different drug classes available to treat hypertension; medications and situations in which a particular agent is most appropriate are listed in Table 11–16.** Generally, the **goal is to normalize BP; systolic BP consistently ≤ 140 mm Hg, and diastolic BP ≤ 90 mm Hg.** The following may **modify these goals:** goal BP with DM is 130/80 mm Hg and with renal disease is 125–130 mm Hg systolic and 75–80 mm Hg diastolic. The **strategies available in the case of failure to achieve goal BP** are to increase the dose of the first drug, add a small dose of a second drug, and switch to a different drug from a different class. **Particularly useful combinations** are an ACE inhibitor and diuretics, an ACE inhibitor and calcium channel blockers, beta-blockers and diuretics, and beta-blockers and dihydropyridine calcium channel blockers.

RX1 Table 11–16

DS1 Table 11–16

SE1 Table 11–16

TX2 **Hypertensive emergencies: These situations require reduction of BP within 1 hour.** The emergencies, treatment of choice, and agents to avoid are listed in Table 11–13. For aortic dissection, the goal BP is 120/70

Table 11–13. Hypertensive Emergencies

Disorder	Drug(s) of Choice	Drug(s) to Avoid*
Accelerated malignant hypertension	Labetalol Nitroprusside	—
Acute coronary syndromes (unstable angina pectoris and myocardial infarction)	Beta-blockers Nitroglycerin	Hydralazine
Acute pulmonary edema	Furosemide Nitroglycerin Nitroprusside	Hydralazine
Aortic dissection	Esmolol and nitroprusside Labetalol and nitroprusside	Hydralazine —

Catecholamine excess
  Clonidine withdrawal
  Cocaine intoxication
  Pheochromocytoma
  Use of monoamine oxidase inhibitor together with tyramine-containing food or a sympathomimetic agent
	Labetalol
	Phentolamine	

Eclampsia	Hydralazine Labetalol	Nitroprusside
Hypertensive encephalopathy	Nitroprusside Labetalol	Methyldopa
Intracranial hemorrhage†	Labetalol Nitroprusside	Methyldopa

*See Table 11–14.

†Treatment of hypertension in the setting of stroke (whether it is ischemic or hemorrhagic) is controversial.

mm Hg, and the goal for pulse rate is < 60 beats per minute. For the other conditions, the goal is a reduction in mean arterial BP of approximately 25% (mean arterial BP is defined as the diastolic BP plus one-third the difference between the systolic and diastolic levels). The diastolic BP should not be reduced to < 100–110 mm Hg acutely.

TX2 Table 11–13 and Table 11–14

DS2 Table 11–13 and Table 11–14

SE2 Table 11–13 and Table 11–14

TX3 **Hypertensive urgencies: These are situations in which one should see a significant reduction in 24–48 hours,** but **more precipitous reductions in these asymptomatic situations should be avoided.** Oral drugs for the treatment of hypertensive urgencies are listed in Table 11–15. Often, more than one of these drugs needs to be used. A useful regimen is the combination of a beta-blocker (particularly labetalol) and

Table 11–14. Drugs for the Treatment of Hypertensive Emergencies

Generic (Brand) Name	Dose	Side Effects	Situations in Which Especially Useful
IV drugs			
Esmolol (Brevibloc) [C/D in second and third trimesters]	200–500 µg/kg/min for 4 minutes, then 50–300 µg/kg/min infusion	Same as for beta-blockers (see Table 11–16)	Aortic dissection Coronary ischemia
Hydralazine (Apresoline) [C]	10–20 mg IV	Worsening of myocardial ischemia Tachycardia	Eclampsia
Labetalol (Normodyne, Trandate) [C/D in second and third trimesters]	2 mg/min infusion until BP controlled, repeat q6–8hr 20–80 mg bolus prn	Same as for beta-blockers (see Table 11–16)	Accelerated malignant hypertension Aortic dissection Catecholamine excess Hypertensive encephalopathy Stroke
Nicardipine (Cardene—*U.S.*; Ridene—*Can.*) [C]	2–8 mg/hr infusion until BP controlled	Flushing Headache Tachycardia	—
Nitroglycerin [C]	5–100 µg/min infusion until BP controlled	Headache Tolerance	Coronary ischemia Left ventricular failure
Nitroprusside (Nitropress—*U.S.*; Nipride—*Can.*) [C]	0.25–10 µg/kg/min infusion until BP controlled	Accumulates with renal failure Cyanide toxicity Thiocyanate toxicity Excessive hypotension (requires monitoring in the ICU)	Any hypertensive emergency except eclampsia
Phentolamine (Regitine—*U.S.*, Rogitine—*Can.*) [C]	5–15 mg IV	Tachycardia	—

BP = blood pressure.

Table 11–15. Drugs for the Treatment of Hypertensive Urgencies

Generic (Brand) Name	Dose	Side Effects
Amlodipine (Norvasc) [C]	5–10 mg PO qd	See Table 11–16
Captopril (Capoten) [C/D in second and third trimesters]	25–50 mg PO tid	See Table 11–16
Clonidine (Catapres, Duraclon—*U.S.*; Dixarit—*Can.*) [C]	0.2 mg PO, then 0.1 mg q1hr (maximum 0.7 mg)	See Table 11–16
Labetalol (Normodyne, Trandate) [C/D in second and third trimesters]	200–400 mg PO q6hr	See Table 11–16
Prazosin (Minipress) [C]	1–2 mg PO q8hr	Dizziness, edema, first-dose syncope, headache, orthostatic hypotension, palpitations, weakness Rarely, angina, blurred vision, bradycardia, dyspnea, tachycardia

a long-acting dihydropyridine calcium channel blocker, which can effectively bring the BP to a reasonable range in the desired time frame of 24–48 hours.

RX3 Table 11–15

DS3 Table 11–15

SE3 Table 11–15. It is important to emphasize that a **precipitous reduction in BP in the setting of asymptomatic hypertension is more likely to cause harm than benefit** to the patient and therefore should be avoided. **In particular, sublingual short-acting nifedipine should not be used because of significant risk of severe hypotension and coronary and/or myocardial ischemia.**

METABOLIC ACIDOSIS

KY Metabolic acidosis exists when a low plasma pH (< 7.40) is present, together with a low plasma bicarbonate concentration (< 24 mEq/L). The causes of metabolic acidosis include alcoholic and diabetic ketoacidosis, lactic acidosis, renal failure, salicylate overdose, diarrhea, and renal tubular acidosis. Several drugs or toxins can lead to metabolic acidosis, including salicylate, ethanol, methanol and ethylene glycol, glue-sniffing, and (in the setting of renal failure) metformin.

TX The details of management of the individual disorders are beyond the scope of this chapter. Two important issues are related to treatment of the acid-base disorder:

- Presence of a coexisting respiratory acidosis; in other words, the failure to observe an appropriate degree of ventilatory compensation in response to the metabolic acidosis, which can lead to a very severe

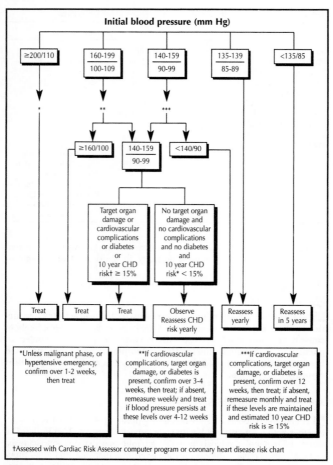

FIGURE 11-1 Blood pressure thresholds and drug treatment in hypertension. Reprinted with permission from Ramsay LE, Williams B, Johnston GD, et al. British Hypertension Society guidelines for hypertension management 1999: summary. *BMJ* 1999;319:630–635.

degree of acidemia and may require tracheal intubation and assisted ventilation (particularly if the cause of the metabolic and respiratory acidoses cannot be rapidly reversed)
- Exogenous alkali, namely, $NaHCO_3$, administration

RX **$NaHCO_3$: Its use is a controversial topic,** and only general guidelines are possible. If the plasma level is extremely low (e.g., < 8 mEq/L), one is more inclined to use $NaHCO_3$. One is also more likely to use $NaHCO_3$ if there is no anion present whose metabolism will lead to the regeneration of $NaHCO_3$; the only such anions are lactate and the anions generated during ketoacidosis (beta-hydroxybutyrate and acetoacetate).

DS The precise dose of $NaHCO_3$ is somewhat difficult to estimate. In general, the more severe the degree of acidosis (and the lower the pH), the greater the amount of $NaHCO_3$ that must be given; a reasonable goal in therapy is to increase the plasma concentration of bicarbonate to 8–10 mEq/L. One should also assume a volume of distribution of approximately half the body weight, and this volume is then multiplied by the desired increment in plasma bicarbonate concentration.

SE **$NaHCO_3$** is contraindicated in the presence of hypokalemia because exogenous $NaHCO_3$ will cause a shift of potassium into cells. **Also contraindicated in the presence of ECF volume overload,** as the sodium load will exacerbate the volume overload.

METABOLIC ALKALOSIS

KY Metabolic alkalosis exists when the pH is > 7.40 and the plasma bicarbonate concentration > 24 mEq/L. The pH may be < 7.40 if there is a coexistent respiratory acidosis or a coexistent metabolic acidosis. Most patients with metabolic alkalosis have either had vomiting or been treated with diuretics. A few patients have primary hyperaldosteronism or some other unusual cause of mineralocorticoid excess. It is important to appreciate that **a variety of factors perpetuates the presence of metabolic alkalosis by preventing the excretion of the excess bicarbonate via the kidneys.** These factors include potassium depletion and ECF volume depletion from diuretic therapy or vomiting, which causes decreased renal reabsorption and increased secretion of bicarbonate.

TX In addition to **treating the underlying cause** of the metabolic alkalosis, it is essential to reverse the conditions that perpetuate it, namely, to **correct the potassium chloride and sodium chloride (NaCl) deficiencies.**

RX1 Correction of **NaCl deficit:** 0.9% NaCl infusions.

DS1 Rate of infusion dictated by the assessment of ECF volume.

SE1 Fluid overload.

RX2 Repletion of **potassium.**

DS2 Table 11–5

SE2 Table 11–5

(Text continues on page 228)

Table 11–16. Drugs Used for the Treatment of Hypertension

Class	Generic (Brand) Name	Dose (PO)
Alpha-1-antagonists	Doxazosin (Cardura) [C]	1–8 mg qd
	Terazosin (Hytrin) [C]	1–8 mg qd
Alpha-beta-blocker	Labetalol (Normodyne, Trandate) [C/D in 2nd and 3rd trimester]	100–400 mg bid
ACE inhibitors	Ramipril (Altace) [C/D in 2nd and 3rd trimester]	2.5–10 mg qd
	Lisinopril (Prinivil, Zestril) [C/D in second and third trimesters]	5–20 mg qd
	Fosinopril (Monopril) [C/D in second and third trimesters]	10–40 mg qd
	Benazepril (Lotensin) [C/D in second and third trimesters]	5–40 mg qd
	Captopril (Capoten) [C/D in secoond and third trimesters]	12.5 mg bid–50 mg tid
	Perindopril (Aceon—*U.S.*; Coversyl—*Can.*) [D]	2–8 mg qd
	Enalapril (Vasotec) [C/D in second and third trimesters]	2.5–20 mg bid
Angiotensin II receptor antagonists	Losartan (Cozaar) [C/D in second and third trimesters]	25–100 mg qd
	Valsartan (Diovan) [C/D in second and third trimesters]	80–320 mg qd
	Irbesartan (Avapro) [C/D in second and third trimesters]	75–300 mg qd
	Candesartan (Atacand) [C/D in second and third trimesters]	8–16 mg qd
Beta-blockers	Atenolol (Tenormin—*U.S.*; Atenol, Tenolin—*Can.*) [D]	25–100 mg qd
	Metoprolol (Lopressor, Toprol—*U.S.*; Betaloc, Durules—*Can.*) [C/D in second and third trimesters]	12.5–100 mg bid

Side Effects	Situations in Which to Avoid Using the Drug Class	Situations in Which the Drug Class Is Especially Helpful
First-dose hypotension Orthostatic hypotension Cardiac arrhythmias Sexual dysfunction	— —	Prostatism
Same as for alpha-1-antagonists and beta-blockers	Same as for beta-blockers	Severe hypertension
Angioedema Cough Hyperkalemia Reduction in GFR (patients with CRF, CHF, bilateral renal artery stenosis, treated with NSAIDs)	Bilateral renal artery stenosis Hyperkalemia	CHF or left ventricular dysfunction Diabetes mellitus Renal disease with proteinuria
Hyperkalemia Reduction in GFR (patients with CRF, CHF, bilateral renal artery stenosis, treated with NSAIDs)	Bilateral renal artery stenosis Hyperkalemia	Same as for ACE inhibitors, but generally the evidence is not yet as strong
Airways constriction Bradycardia, heart block Impotence Left ventricular dysfunction* Peripheral vascular disease Reduced awareness of hypoglycemia	Asthma Bradycardia Chronic obstructive lung disease Uncontrolled CHF Peripheral vascular disease (relative)	Coronary artery disease Left ventricular dysfunction (great care required)

(continued)

Table 11–16. Drugs Used for the Treatment of Hypertension *(Continued)*

Class	Generic (Brand) Name	Dose (PO)
Dihydropyridine calcium channel blockers	Amlodipine (Norvasc) [C]	2.5–10 mg qd
	Felodipine (Plendil—*U.S.*; Renedil—*Can.*) [C]	2.5–10 mg qd
	Nifedipine (long-acting) (Adalat, Procardia) [C]	30–120 mg qd
Nondihydropyridine calcium channel blockers	Diltiazem (long-acting) (Cardizem) [C]	120–360 mg qd
	Verapamil (long-acting) (Calan, Isoptin, Verelan) [C]	180–360 mg qd
Centrally acting sympatholytic agents	Clonidine (Catapres, Duraclon—*U.S.*; Dixarit—*Can.*) [C]	0.1–1 mg bid
	Methyldopa (Aldomet—*U.S.*; Dopamet—*Can.*) [B]	250 mg bid–500 mg qid
Diuretics	Hydrochlorothiazide (Aquazide, Esidrix, Ezide, Hydrocot, HydroDIURIL, Microzide, Oretic—*U.S.*; Hydrazide, Urozide—*Can.*) [B/D]	12.5–25 mg qd
	Indapamide (Lozol—*U.S.*; Lozide—*Can.*) [B/D]	1.25–2.5 mg qd
Direct vasodilator	Hydralazine (Apresoline) [C]	10–50 mg tid
	Minoxidil (Loniten) [C]	2.5 mb bid

ACE = angiotensin-converting enzyme; CHF = congestive heart failure; CRF = chronic renal failure; GFR = glomerular filtration rate; NSAID = nonsteroidal anti-inflammatory drug.

*The use of beta-blockers in CHF is detailed in Ch 3 Cardiology.

Side Effects	Situations in Which to Avoid Using the Drug Class	Situations in Which the Drug Class Is Especially Helpful
Peripheral edema Palpitations Sexual dysfunction Gastrointestinal upset Pulmonary edema Cardiac arrhythmias	—	—
—	—	—
Bradycardia and heart block Constipation Hematologic dyscrasias Allergic reactions Left ventricular dysfunction Peripheral edema	Bradycardia and heart block Left ventricular dysfunction	Patients who are elderly Patients who are of black or African descent
Hemolytic anemia (methyldopa) Hypertensive crisis if abruptly withdrawn (clonidine) Orthostatic hypotension Sedation	Hypertensive crises with neurologic involvement	—
Glucose intolerance Hyperuricemia and gout Hypokalemia Hyponatremia Impotence Metabolic alkalosis	Gout	Patients who are elderly Patients of black or African descent Patients whose blood pressure is not controlled while taking two other drug classes
Fluid retention (Hypertrichosis for minoxidil) Tachycardia	—	—

TUBULOINTERSTITIAL RENAL DISORDERS

Acute Interstitial Nephritis

KY **The major causes of this syndrome are drug reactions.** The most commonly implicated agents include antibiotics (e.g., beta-lactam antibiotics, sulfonamides, quinolones, rifampin), allopurinol, diuretics (e.g., hydrochlorothiazide, furosemide), and NSAIDs. **Other etiologic factors are mainly infectious.** The diffuse tubular inflammation causes tubular dysfunction and ultimately may lead to reduced GFR, at least partly via tubular obstruction. Patients present with a variable degree of renal insufficiency (with an elevation in the plasma creatinine level), there may be evidence of abnormal tubular function such as hyperkalemia or renal tubular acidosis, and the urinalysis reveals pyuria with white blood cell casts, hematuria, and eosinophils in the urine. Definitive diagnosis requires a renal biopsy.

TX **The mainstay is removal of the offending agent (or treatment of the underlying infection).** In addition, a course of prednisone is warranted if there is severe renal insufficiency or the renal failure is not responding to withdrawal of the presumed causative medication.

RX **Prednisone** [B]: Drug has multiple immunosuppressive and antiinflammatory effects.

DS Starting dose 1 mg/kg PO once daily, tapered over about 3 months

SE Adrenal suppression. Predisposes to a variety of infections. Osteoporosis. Proximal muscle weakness. Avascular necrosis of long bones. Easy bruising. Cushingoid appearance with round face and dorsal fat pad as well as abdominal striae. Hypertension, fluid retention, and glucose intolerance. May impair healing of peptic ulcer. Cataracts and glaucoma.

Acute Tubular Necrosis (ATN)

KY **ATN leads to ARF.** The diagnosis depends on recognizing predisposing factors in the clinical context and on the urinalysis, which reveals the presence of pigmented granular casts. **The causes of ATN are categorized as ischemic** or **toxic;** the major toxins implicated are exogenous and endogenous (free hemoglobin resulting from intravascular hemolysis and myoglobin, released from skeletal muscle in the setting of rhabdomyolysis). **The management of ATN is essentially treatment of the underlying condition, including withdrawal of any offending nephrotoxins, and supportive care** for the ARF.

TX1 **Dye nephrotoxicity:** The risk of contrast dye–induced acute renal injury can be reduced by IV fluid therapy for 12 hours before and 12 hours after contrast administration.

RX1a 0.45% NaCl

DS1a 0.45% NaCl 1 mL/kg/hr IV

SE1a Fluid overload.

or

RX1b **Acetylcysteine** (Mucomyst, Mucosil—*U.S.*; Parvolex—*Can.*) [B]: Seems to work by reducing oxidative damage and improving renal hemodynamics.

DS1b 600 mg PO bid the day before and the day of contrast administration.

SE1b Fever, drowsiness, and dizziness. Rarely, bronchospastic allergic reaction.

TX2 **Myoglobinuria:** The severity of renal injury may be reduced by inducing an alkaline diuresis using NaHCO$_3$ IV.

RX2 **NaHCO$_3$** (Neut—*U.S.*; Brioschi—*Can.*) [C]

DS2 Solution of 135 mEq/L of NaHCO$_3$ infused at a rate of 150–300 mL/hr.

SE2 Focal tissue necrosis can occur with extravasation. May cause sodium retention, edema, cerebral hemorrhage, tetany, metabolic alkalosis, hypernatremia, hypokalemia, hypocalcemia, and hyperosmolality. **Use with caution in CHF, edema, cirrhosis, or renal failure.**

12

Neurology

COLIN D. LAMBERT

This chapter focuses on commonly encountered situations in adult clinical neurology, in which relatively prompt intervention by pharmacotherapy is indicated in office or hospital practice. Three situations are addressed: stroke, headache, and seizure disorders.

ACUTE STROKE SYNDROMES

KY *Stroke* is the term applied to an acute focal neurologic deficit of ischemic or hemorrhagic origin. Imaging, usually an unenhanced computed tomographic image of the head, is required to detect blood and other pathologies and to assess early signs of ischemic infarction. Ischemic stroke can be subdivided into five etiologic groups:

- Atherosclerotic disease of large arteries (aorta, carotid, vertebral)
- Disease of small penetrating arteries (lacunar infarction)
- Cardioembolic (multiple potential sources)
- Stroke of other known cause (e.g., dissections)
- Stroke of unknown cause

TX **Intravenous thrombolysis:** Tissue plasminogen activator (t-PA) is the first treatment proven effective for acute stroke. All ischemic strokes should be urgently considered for thrombolysis. Strict adherence to exclusion criteria is advised (Table 12–1). The time window for treatment (onset of stroke symptoms to intervention) is 3 hours.

Intra-arterial thrombolysis: An option in some centers. Consider in selected patients with occlusion of the middle cerebral artery (MCA) or in basilar artery thrombosis. The time window to intervention is longer than for IV therapy; up to 6 hours for MCA infarcts, and longer for basilar artery disease.

Anticoagulant drugs: Anticoagulation therapy is primarily indicated for prevention of stroke of cardiac origin, excluding events caused by tumor (e.g., atrial myxoma) or infection (e.g., infective endocarditis). Primary prevention must be considered for those in atrial fibrillation (intermittent or chronic), and secondary prevention after a cerebral event has occurred. Treatment is indefinite, and long-term supervision is mandatory to minimize hemorrhagic complications. The timing of initiation of therapy after an acute stroke remains controversial. If thrombolysis has been performed, heparin cannot be administered for 48 hours. Other possible indications for anticoagulation in stroke include antiphospholipid antibody syndromes and other hypercoagulable states, intracranial occlusive vascular disease, extracranial arterial dissections, and cerebrovenous thrombosis. In cerebrovenous thrombosis, the existence of intracranial hemorrhage does not necessarily contraindicate the use of an anticoagulant.

Table 12–1. Contraindications to Thrombolysis in Stroke

- Age < 18 years
- History
  - Previous intracerebral hemorrhage
  - Stroke or head trauma within 3 months
  - Intracranial or intraspinal surgery within 2 months
  - Gastrointestinal or urinary tract hemorrhage within 3 weeks
  - Major surgery within 2 weeks
  - Arterial puncture at a noncompressible site, or lumbar puncture, within 7 days
- Clinical signs
  - "Stroke" signs minor or resolving
  - Seizure at onset
  - Features suggestive of subarachnoid hemorrhage or encephalitis
  - Blood pressure > 185 mm Hg systolic or > 110 mm Hg diastolic
- Laboratory data showing
  - PT > 15 sec or INR > 1.7
  - PTT above normal range
  - Platelet count < 100,000/μL

Blood glucose < 50 or > 400 mg/dL

PT = prothrombin time; PTT = partial thromboplastin time; INR = international normalized ratio.

Antiplatelet drugs: These are the mainstays of treatment for prevention of recurrent cerebrovascular events after transient ischemic attacks (TIAs) or stroke. The commonly used drugs include aspirin, extended-release dipyridamole plus aspirin (Aggrenox), and clopidogrel (Plavix) (Table 12–2). Ticlopidine (Ticlid) is no longer used to initiate therapy because of concerns for neutropenia and thrombotic thrombocytopenic purpura. It is recommended that aspirin 75–325 mg PO qd be started within 48 hours of onset of ischemic stroke in patients not receiving anticoagulation or thrombolytic agents. High-dose aspirin (> 325 mg) is no longer considered more beneficial than lower doses. Failure of aspirin alone suggests switching to dipyridamole or clopidogrel. The benefit and safety of combining aspirin (50–81 mg PO qd) with clopidogrel is not known in stroke.

Carotid endarterectomy: Indications for this procedure include TIA or minor stroke in the distribution of the internal carotid artery when the stenosis at the origin of the internal carotid artery is 70%–99% by angiography (according to criteria set by NASCET, the North American Sympto-

Table 12–2. Antiplatelet Drug Options

Generic (Brand) Name	Dose (PO)	Major Side Effects
Aspirin [C/D in third trimester]	50–325 mg qd	Bleeding, rash, thrombotic thrombocytopenic purpura (TTP), headache, GI side effects
Clopidogrel (Plavix) [B]	75 mg qd	Bleeding, rash, TTP
Dipyridamole (extended-release) plus aspirin (Aggrenox)*	25–200 mg bid	Bleeding, headache, diarrhea

*Should not be used in the third trimester of pregnancy.

matic Endarterectomy Trial). Surgery is not beneficial for low-grade steno-sis (< 50%) or once occlusion has occurred. Surgery is additive to best medical therapy.

RX1 **Tissue plasminogen activator** (t-PA): Targets plasminogen, which contains an enzymatically active site. Plasminogen is transformed to plas-min when a cut is made at its enzymatic site (Arg^{500}–Val^{561}), rendering it active, at which time fibrinolysis can occur.

DS1 Do not use cardiac dose.

The dosage for stroke: 0.9 mg/kg to a maximum dose of 90 mg: 10% of total t-PA dose IV over 1 minute; continue IV infusion of the remaining 90% of the total dose over 1 hour. Maintain systolic blood pressure at < 185 mm Hg and diastolic blood pressure at < 110 mm Hg. Postinfusion of t-PA, patients should ideally be monitored in an ICU setting with adher-ence to treatment protocols for management of elevated blood pressure.

SE1 This **risk of symptomatic intracranial** hemorrhage with t-PA is increased 10-fold compared with placebo (NINDS trial). Adherence to published guidelines is strongly recommended. Risk is higher in large infarcts and in individuals > 75 years of age. Most hemorrhages occur within the first 24 hours of treatment, and nearly half of these are fatal. **Allergic reactions** have been demonstrated after infusion of t-PA: 45–60 minutes after t-PA infusion, the patient complains of difficulty swallow-ing, and examination shows swelling of the tongue on the side of the hemiplegia. **There is an association between allergic reaction to t-PA and angiotensin-converting enzyme inhibitors** (see Ch 3 Cardiology), so **caution** in this group is recommended.

ANTIDOTE

Interventions in the case of an allergic reaction to t-PA include ranitidine (Zantac) 50 mg IV plus diphenhydramine (Benadryl) 50 mg IV; hydrocortisone may occasionally be required.

Side effects are also described in Ch 3 Cardiology. **Contraindications to thrombolysis in stroke are listed in** Table 12-1.

or

RX2 **Antiplatelet drugs** (Table 12–2)

DS2 Table 12–2

SE2 Table 12–2

plus/minus

RX3 **Heparin:** See Ch 9 Hematology.

DS3 See Ch 9 Hematology.

SE3 See Ch 9 Hematology.

or

RX4 **Warfarin** (Coumadin) [D]: See Ch 9 Hematology.

DS4 See Ch 9 Hematology.

SE4 See Ch 9 Hematology.

HEADACHES

Headaches are common, and most are benign, but the differential diagnosis is extensive. Initial management aims to identify those headaches that are indicative of a serious illness (secondary headaches). This may require specific therapy directed at that process. Such processes may be surgical (such as subarachnoid hemorrhage, subdural hematoma, and cerebral tumor) or medical (such as meningitis, giant cell [temporal] arteritis, idiopathic [benign] intracranial hypertension, cerebral venous thrombosis, and extracranial artery dissections).

Giant Cell (Temporal) Arteritis

KY Usually occurs in those > 50 years of age, with persistent, often localized, headache refractory to the usual analgesics and other systemic symptoms (myalgia, fever, weight loss). Jaw claudication is a very suggestive symptom. The erythrocyte sedimentation rate (ESR) is usually elevated. A temporal artery biopsy is indicated to confirm diagnosis.

TX **Giant cell arteritis requires long-term (approximately 2 years) steroid therapy,** which produces substantial side effects in the elderly. Diagnosis, therefore, should be clearly established. Biopsy should be undertaken within the first 2 weeks after initiation of therapy to avoid false negatives. The ESR can be helpful as a surrogate marker of control.

RX **Prednisone** [B]

DS 60–80 mg PO qd, tapering to the lowest maintenance dose that controls symptoms. If monocular visual loss has already occurred, consider treating with high-dose methylprednisolone [C] 1 g IV qd for 5 days initially.

SE Glucose intolerance, hypertension, osteoporosis, osteonecrosis, cataract, skin fragility, increased susceptibility to infections, peptic ulcer, cushingoid features, avascular necrosis, myopathy, cataract, glaucoma, and mood changes.

Idiopathic (Benign) Intracranial Hypertension

KY Usually young female, overweight, papilledema, and transient brief losses of vision. Permanent visual impairment is the feared complication. Cerebrospinal fluid examination confirms elevation of pressure without alteration in cell count or glucose. Idiopathic (benign) intracranial hypertension can occur without papilledema.

TX Treatment is by a combination of weight reduction and diuretic therapy with acetazolamide or furosemide. Surgical therapy to be considered only in refractory cases.

RX1 **Acetazolamide** (Diamox) [C]: Carbonic anhydrase inhibitor.

DS1 250 mg PO bid

SE1 No significant side effects.

or

RX2 **Furosemide** (Lasix) [C]: A loop diuretic that inhibits sodium reabsorption in the ascending loop of Henle.

DS2 20–120 mg orally

SE2 Volume depletion and hypokalemia.

Migraine

KY Diagnostic criteria include the following:

- At least five attacks that fulfill the next three criteria
- Headache lasts 2–72 hours (untreated or unsuccessfully treated)
- Two of the following features present: (1) unilateral, (2) pulsating, and (3) moderate to severe intensity, aggravation by physical activity
- During the headache, at least one of the following: (1) nausea or vomiting or (2) photophobia or phonophobia

TX Treatment of migraine has three components: avoidance of precipitating factors when possible, termination of the acute migraine headache, and prophylaxis.

RX1 **Triptans:** Class of drugs specifically tailored to target the serotonin receptors 5HT1b/1d, which are considered to have a major role in the genesis of migraine both at vascular (5HT1b) receptors (which are also expressed on coronary arteries) and at the neuronal (5HT1d) level. The triptans are analogs of serotonin (5 hydroxytryptamine). Several formulations are available (Table 12–3). All triptans are metabolized by the liver. Some triptans are metabolized by monoamine oxidase A and should not be used in patients who are taking that class of drugs (e.g., moclobemide, phenelzine, or tranylcypromine) or within 2 weeks of their discontinuation.

Sumatriptan, administered SC, has the most rapid onset of action and is most likely to result in pain relief in 1 hour. These advantages are offset by a higher incidence of side effects and higher cost. This formulation is most appreciated by those with cluster headaches. Naratriptan has the slowest mode of onset but has the least side effects. Lack of response to respond to one triptan does not preclude response to another.

DS1 Table 12–3

SE1 Flushing; paraesthesia; dizziness; somnolence; and throat, neck, and chest tightness (mimicking angina). Potential for summation of action with other drugs that increase serotonin levels (e.g., serotonin selective drugs, ergot preparations). Propranolol (but not metoprolol or nadolol) increases the bioavailability of rizatriptan and zolmitriptan; a lower dose of rizatriptan is recommended with concomitant propranolol administration. **Contraindicated** in coronary artery disease and uncontrolled hypertension.

or

RX2 **Dihydroergotamine** (DHE) (Migranal) [X]: Acts on serotonin receptors and at the adrenergic and dopaminergic receptors. Has vasoconstrictive and venoconstrictive effects. Nasal spray is available.

Table 12–3. Triptan Formulations and Doses

Generic (Brand) Name	Formulation and Dose
Frovatriptan (Frova) [C]	PO: 2.5 mg
Naratriptan (Amerge) [C]	PO: 1–2.5 mg
Rizatriptan (Maxalt) [C]	PO 5–10 mg
Sumatriptan (Imitrex) [C]	PO: 25–100 mg
	Intranasal: 5–20 mg
	SC: 6 mg
Zolmitriptan (Zomig) [C]	PO: 2.5 mg

DS2 At onset, 1 spray is delivered to each nostril; if necessary, this is repeated in 15–30 minutes. **As with other ergots, there is a maximum limit suggested of 12 mg weekly.** Alternate method (which can be used in an emergency department setting): metoclopramide 10 mg IV, followed by DHE of 0.5 mg (diluted in 10 mL of normal saline) IV given over 2–3 minutes.

SE2 DHE should not be used for patients with coronary or peripheral vascular disease, hypertension, or pregnancy or within 24 hours of a triptan.

or

RX3 **Butorphanol** (Stadol) [C/D with high doses or prolonged use]: Acts as an agonist at kappa-opioid receptors and as a mixed agonist-antagonist at mu-opioid receptors in the central nervous system to alter the perception of pain.

DS3 Onset of effect is within 15–30 minutes and **requires individualization of dosage based on clinical response.** The usual recommended adult dose for initial nasal administration is 1 spray in one nostril (1 mg). If adequate pain relief is not achieved within 60–90 minutes, an additional 1-mg dose may be administered. Repeat administration is recommended only after 3–4 hours from last dose. Total maximum dose is 16 mg/day.

SE3 Major side effects include sedation and dysphoria. Opiate withdrawal symptoms can be precipitated in those taking opiate analgesics on a regular basis. A patient should not drive or work with machinery until sedation has cleared. **Strict control over prescriptions is recommended** to avoid overuse and dependence. **Caution** in those with hepatic or renal impairment.

SEIZURE DISORDERS

Epilepsy

KY Epilepsy is a chronic condition characterized by the tendency to recurrent unprovoked seizures. A seizure is a symptom resulting from paroxysmal excessive discharges from neuronal cell populations, which are usually self-limiting. Such discharges may be focal (resulting in partial seizures) or generalized. Generalized (tonic-clonic) seizures may either be primarily generalized or result from extension of a partial seizure (secondarily generalized). The secondary nature of a generalized seizure is suggested by the preceding occurrence of an aura, a focal onset, focal discharges recorded during an interictal electroencephalogram (EEG), or by demonstration of a relevant structural lesion by brain imaging.

TX Antiepileptic drugs (AEDs) are the mainstay of treatment in most cases. Monotherapy is preferred but is not always sufficient. In some situations, long-term drug therapy is often not indicated, for example, seizures related to acute drug intoxication or withdrawal and seizures related to transient metabolic disturbances. The introduction of AED therapy carries with it the consequence of prolonged treatment over years. The decision to start medication, therefore, requires consideration of the risk-to-benefit ratio in terms of likelihood of recurrence of seizures, efficacy, and implications for lifestyle balanced against side effects and cost. The risk of recurrence after a first unprovoked generalized tonic-clonic seizure is approximately 40% at 2 years, being less in the absence of an underlying identifiable cause and with normal EEG findings, but higher in the converse situation. Partial seizures, which are usually of complex type in adult life, show a high recurrence rate of approximately $\geq 60\%$. This increases toward 80% after a second event. Table 12–4 lists some factors involved when choosing an AED.

Blood tests (complete blood cell count, creatinine, glucose, electrolytes, and liver function tests) should be conducted before therapy to provide a baseline.

Primidone (Mysoline) is the least-tolerated AED. Phenobarbital (Donnatal) is effective but may not be well tolerated; it acts at the chloride (γ-aminobutyric acid-A [GABA-A] channel. The three commonly used drugs are phenytoin, carbamazepine , and valproic acid (also called valproate). Table 12–5 lists commonly used AEDs.

Table 12–4. Factors in Choosing an Antiepileptic Drug (AED)*

- Seizure type or epileptic syndrome
- Individual patient characteristics and side effect profiles
- Immediacy of effect, as in status epilepticus or with serial seizures (some drugs require very slow titration [e.g., lamotrigine, topiramate])
- Spectrum of action of drug: broad versus narrow
- Frequency of dosing (e.g., greater compliance if dosing is once daily)
- Special situations: safety of the newer AEDs has not been established in pregnancy. The risk of teratogenicity must be considered in all women who may become pregnant. All AEDs are to some extent teratogenic. Valproic acid and carbamazepine are especially associated with spina bifida, which occurs in 1%–2% of fetuses. Folic acid supplement 1–5 mg/day is recommended for all women taking AEDs who could become pregnant.
- Drug interactions: some AEDs (carbamazepine, phenobarbital, phenytoin, primidone, topiramate) are hepatic enzyme inducers and therefore may reduce the effectiveness of other medications, including oral contraceptive pills.
- Cross-reactivity: hypersensitivity to phenytoin is frequently associated with a similar reaction to carbamazepine or phenobarbital or primidone. Valproic acid and clobazam are alternatives in this context. Lamotrigine carries the highest incidence of severe skin allergic reactions. Patients should be advised of the rare possibility of severe allergic reactions.

*Compliance should be monitored: therapeutic ranges are established for carbamazepine, phenobarbital, phenytoin, and valproic acid but not for the new-generation AEDs. Allow five times the drug's half-life to elapse before estimating the new level.

Table 12–5. Commonly Used Antiepileptic Drugs

Generic (Brand) Name	Half-life	Therapeutic Ranges	Major Side Effects
Carbamazepine (Tegretol) [D]	10–25 hours	4–12 µg/mL (SI: 25–51 µmol/L)	Dizziness, double vision, lethargy, unsteadiness Rarely, hematologic depression
Phenobarbital (Luminal Sodium—*U.S.*; Barbilixir—*Can.*) [D]	2–5 days	20–40 µg/mL (SI: 86–172 µmol/L)	Sedation, blood dyscrasias
Phenytoin (Dilantin) [D]	8–40 hours	10–20 µg/mL (SI: 40–80 µmol/L)	Gum hypertrophy, nystagmus, slurred speech, unsteadiness
Valproic acid (Depacon, Depakene, Depakote—*U.S.*; Epival—*Can.*) [D]	8–15 hours	50–100 µg/mL (SI: 350–690 µmol/L)	Gastrointestinal upset, hair loss, hepatotoxicity at toxic levels, tremor, weight gain

New-Generation AEDs: These agents do not require estimation of serum levels. There are no recommended therapeutic ranges. Hematologic or hepatic toxicity is rare. **Safety in pregnancy has not been established.** Several new drugs are currently available: clobazam, lamotrigine, gabapentin, vigabatrin, topiramate, oxcarbazepine, levetiracetam, tiagabine, zonisamide, and fosphenytoin.

RX1 **Phenytoin** (Dilantin) [D]: Blocks sodium channels. Can be given IV, and once-daily dose is possible. Exhibits nonlinear kinetics; > 300 mg daily, dosage must be increased by small increments (e.g., 30–50 mg steps) to avoid overshooting therapeutic range.

DS1 Initial dose: 300 mg PO/IV qd. If quicker induction is required, then loading can be achieved with 300 mg PO tid on the first day, followed by 300 mg PO qd.

SE1 Unsteadiness, slurred speech, nystagmus, gum hypertrophy, and hirsutism. Concomitant use decreases efficacy of oral contraceptive pills (OCPs).

or

RX2 **Carbamazepine** (Tegretol) [D]: Blocks sodium channels. Twice-daily dosage is possible with a controlled-release preparation. Carbamazepine induces its own metabolism, sometimes necessitating a further dose increase; low initial doses (100–200 mg PO bid) are recommended, with increases at approximately weekly intervals.

DS2 Build up to a maximum level of 1,600 mg/day. Usual dose is 300–400 mg PO bid.

SE2 Hyponatremia, cardiac conduction defects, dizziness, unsteadiness, double vision, lethargy, and hematologic depression. Concomitant use decreases efficacy of OCPs. **Contraindicated** in pregnancy because of the possibility of spina bifida in the fetus.

or

RX3 **Oxcarbazepine** (Trileptal) [C]: Activity primarily caused by a metabolite (MHD). Similar mode of action as carbamazepine.

DS3 Doses range from 900–2400 mg/day; average dose is 600 mg PO bid.

SE3 Similar but lower incidence as carbamazepine, except hyponatremia is more common. Patients with hypersensitivity to carbamazepine show up to 30% cross-reactivity with oxcarbazepine.

or

RX4 **Valproic acid (also called valproate)** (Depacon, Depakene, Depakote—*U.S.*; Epival—*Can.*) [D]: Blocks sodium channels and also probably acts at the GABA-A receptor and blocks calcium channels. Broad spectrum; available in IV, liquid, and sprinkle formulations. Valproic acid does not interfere with OCPs.

DS4 Initial dose is usually 125–250 mg PO/IV/IM bid.

SE4 Teratogenicity (spina bifida, 2%) in pregnancy. Concomitant administration with phenobarbital can result in profound sedation. Gastrointestinal upset, weight gain, tremor, hair loss, polycystic ovarian syndrome, and hepatotoxicity have also been reported.

or new-generation AED

RX5 **Clobazam** (Frisium—*Can.*; not commercially available in the United States): A benzodiazepine with a broad spectrum of action. Can be readily used as add-on therapy.

DS5 Initial dose 5–10 mg PO qhs and increasing to 20–30 mg PO qhs.

SE5 Tolerance may develop. Causes sedation.

or

RX6 **Lamotrigine** (Lamictal) [C]: Broad-spectrum drug that blocks sodium channels and suppresses the release of glutamate.

DS6 Therapy must be instituted slowly. Initial dose: 50 mg PO qd, increasing to 50 mg PO bid in weeks 3 and 4. In patients who are taking valproic acid, which inhibits the hepatic metabolism of lamotrigine, induction of therapy must be as slow as 25 mg PO every other day. Hepatic enzyme–inducing drugs (phenytoin, carbamazepine, phenobarbital) reduce elimination half-life by about 50%. Standard dose is 300 mg PO qd to a maximum of 600 mg.

SE6 Associated with **severe and potentially life-threatening cutaneous reactions,** including Stevens-Johnson syndrome; incidence is 1 in 1,000 in adults and can be as high as 1%–2% in children.

or

RX7 **Gabapentin** (Neurontin) [C]: Undetermined mode of action. May block amino acid transport across the blood-brain barrier. Indications are partial seizures with or without secondary generalization.

DS7 Drug half-life is short (6 hours), and tid dosage is required. Titration of therapy can be rapid: 300 or 400 mg PO qd, increasing every 2–3 days to a maximum of 3,600 mg PO qd.

SE7 Somnolence is the major side effect. Often used for chronic neuropathic pain.

or

RX8 **Vigabatrin** (Sabril—*Can.*; not available in the United States): Inhibits the breakdown of the inhibitory neurotransmitter GABA. Indications are partial seizures with or without secondary generalization. Absence and myoclonic seizures may be aggravated.

DS8 Titration of therapy is slow. Initial dose is 500 mg PO bid, increasing to a total of 2,000–4,000 mg PO qd in 4–6 weeks.

SE8 Somnolence is the most common side effect. Occasionally, behavioral disturbances (e.g., depression, psychosis) occur. Vigabatrin is seldom used in adult patients because it can cause **ophthalmologic abnormalities, disc pallor, optic atrophy, and irreversible visual field defects.** Visual field assessment is recommended every 3 months.

or

RX9 **Topiramate** (Topamax) [C]: Acts by several mechanisms: sodium channel blockade, attenuation of glutamate responses, carbonic and anhydrase inhibition, and enhancement of GABA activity. Excretion is primarily renal. Half-life is approximately 20–30 hours.

DS9 Titration of therapy is slow; initial dose is 25–50 mg PO qd, with incremental increases of 25–50 mg at weekly intervals to a total of 400–600 mg/day.

SE9 Can cause reversible cognitive disturbances, and renal calculi can occur in up to 2%. Weight loss occurs in some. An acute ocular syndrome can occur, usually within the first month of treatment. Enzyme-inducing drugs (e.g., phenytoin, carbamazepine) reduce topiramate concentration by 40%–60%. Topiramate may increase phenytoin levels and decrease the effectiveness of OCPs.

or

RX10 **Levetiracetam** (Keppra) [C]: Unknown mode of action. **Used as adjunctive therapy for partial seizures.** No significant drug interactions.

DS10 Starting dose 500 mg bid, and increase to 1,000–3,000 mg/day as required.

SE10 Usually occur in the first month of treatment: somnolence, asthenia, and dizziness.

or

RX11 **Tiagabine** (Gabitril) [C]: Blocks GABA reuptake. Used as adjunctive therapy for partial or secondarily generalized seizures. May aggravate some primary generalized seizure disorders. Short half life.

DS11 Starting dose 4 mg PO qd; then increase at 2-week intervals as bid or tid doses. Maximum dose: 56 mg/day.

SE11 Somnolence, cognitive or behavioral changes. Severe weakness or difficulty walking in 1%. Abdominal pain can occur.

or

RX12 **Zonisamide** (Zonegran) [C]: Several postulated mechanisms of action. Broad-spectrum activity but approved for adjunctive therapy of partial or secondarily generalized seizures. Metabolized by the liver to inactive compounds excreted normally.

DS12 100–600 mg daily qd or bid; Starting dose 100 mg PO qd; increase to 50–300 mg PO qd–bid as needed.

SE12 Sulfonamide derivative. **Severe idiosyncratic reactions** (cutaneous, hematologic, hepatic) have occurred. Renal calculi and **significant psychiatric symptoms** have been reported.

Status Epilepticus

KY Defined as > 30 minutes of seizure activity or lack of recovery between discrete seizures.

Table 12–6. Management Sequence in Status Epilepticus

1. Check airway, breathing, circulation, and temperature.
2. Obtain blood tests: complete blood cell count, glucose, creatinine, electrolytes, LFT, calcium, magnesium, and appropriate AED level if the patient is a known epileptic. Toxicology screen and blood cultures to be considered.
3. Give a 50-mL ampule of 50% glucose (if patient is hypoglycemic) plus 100 mg of thiamine (Thiamilate) IV.
4. Perform rapid clinical assessment to address cause: head injury, CNS infection or tumor, alcohol or drug abuse, or other cause.
5. Correct abnormalities of STAT blood work where possible.
6. Administer AEDs **IV** (see Table 12–7 for doses)
   - Lorazepam/diazepam first-line treatment
   - Phenytoin/fosphenytoin second-line treatment (unless the patient is a known hypersensitive); if the patient is known to be taking phenytoin, assume non-compliance and administer full loading dose
   - Additional infusion of phenytoin at 10 mg/kg IV after 20 minutes from initial dose if seizures continue
7. Obtain head CT and consider LP.
8. Transfer the patient to the ICU for ongoing management if status epilepticus continues.
   - Consider propofol, midazolam, thiopental, or phenobarbital infusion

AED = antiepileptic drug; CNS = central nervous system; CT = computed tomography; LFT = liver function test; LP = lumbar puncture; ICU = intensive care unit.

TX Immediate intervention with an AED at full dosage, given IV, is mandatory. Delayed therapy may result in poor outcome or mortality. Table 12–6 describes the steps that should be initiated in the case of status epilepticus.

RX1 Table 12–5, Table 12–6, and Table 12–7

DS1 Table 12–7 and Table 12–8

SE1 Table 12–7 and Table 12–8

or

RX2 **Fosphenytoin sodium** (Cerebyx) [D]: A prodrug of phenytoin and represents an alternative to IV phenytoin. It is used for short-term parenteral administration, or it can substitute for oral phenytoin on a short-term basis. Indications are generalized status epilepticus and the treatment or prevention of seizures that occur during neurosurgery. Fosphenytoin is rapidly and completely converted to phenytoin, and its mechanism of action, drug interactions, and systemic side effects are the same as for phenytoin.

DS2 **Fosphenytoin:** 75 mg is equivalent to phenytoin 50 mg. Dose and infusion rates are expressed as phenytoin sodium equivalents (PE). Status epilepticus **loading dose:** PE 15–20 mg/kg IV at 100–150 mg/min. Cardiovascular monitoring is required during IV loading. **Maintenance dose:** PE 4–6 mg/kg/day IV/IM. Advantages of fosphenytoin over phenytoin include greater aqueous solubility, fewer local side effects at the injection site, and better absorption.

Table 12–7. Antiepileptic Drugs Available for Parenteral Administration

Generic (Brand) Name	Route(s) of Administration	Dose (mg/kg)	Maximum Infusion Rate (mg/min)
Diazepam (Valium) [D]	IV PR*	0.20	5
Fosphenytoin (Cerebyx) [D]†	IV, IM	PE 4–6 mg/kg/day	150
Lorazepam (Ativan) [D]	IV	0.1	2
Phenobarbital (Luminal Sodium—*U.S.*; Barbilixir—*Can.*) [D]	IV	10–20	100
Phenytoin (Dilantin) [D]	IV	20	50
Valproate (Depacon, Depakene, Depakote—*U.S.*; Epival—*Can.*) [D]	IV	20	20

*Rectal gel: initial dose is 0.2 mg/kg PR (see text for additional information).

†The dose, concentration in solutions, and infusion rates for fosphenytoin are expressed as phenytoin equivalents (PEs).

SE2 Dizziness, somnolence, ataxia, pruritus, nystagmus, hypotension, vasodilation, tachycardia, tremor, and blood dyscrasias.

with or without

RX3 **Diazepam** (Diastat) [D]: Available as a gel for rectal administration. Usage is as **adjunctive therapy** in known epileptic patients in whom clusters of seizures occur in a relatively predictable manner.

DS3 Prefilled syringes are available in doses of 10, 15, and 20 mg. For adults, 0.2 mg/kg PR is indicated. A second dose may be given but not to exceed 2 doses in 5 days, or 5 doses per month.

SE3 Drowsiness, fatigue, confusion, amnesia, cognitive impairment, incoordination, ataxia, disinhibition, and dizziness. Withdrawal syndrome and dependence occur with prolonged use.

Table 12–8. Compatibility of Medications With Infusion Fluids

Generic (Brand) Name	Compatibility
Diazepam (Valium) [D]	NS, RL, D-5-W
Fosphenytoin (Cerebyx) [D]	NS, RL, D-5-W
Lorazepam (Ativan) [D]	NS, RL, D-5-W
Phenytoin (Dilantin) [D]	NS, RL (*not* D-5-W)
Valproic acid (Depacon, Depakene, Depakote—*U.S.*; Epival—*Can.*) [D]	NS, RL, D-5-W

D-5-W = 5% dextrose in water, supplied ready mixed; NS = normal saline (0.9% sodium chloride); RL = Ringer's lactate (solution).

or

RX4 **Valproic acid** (Depacon, Depakene, Depakote) [D]: An IV formulation. Experience in status epilepticus is limited.

DS4 Dosage is equivalent to that of the oral form. The recommended rate of infusion (20 mg/kg) is too slow in status epilepticus; faster infusion rates, up to 500 mg/min, have been given and seem well tolerated, but hypotension may occur.

SE4 See the Epilepsy section.

Obstetrics

MICHELLE R. WISE, KERRY A. WILSON, CHRISTINE M. DERZKO

CHORIOAMNIONITIS

KY Intrapartum polymicrobial infection of the amniotic fluid, membranes, placenta, or uterus that occurs in 4%–10% of all deliveries and is associated with maternal and neonatal infectious morbidity. Diagnose by fever of 37.8°C and two of the following symptoms: maternal or fetal tachycardia, tender uterus, maternal leukocytosis, or malodorous amniotic fluid.

TX Broad-spectrum IV antibiotics should be started as soon as diagnosed and continued until the patient is afebrile for 24 hours. Combinations include ampicillin and gentamicin or, if the patient has a penicillin allergy, clindamycin and gentamicin. Other regimens include cefazolin and gentamicin, and ampicillin and sulbactam, cefuroxime, and piperacillin. There is no benefit to follow-up oral antibiotic therapy. Acetaminophen (Tylenol) will decrease hyperthermic stress on the fetus.

RX1 **Ampicillin** (Marcillin—*U.S.*; Ampicin—*Can.*) [B]: Broad-spectrum penicillin.

DS1 2 g PO q6hr

SE1 Hypersensitivity, which is increased in patients with infectious mononucleosis and lymphatic leukemia.

or

RX2 **Clindamycin** (Cleocin—*U.S.*; Dalacin—*Can.*) [B]: Exerts its antibacterial effect by causing cessation of protein synthesis and also by causing a reduction in the rate of synthesis of nucleic acid. Use in cases of ampicillin allergy.

DS2 600 mg PO q8hr

SE2 **Safety in pregnancy has not been established,** and its use is left to the judgment of the physician.

plus

RX3 **Gentamicin** (Garamycin—*U.S.*; Cidomycin—*Can.*) [C]: Bacteriocidal antibiotic that affects bacterial growth by specific inhibition of protein synthesis in susceptible bacteria.

DS3 Start at 1.5 mg/kg PO q8hr. Once postpartum, then can change dose to 5–7 mg/kg q24hr.

SE3 Hypersensitivity, ototoxicity, and nephrotoxicity.

DIABETES MELLITUS, GESTATIONAL (GDM)

KY GDM is glucose intolerance present only during pregnancy, and it occurs in 2%–4% of pregnancies. There is a relative insulin resistance during the second and third trimesters. High cortisol and human placental lactogen in pregnancy also produce hyperglycemia. Screening for GDM can be offered routinely or to women at high risk. It is performed at 24–28 weeks and involves a 1-hour 50-g glucose challenge test (Table 13–1). A positive screen should be followed up with a 2-hour 75-g oral glucose tolerance test (OGTT) (Canadian Diabetes Association) or a 3-hour 100-g OGTT (American College of Obstetricians and Gynecologists). GDM is associated with macrosomic infants, which is associated with morbidity and mortality. There is no increased risk of congenital malformations.

TX Once diagnosis of GDM is made, the patient is advised to follow a diabetic diet and to exercise regularly. If fasting blood sugar is consistently greater than 105 mg/dL, or 2-hour postprandial glucose is greater than 120 mg/dL, insulin should be initiated. **Sulfonylurea drug therapy, with tolbutamide and chlorpropamide, which cross the placenta, is considered to be contraindicated** in the treatment of GDM because of the drugs' ability to cause fetal hyperinsulinemia and therefore macrosomia and prolonged neonatal hypoglycemia. Glyburide (DiaBeta) only has minimal transplacental passage ability, and teratogenicity is not a concern in women in whom treatment is begun after organogenesis. **Metformin (Glucophage) has been used in the treatment of GDM; however, it is associated with an increased risk of preeclampsia and stillbirth.** At this time, oral hypoglycemic agents are not routinely used in pregnancy. After delivery, insulin is stopped. An OGTT is conducted at 6 weeks to 6 months postpartum. Half of the patients with GDM develop overt type 2 DM in the next 20 years.

RX Insulin [B]: The type and dose of insulin used is dependent on the abnormality of blood glucose noted during monitoring. See Ch 5 Endocrinology for more information on the insulins.

DS If insulin is required because the fasting blood glucose concentration is high, an intermediate-acting insulin, such as NPH insulin, is given before bedtime; initial dose should be 0.15 U/kg body weight.

If postprandial blood glucose concentrations are high, then regular insulin or insulin lispro should be given before meals in a dose calculated to be 1.5 U per 10 g of carbohydrate in the breakfast meal and 1 U per 10 g of carbohydrate in the lunch and dinner meals.

Table 13–1. Interpretation of Oral Glucose Challenge Test Results

1-hour Blood Sugar Level	Interpretation
< 7.8 mmol/L (< 140 mg/dL)	Normal
7.8–10.3 mmol/L (140–200 mg/dL)	Impaired glucose tolerance
> 10.3 mmol/L (> 200 mg/dL)	Diagnostic for GDM

GDM = gestational diabetes mellitus.

If both preprandial and postprandial blood glucose concentrations are high, then a regimen of four injections per day should be initiated. According to this regimen, the total daily dose is 0.7 U/kg for weeks 6–18; 0.8 U/kg for weeks 19–26; and 1.0 U/kg for weeks 37–term. The insulin should be divided in the following schedule: **about 45% as NPH insulin** (30% before breakfast and 15% before bedtime) and about **55% as preprandial regular insulin** (22% before breakfast, 16.5% before lunch, and 16.5% before dinner).

Adjustments in insulin doses are based on the results of self-monitoring of blood glucose (Table 13–2). Insulin resistance increases as gestation proceeds, requiring an increase in insulin dose.

SE Hypoglycemia, palpitation, tachycardia, fatigue, mental confusion, loss of consciousness, headache, hypothermia, urticaria, muscle weakness, paresthesia, tremors, transient presbyopia, anaphylaxis.

DIABETES MELLITUS (DM), PREEXISTING

Also covered in Ch 5, Endocrinology.

KY **Preexisting DM is associated with increased risk** of spontaneous abortion, congenital anomalies, stillbirth, fetal macrosomia and shoulder

Table 13–2. Insulin Adjustments Related to Self-Measured Blood Glucose Concentrations

Time Blood Glucose Is Monitored	Blood Glucose Concentration (mg/dL)	Insulin Adjustments
07:30 AM	> 90	Monitor at bedtime and at 03:00 AM. If the bedtime value is elevated, then increase the dinner regular insulin or decrease the evening snack. If the bedtime value is normal but the 03:00 AM value is > 100 mg/dL, then increase bedtime NPH insulin by 2 U.
	< 60	Reduce bedtime NPH insulin by 2 U.
10:00 AM	> 140	Increase next morning regular insulin dose by 2 U.
	< 110	Decrease next morning regular insulin dose by 2 U.
13:00 PM	> 140	Increase next day lunch regular insulin dose by 2 U.
	< 110	Decrease next day lunch regular insulin dose by 2 U.
16:30 PM	> 90	Increase morning NPH insulin dose by 2 U.
	< 60	Increase morning NPH insulin dose by 2 U.
18:00 PM	> 140	Increase dinner regular insulin dose by 2 U.
	< 110	Decrease dinner regular insulin dose by 2 U.

dystocia, preterm labor, restricted growth, and delayed fetal lung maturity (decreased surfactant synthesis). **Neonatal complications** include those related to birth trauma, hypoglycemia, and hyperbilirubinemia. **Maternal complications** include rapid progression of disease (e.g., retinopathy and nephropathy) and gestational hypertension with or without proteinuria.

TX **The management of DM in pregnancy involves a multidisciplinary team and is individualized. Oral hypoglycemics should be discontinued, because they cause fetal hyperinsulinemia and have been associated with congenital malformations.** Insulin is safe and should be adjusted to maintain tight glycemic control in order to minimize the above complications.

RX **Insulin (Humulin R)**

DS **During labor,** an intravenous insulin and glucose drip should be started and titrated to maintain blood glucose between 63 and 117 mg/dL. **After delivery,** insulin dose should be decreased to minimize the risk of postpartum hypoglycemia.

SE Avoid hypoglycemics. Monitor glucose. (See Ch 5 Endocrinology.)

ECLAMPSIA

KY Characterized by **generalized tonic-clonic seizures** that develop in women with **gestational hypertension,** usually with **proteinuria. Risks to mother and fetus are severe.**

TX Management includes **seizure control, correction of hypoxia and acidosis, blood pressure control, and delivery of fetus once mother is stabilized.**

RX **Magnesium sulfate [B]:** Prevents or controls convulsions by blocking neuromuscular transmission and by decreasing the amount of acetylcholine liberated at the end plate by the motor nerve impulse.

DS **For seizure prophylaxis:** 4 g IV bolus over 20 minutes followed by continuous infusion of 1–2 g/hr, and continue until 24 hours postpartum.

For seizure control: 4 g IV bolus over 4 minutes followed by continuous infusion of 2 g/hr until 24 hours postpartum. Monitor reflexes, urine output, respiratory rate, and serum magnesium levels.

SE **Minor adverse effects** include hot flashes and dyspnea. **Major adverse effects** include respiratory depression caused by overdose or renal insufficiency. May also cause decrease in fetal heart rate variability. **Concomitant use with nifedipine (Adalat) can cause severe hypotension and fetal distress.** As the plasma magnesium level rises above 4 mEq/L, the deep tendon reflexes are first decreased and then disappear as the level approaches 10 mEq/L; this can ultimately lead to respiratory depression.

ANTIDOTE

Antidote for magnesium sulfate overdose: 10 mL 10% calcium gluconate 1 g IV push over 3 minutes.

ERYTHROBLASTOSIS FETALIS

See ISOIMMUNIZATION—ERYTHROBLASTOSIS FETALIS.

GESTATIONAL DIABETES MELLITUS (GDM)

See DIABETES MELLITUS, GESTATIONAL (GDM).

GESTATIONAL HYPERTENSION WITH OR WITHOUT PROTEINURIA

KY **Hypertension in pregnancy is diastolic blood pressure (dBP) > 89 mm Hg in the sitting position on two occasions** (Canadian Hypertension Society). **Proteinuria is the excretion of protein in urine in excess of 300 mg in 24 hours.** Pathophysiology is secondary to vasospasm, leading to arterial hypertension and blood vessel damage. **Gestational hypertension is associated with many maternal and fetal adverse conditions,** including eclamptic seizures.

TX **Definitive treatment is delivery;** however, there is the need to take into account gestational age. If dBP is > 89 mm Hg, consider short-term hospitalization to assess maternal and fetal well-being, and consider initiation of pharmacologic treatment. **If dBP is > 109 mm Hg, pharmacologic treatment is definitely indicated to prevent maternal cerebral hemorrhage** (Table 13–3). Anti-convulsants may be used to prevent primary or recurrent seizures (see Eclampsia).

RX Table 13–3

DS Table 13–3

SE Table 13–3. **Angiotensin-converting enzyme inhibitors are contraindicated in pregnancy** owing to association with hypocalvaria, oligohydramnios, renal anomalies, neonatal renal failure, pulmonary hypoplasia, and death.

GROUP B STREPTOCOCCAL (GBS) INFECTION

See PREVENTION OF GROUP B STREPTOCOCCAL (GBS) INFECTION.

HYPEREMESIS GRAVIDARUM

KY **Intractable vomiting** in pregnancy that **results in weight loss, dehydration, electrolyte imbalance, and acid-base disturbance.** It occurs in 1% of pregnant women and is related to high or rapid rise in β–human chorionic gonadotropin levels.

TX Management includes intravenous fluids, correction of metabolic changes, and antiemetics (Table 13–4).

RX Table 13–4

DS Table 13–4

SE Table 13–4

Table 13-3. Antihypertensive Medications* Used in Pregnancy†

Generic (Brand) Name	Dose	Mechanism of Action	Side Effects and Cautions
Hydralazine (Apresoline) [C]	10 mg PO qid then titrate up to 50 mg PO qid or 5–10 mg IV q20min	Vasodilator, reflex increase in cardiac output	Maternal tachycardia
Labetalol (Normodyne, Trandate) [C]‡	100 mg PO bid or 5–20 mg IV q10–20min	Beta-blocker	Maternal bradycardia, less benefit if in heart failure
Methyldopa (Aldomet—U.S.; Dopamet—Can.) [B]	250 mg PO tid	Aromatic amino acid decarboxylase inhibitor	Maternal bradycardia
Nifedipine (Adalat, Procardia) [C]	Adalat XL: 30–60 mg PO daily or Adalat PA: 5–10 mg PO q30min	Calcium channel blocker	Maternal tachycardia

*Also see Ch 11 Nephrology.
†**Angiotensin-converting enzyme inhibitors are contraindicated in pregnancy** owing to association with hypocalvaria, oligohydramnios, renal anomalies, neonatal renal failure, pulmonary hypoplasia, and death.
‡Labetalol is considered first-line drug choice in this situation.

Table 13–4. Antiemetic Medications Used in Pregnancy

Generic (Brand) Name	Dose
Dimenhydrinate (Dramamine, Dymenate, Hydrate—*U.S.*; Gravol—*Can.*) [B]	25–50 mg PO/IM/IV or 50–100 mg PR q4hr prn or 100 mg/L in normal saline infused at 100 mL/hr IV
Doxylamine succinate/ pyridoxine hydrochloride (Bendectin, Diclectin)*	1 tablet in morning + 1 tablet in afternoon + 2 tablets in evening
Metoclopramide (Reglan—*U.S.*; Maxeran—*Can.*) [B]	10 mg IM/IV q2–3hr prn or 10–30 mg PO before meals and bedtime (total dose must not exceed 0.5 mg/kg body weight)
Prochlorperazine (Compazine, Compro—*U.S.*; Prorazin, Stemetil—*Can.*) [C]	5–10 mg PO/IM/IV q4hr or 25 mg PR q12hr prn
Systemic corticosteroids, e.g., prednisone (Deltasone—*U.S.*; Winpred—*Can.*) [B]	Individualized (e.g., 5 mg PO qd)

CNS = central nervous system; GI = gastrointestinal.

*Not available in the United States.

INDUCTION AND AUGMENTATION OF LABOR

KY Labor can be induced before its spontaneous onset for a variety of maternal and fetal indications. **Induction is contraindicated if a vaginal birth is unsafe** (e.g., placenta previa, cord prolapse, active genital herpes) **or if forceful uterine contractions cannot be tolerated** (e.g., nonreassuring fetal status, previous uterine surgery). **Labor augmentation** improves the frequency and strength of contractions when spontaneous contractions are inadequate to produce cervical dilatation and descent of the fetus.

TX A favorable cervix is associated with a higher likelihood of successful induction. Cervical ripening can be achieved by mechanical techniques (e.g., intra-cervical Foley catheter) or pharmacologically. Intravenous oxytocin is used to induce periodic uterine contractions.

RX1 Dinoprostone (Cervidil vaginal insert, Prepidil Vaginal Gel, Prostin E$_2$ Vaginal Suppository—*U.S.*) [C]: Simulates natural prostaglandins in the amniotic fluid, leading to biochemical and structural alterations of the cervix.

Mechanism of Action	Side Effects and Cautions
Antihistamine and antiemetic	Drowsiness, dizziness, dry mouth **Contraindicated** in glaucoma and chronic lung disease.
Antihistamine; delayed onset of action	Drowsiness, vertigo, nervousness, epigastric pain, headache, palpitations, diarrhea, disorientation, irritability, convulsions, urinary retention, insomnia
Stimulates upper GI motility; central antagonism of dopamine receptors	Drowsiness, fatigue, insomnia, headache, dizziness, bowel disturbances, and extrapyramidal side effects. **Metoclopramide elevates prolactin levels, and the elevation persists during chronic administration; this may stimulate prolactin-dependent breast cancer.**
Antipsychotic; stimulates chemoreceptor trigger zone	**Safety during pregnancy has not been established,** and its use is left to the judgment of the physician. Causes hypotension and potentiates effects of CNS depressants and anesthetics. **Contraindicated** in severely depressed patients, in the presence of blood dyscrasias, liver disease, renal insufficiency, pheochromocytoma, severe cardiovascular disorders, or history of hypersensitivity to phenothiazine derivatives.
Antiemetic effect is not well established	Side effects depend on the duration of administration and can include glucose intolerance, hypertension, osteoporosis, osteonecrosis, cataract, skin fragility, increased susceptibility to infections, gastric ulcer, cushingoid features, avascular necrosis, myopathy, cataract, glaucoma, and mood changes.

DS1 Prepidil Vaginal Gel contains 2.5 mg of dinoprostone and lasts approximately 6 hours. Cervidil vaginal insert contains 10 mg of dinoprostone released at 0.3 mg/hr over 12 hours; it should be removed after 12 hours or earlier if active labor begins.

SE1 **The major risk is uterine hyperstimulation** (more than five contractions in 10 minutes). An advantage of the vaginal insert is that it can be removed should hyperstimulation occur, with uterine relaxation over the next few minutes. **Side effects** include fever, vomiting, and diarrhea. **Prostaglandins should not be used concomitantly with oxytocin.** The risk of uterine hyperstimulation is increased owing to a synergistic effect.

with or without

RX2 **Oxytocin** (Pitocin—*U.S.*; Toesen—*Can.*): Directly stimulates uterine activity by acting on oxytocin receptors. Its half-life is 3–5 minutes, and a steady state is achieved in 20–40 minutes. Sensitivity varies among individuals, so response must be monitored closely.

DS2 Titrated for a goal of three to five contractions per 10 minutes, with each contraction measuring 25–75 mm Hg above baseline.

Low-dose regimen: Start at 0.5–2 mU/min and increase by 1–2 mU/min every 20–30 minutes to a maximum of 20 mU/min.

High-dose regimen: Start at 6 mU/min and increase by 6 mU every 15 minutes to a maximum of 44 mU/min.

SE2 Contraindicated in the presence of significant cephalopelvic disproportion, severe toxemia, malpresentation, unripe cervix, and grand multiparity. **Side effects** are usually dose related. The most common is nonreassuring fetal status associated with uterine hyperstimulation. **Other risks** include abruptio, uterine rupture, and uterine fatigue with postpartum atony. **Management of hyperstimulation** involves decreasing or stopping the oxytocin infusion, changing maternal position, applying oxygen, and administering IV fluids. If no response, consider magnesium sulphate 2–6 g IV, albuterol or salbutamol (Proventil, Ventolin) 2–6 puffs, or nitroglycerin 50 μg IV.

ISOIMMUNIZATION—ERYTHROBLASTOSIS FETALIS

KY The maternal-fetal circulation is normally separated by the placental barrier. When any fetal blood group factor—most commonly Rhesus (Rh) Factor D—is inherited from the father but not possessed by the mother, a maternal immune response may occur after exposure to this foreign antigen. IgM and then IgG are formed; the latter crosses the placenta and causes fetal red blood cell hemolysis. **This can lead to fetal anemia, heart failure, and hydrops, with death in severe cases.**

TX The administration of anti-D immune globulin (RhoGAM, WinRho) to Rh-negative mothers decreases the risk of sensitization to the D antigen. Thus, all women should be screened for Rh status at the initial prenatal visit, along with ABO blood group and an antibody screen for other more rare antibodies.

RX **Anti-D immune globulin** (RhoGAM, WinRho) [C]: Prevents Rh on fetal red blood cells from sensitizing the Rh-negative mother.

DS **Standard dose: 300 μg IM,** which protects from 30 mL of fetal blood. If exposure greater than this is suspected, the Kleihauer-Betke test is used to quantitate the exposure and the necessary dose of anti-D immune globulin calculated. **If anti-D immune globulin is indicated in the first trimester, only 50 μg is necessary** owing to the small fetal red blood cell mass. It is routinely administered to Rh-negative patients at 28–32 weeks' gestation and within 72 hours after delivery of an Rh-positive baby. **It is indicated** after invasive procedures during pregnancy (amniocentesis, chorionic villous sampling), with ectopic pregnancy, after spontaneous or therapeutic abortion, antepartum hemorrhage, molar pregnancy, intrauterine fetal death, abdominal trauma, and external cephalic version.

SE Risk of transmission of viral infections (human immunodeficiency virus, hepatitis B and C) to mother and fetus.

PAIN MANAGEMENT IN LABOR AND DELIVERY

KY **Early stage 1 pain** occurs from dilatation of the cervix, lower uterine distension, and uterine contraction. Pain impulses travel via visceral afferents and enter the spinal cord at levels T10–L1. **Late stage 1 and stage 2 pain** occurs from contraction of the uterus and from distension and stretching of the pelvic floor, vagina, and perineum. Pain impulses travel via visceral and somatic afferents (pudendal nerve) and enter the spinal cord at levels S2–S4.

TX Pharmacologic relief of pain experienced during labor and delivery include systemic (IV, IM, inhalational routes) and locoregional approaches.

RX1 **Opioids:** See Ch 17 Pain Management. Commonly used agents include Fentanyl (Actiq, Sublimaze), morphine, and nalbuphine (Nubain). Fentanyl is highly lipophilic, with a rapid onset of action.

DS1 Fentanyl: 50–100 mg IV q1hr prn, or administered as patient-controlled analgesia

> Morphine: 5–15 mg IM
> Nalbuphine: 20 mg IM

SE1 Maternal sedation, neonatal respiratory depression (except with fentanyl), nausea, vomiting, pruritus, hypotension, decreased fetal heart rate variability, and impaired early breastfeeding.

ANTIDOTE

For opioid overdose, the antidote is naloxone hydrochloride (Narcan). For the mother, start with 0.4 mg IV and titrate up every 3–5 minutes. **For the newborn,** start at 0.1 mg/kg. Naloxone has a short half-life, and dosages may have to be repeated to maintain reversal.

---

or

RX2 **Nitrous oxide:** See Ch 2 Anesthesiology. Provides modest analgesia during labor and delivery. Not used widely in the United States.

DS2 Patient-controlled inhalational of 40%–50% nitrous oxide.

SE2 Variable effect, maternal amnesia, loss of protective airway reflexes, and pulmonary aspiration of gastric contents.

or

RX3 Anesthetic agents: Can be administered by epidural, general, pudendal block, or spinal anesthesia (Table 13–5).

DS3 Beyond the scope of this chapter.

SE3 Table 13–5

POSTPARTUM HEMORRHAGE (PPH)

KY PPH is defined as any amount of blood loss after delivery that threatens the woman's hemodynamic stability. Early PPH occurs within 24 hours of delivery; late PPH occurs after 24 hours and within 6 weeks.

Table 13–5. Anesthesia Used in Labor and Delivery

Anesthetic Agent		Side Effects and Cautions
Epidural: Injection of local anesthetic with or without opioid into epidural space	Adding narcotics reduces the dose of local anesthetic required for pain relief, thus decreasing motor blockade.	May decrease maternal expulsive effort, thus prolonging stage 2 of labor. Risk of maternal hypotension, which can be reduced by administering 1 L IV bolus.
General anesthetic	Used in cases of emergency caesarian section.	In emergency situations there is an increased risk of maternal aspiration, which can be reduced by using a rapid-sequence induction.
Pudendal block: Local anesthetic injected at the pudendal nerve	Used in late stage 1 and stage 2 of labor.	High failure rate. Local anesthetic toxicity, vaginal laceration, hematoma or abscess formation, direct fetal needle trauma
Spinal: Injection of opioid into sub-arachnoid space	Provides intense motor blockade, rapid onset, lasts 90 minutes.	Hypotension, nausea, vomiting, pruritus, headache

TX Routine oxytocic administration in the third stage of labor after the delivery of the anterior shoulder reduces the risk of PPH. In the event of early PPH, need to explore the lower genital tract (to rule out trauma) and uterus (to rule out retained tissue or uterine inversion); obtain large bore intravenous access; give crystalloids; and send blood for complete blood cell count, coagulation screen (to rule out coagulopathy), and cross-matching. Uterine atony is the most common cause, and it can be treated immediately by uterine massage/compression, removal of clots, and oxytocic agents (Table 13–6). In cases of intractable PPH, surgical management or interventional vascular embolization may be necessary.

RX Table 13–6

DS Table 13–6

SE Table 13–6

PRETERM LABOR

Antenatal Corticosteroid Therapy for Fetal Maturation

KY The benefit of corticosteroid therapy is **risk reduction of neonatal complications** (respiratory distress syndrome, intraventricular hemorrhage, and death).

Table 13–6. Oxytocic Medications Used in the Treatment of Postpartum Hemorrhage

Generic (Brand) Name	Dose	Mechanism of Action	Side Effects and Cautions
Carboprost, tromethamine (Hemabate)	0.25 mg IM/IMM q15min to a maximum 8 doses	Prostaglandins induce smooth muscle contraction.	Fever, nausea, vomiting, diarrhea **Contraindicated** in patients with major cardiac, pulmonary, hepatic, or renal disease.
Ergonovine (Ergotrate maleate) Methylergonovine (Methergine)	0.25 mg IM/IMM q5min to a maximum 5 doses or 1.25 mg IV	Ergots produce tetanic contraction of the uterus.	Causes peripheral vasospasm. **Contraindicated** in patients with hypertension.
Oxytocin (Pitocin—*U.S.*; Toesen—*Can.*)	Prophylaxis: 10 U IM, 5 U IV push, or 20 U/L NS at 125 mL/hr Treatment: 10 U IMM or 20 U/L IV NS at 125 mL/hr	Synthetic posterior pituitary hormone—causes contraction of the uterus.	Theoretical risk of water intoxication at high doses owing to vasopressinlike antidiuretic activity.

TX Treat all women of 24–34 weeks' gestation who are at risk for preterm birth. Optimal benefits begin 24 hours after initiating therapy and last 7 days.

RX **Betamethasone** (Celestone) or **dexamethasone** (Decadron)

DS Betamethasone: two doses of 12 mg IM q12hr or q24hr or

Dexamethasone: four doses of 6 mg IM q6hr or q12hr

SE Little or no mineralocorticoid activity and no significant side effects.

Spontaneous Preterm Labor

KY The etiology of spontaneous onset of labor before 37 weeks' gestation is unknown. It is a major contributor to the 6%–8% incidence of preterm birth, which is a major cause of neonatal morbidity and mortality.

TX There is no effective method of preventing preterm labor. Bed rest, hydration, and sedation are ineffective. Tocolytics may delay delivery by 24–48 hours (Table 13–7), enabling maternal transfer to a tertiary care center and administration of corticosteroids for fetal maturation. Tocolytics have not been shown to improve perinatal outcome and are **contraindicated** in the presence of chorioamnionitis, severe gestational hypertension or eclampsia, fetal demise, nonreassuring fetal or maternal status, or fetal maturity.

RX **Tocolytics:** Include beta-adrenergic receptor antagonists, magnesium sulfate, calcium channel blockers, cyclooxygenase inhibitors, and nitric oxide donors.

DS Table 13–7

SE Table 13–7

PREVENTION OF GROUP B STREPTOCOCCAL (GBS) INFECTION

KY GBS is a major cause of bacterial sepsis in the newborn. Infection occurs before or during the birth process via the colonized mother's genital tract.

TX Intrapartum maternal chemoprophylaxis is the best strategy to reduce neonatal morbidity and mortality. One strategy involves universal screening at 35–37 weeks' gestation with a single rectovaginal GBS culture swab and offering prophylaxis to all GBS-positive women. Another involves offering prophylaxis to women with identified risk factors or with documented GBS bacteriuria during pregnancy or with a previous GBS-infected infant. Intravenous antibiotics should be continued until delivery.

RX Table 13–8

DS Table 13–8

SE Table 13–8

Table 13–7. Tocolytic Medications Used to Delay Preterm Labor

Class	Generic (Brand) Name	Dose	Mechanism of Action	Side Effects and Cautions
Betamimetic	Ritodrine (Yutopar) [B]	50 µg/min continuous IV	Binds to beta-2 adrenergic receptors in myometrium.	Maternal: tachycardia, pulmonary infusion edema, chest pain, nausea, electrocardiographic changes, hyperglycemia, hypokalemia, **death**
	Terbutaline (Brethaire, Brethine, Bricanyl) [B]	0.25 mg SC q1–4hr		
Calcium channel blocker	Nifedipine (Adalat, Procardia) [C]	30 mg PO, then 10–20 mg q4–8hr	Reduces intracellular calcium.	Maternal: hypotension
Prostaglandin synthase inhibitor	Indomethacin (Indocin—*U.S.*; Indocollyre, Indotec—*Can.*) [B/D depending on trimester]	100 mg PR, then 25 mg PO q6hr to a maximum of 8–12 doses	Inhibits both isoforms of cyclooxygenase (COX_1 and COX_2).	Fetal: transient patent ductus arteriosus Neonatal: transient oliguria

Table 13–8. Intravenous Antibiotics Used to Prevent Intrapartum Group B Streptococcal Infection

Generic (Brand) Name	Dose (IV)	Side Effects and Cautions
Ampicillin (Marcillin, Polycillin-N, Principen—*U.S.*; Ampicin, Penbritin—*Can.*) [B]	2 g loading dose, then 1–2 g q4–6hr	Hypersensitivity, which is increased in patients with known infectious mononucleosis or lymphatic leukemia.
Clindamycin (Cleocin—*U.S.*; Dalacin—*Can.*) [B]	600 mg q8hr	Used in cases of penicillin G or ampicillin allergy.
Penicillin G benzathine (Bicillin, Permapen—*U.S.*; Megacillin—*Can.*) [B]	5 MU loading dose, then 2.5–5 MU q4hr	Narrow spectrum of action, less likely to select for antibiotic-resistant organisms. Anaphylaxis reported as 4 in 10,000–100,000.

URINARY TRACT INFECTIONS (UTIs) IN PREGNANCY

KY **UTI is the most common medical complication of pregnancy.** A screening urine culture should be done at the first prenatal visit and repeated in high-risk women at follow-up visits. Given the high risk of developing pyelonephritis in pregnancy, asymptomatic bacteriuria should be treated. Predisposition to UTI in pregnancy is caused by increased urinary stasis related to hormonal and mechanical obstruction. The gravid uterus compresses the ureters, causing dilatation of the ureters, renal pelves, and renal calyces. Increased bladder volume, decreased tone, and increased ureterovesical reflux promote stasis. Increased urinary progestins lead to decreased resistance to invading organisms. Glycosuria provides a habitable milieu for bacteria.

TX The causative organisms are the same as in nonpregnant women, with *Escherichia coli* being most common. **Empiric antibiotics should be started promptly.** Therapy may be modified once the sensitivities are available. **For a simple UTI,** a 7-day course of oral antibiotics is appropriate (Table 13–9). **For pyelonephritis, intravenous antibiotics are indicated** (Table 13–10). **Once the fever and pain have resolved for 24–48 hours, convert to oral antibiotics for a total of 7–10 days.** A follow-up culture should be done 10 days after treatment.

Antibiotic prophylaxis (nitrofurantoin 100 mg PO nightly) is indicated in women with more than two episodes of treated asymptomatic bacteriuria or acute cystitis or one episode of pyelonephritis.

RX Table 13–9 and Table 13–10

DS Table 13–9 and Table 13–10

SE Table 13–9 and Table 13–10

Table 13–9. Oral Antibiotics Used for Urinary Tract Infection During Pregnancy

Generic (Brand) Name	Dose	Side Effects
Nitrofurantoin (Furodantin, Macrobid, Macrodantin—*U.S.*; Nephronex—*Can.*) [B]	100 mg PO bid	Common: nausea, headache, flatulence Rarely, acute pulmonary reactions, hepatitis, peripheral neuropathy
TMP-SMX (Bactrim, Septra) [C/D depending on trimester]	160–800 mg PO bid (equivalent to 1 double-strength tablet PO bid)	Common: nausea, vomiting, rash, urticaria, anorexia Rarely, Stevens-Johnson syndrome, toxic epidermal necrolysis **Caution in first trimester** (TMP is a folate antagonist) **and in the last 6 weeks** (sulfa displaces bilirubin from albumin, giving a risk of kernicterus).
Cephalexin (Keflex) [B]	250–500 mg PO qid	Diarrhea, nausea, vomiting, rash
Erythromycin (Eryc, Erythrocin—*U.S.*; Diomycin, Erybid—*Can.*) [B]	250–500 mg PO qid	Nausea, vomiting, cramps, diarrhea, cholestasis
Amoxicillin-clavulanic acid (Augmentin—*U.S.*; Clavulin—*Can.*) [B]	250 mg PO qid	Nausea, vomiting, cramps, diarrhea, constipation

TMP-SMX = trimethoprim-sulfamethoxazole.

VENOUS THROMBOEMBOLUS (VTE) IN OBSTETRICS

KY **VTE is a leading cause of maternal morbidity and mortality,** occurring in 0.5–3/1,000 pregnancies, with equal frequency in each trimester and postpartum. A hypercoagulable state is physiologic in pregnancy, based on the increase in procoagulants and decrease in anticoagulants. Stasis occurs because of increased venous distensibility and tone, decreased venous flow in lower limbs, and decreased venous return owing to mechanical compression from the enlarging uterus. Endothelial damage occurs at delivery.

TX **Thromboprophylaxis in pregnancy has been controversial, and surveillance can be appropriate for certain groups:**

Patients with **previous VTE associated with transient risk factors** and no current risk factor can be watched and given anticoagulants postpartum.

Table 13–10. Antibiotics Used for the Treatment of Pyelonephritis During Pregnancy

Generic (Brand) Name	Dose	Side Effects
Cefazolin (Ancef, Kefzol) [B]	1–2 g IV q8hr	GI complaints, oral thrush, rash, hypersensitivity reactions
Ampicillin (Marcillin, Polycillin, Principen—*U.S.*; Ampicin—*Can.*) [B] plus	1–2 g IV q6hr plus 1.5 mg/kg IV q8hr	GI complaints, rash, urticaria, hypersensitivity reactions
Gentamicin (Garamycin, Gentacidin—*U.S.*; Cidomycin, Garatec—*Can.*) [C]		Gentamicin is associated with ototoxicity and nephro-toxicity.
Ceftriaxone (Rocephin) [B]	1–2 g IV or IM qd	GI complaints, hypersensitivity reactions

GI = gastrointestinal.

Patients with **either previous episodes of idiopathic VTE or associated with confirmed thrombophilia** (not transiently low free protein S) can either be watched or given a mini-dose of unfractionated heparin (UFH), moderate-dose UFH, or prophylactic low-molecular-weight heparin (LMWH); all with postpartum anticoagulants.

Patients with **thrombophilia without previous VTE** can either be watched or given a mini-dose of UFH or prophylactic LMWH. Prophylaxis indication is stronger in antithrombin-deficient women. Postpartum anticoagulants are indicated.

Patients with **two or more episodes of VTE or undergoing long-term anticoagulation therapy** can undergo adjusted-dose UFH, prophylactic LMWH, or adjusted-dose LMWH; plus postpartum anticoagulants (may be long term).

Treatment options for VTE during pregnancy include adjusted-dose LMWH, or IV UFH bolus followed by infusion followed by adjusted-dose UFH after 5 days; plus postpartum anticoagulants. Heparin can be discontinued 24 hours before induction of labor or whenever true labor begins. Patients at very high risk of recurrence can be switched to IV heparin, which can be discontinued 4–6 hours before expected time of delivery.

RX Table 13–11

DS Table 13–11

SE See Ch 9 Hematology. **UFH is relatively contraindicated** in women with inherited bleeding diathesis or anatomic lesions at risk for bleeding. Complications include bleeding and immune thrombocytopenia. **Avoid concomitant use of antiplatelet agents.**

Table 13–11. Management Options for Venous Thromboembolism in Pregnancy*

Options	Details
UFH [C]	
Mini-dose	5,000 IU SC q12hr
Moderate dose	Adjusted doses, SC q12hr to target anti-Xa level of 0.1–0.3 IU/mL
Adjusted dose	Adjusted doses, SC q12hr to target mid-interval APTT within therapeutic range
	IV schedule: bolus (e.g., 70–80 U/kg), then continuous infusion (e.g., 18 U/kg/hr starting dose) aiming at the therapeutic range.
LMWH [C]	
Prophylactic	Dalteparin (Fragmin) 5,000 IU SC q24hr or enoxaparin (Lovenox) 40 mg SC qd or tinzaparin (Innohep) 75–100 IU/kg SC qd. When in doubt of dose, target peak anti-Xa level of 0.2–0.6 IU/mL.
Adjusted dose	Dalteparin 200 IU/kg SC qd or enoxaparin 1 mg/kg SC q12hr or tinzaparin 175 IU/kg SC qd. Monitoring probably necessary in these patients (e.g., anti-Xa level of 0.5–1 IU/mL).
Postpartum anticoagulation	Warfarin (Coumadin) targeting INR 2–3 for 4–6 weeks with initial overlaps with UFH or LMWH until therapeutic INR.
Surveillance	Clinical observation and aggressive investigation of symptoms suggesting DVT or PE.

anti-Xa = anti–factor Xa; APTT = activated partial thromboplastin time; DVT = deep vein thrombosis; INR = international normalized ratio; LMWH = low-molecular-weight heparin; PE = pulmonary embolus; UFH = unfractionated heparin.

*Also see Ch 9 Hematology.

Heparin effects can be reversed with protamine sulfate (IV push over 10 minutes of 1 mg per 100 IU circulating heparin to a maximum of 250 mg). LMWH complications are the same as for UFH, but the incidence is lower.

Warfarin (Coumadin) is contraindicated in pregnancy owing to fetal warfarin syndrome (nasal hypoplasia and stippled bone epiphyses). Safe in breastfeeding. Major complication is bleeding.

The effects of warfarin can be reversed with vitamin K (0.5–2 mg SC, or 2.5–5 mg PO, or 10–15 mg IV).

VITAMIN SUPPLEMENTATION

KY Supplementation is administered to reduce the risk of neural tube defects and to meet demands of increased requirements during pregnancy.

TX **Folic acid** decreases the risk of neural tube defects. **Iron** requirements increase because of fetal and placental growth and increased maternal red blood cell mass. Supplementation is needed because requirements exceed normal stores and dietary intake.

RX1 **Folic acid** (Folvite—*U.S.*; Flodine—*Can.*) [A] Folic acid is required for the synthesis of purine and pyrimidine.

DS1 The recommended dose is 0.4 mg PO daily (4.0 mg PO daily in high-risk women). Supplementation should ideally start preconceptually and continue throughout the first trimester.

SE1 No significant side effects. Contraindicated in patients with pernicious, aplastic, or normocytic anemia.

RX2 **Iron supplements: Ferrous fumarate** (Femiron, FeoState, Hemocyte, Ircon—*U.S.*; Palafer—*Can.*), **ferrous gluconate** (Fergon—*U.S.*) [A], and **ferrous sulfate** (Feosol, Feratab, Fer-Iron, Slow FE—*U.S.;* Ferodan—*Can.*) [A]

DS2 Ferrous fumarate and ferrous gluconate: 60 mg PO qd, then increased to 60 mg PO bid in later pregnancy or if anemia is identified.

Ferrous sulfate: 300 mg PO qd, then increased to 300 mg PO bid in later pregnancy or if anemia is identified.

SE2 Nausea, epigastric pain, vomiting, abdominal cramps, constipation, and diarrhea. Contraindicated in patients with hemochromatosis or hemolytic anemia.

14
―――――

Oncology

RENAUD WHITTOM, AMIT M. OZA, DAVID
W. HEDLEY, IAN C. QUIRT

This chapter describes some general principles applied in the treatment
of solid tumors, leukemia, and related disorders. The drugs used often
have a narrow therapeutic window, and dosages have to be tailored to
different situations. Thus, individual dosages are beyond the scope of
this chapter.

HEMATOPOIETIC NEOPLASMS

These neoplasms include acute lymphoblastic leukemias, acute myeloblas-
tic leukemias, chronic lymphocytic leukemia and other chronic lymphoproliferative disorders, chronic myelogenous leukemia (CML) and other
myeloproliferative disorders, plasma cell disorders, Hodgkin's lymphoma,
and non-Hodgkin's lymphoma. The lymphomas also have features of solid
tumors.

KY Hematopoietic tissue is widely disseminated in the body. The bone marrow and, in certain circumstances, the spleen and liver can all produce
blood cells. Both mature cells and stem cells can naturally travel through
the organs of the body. Lymphoid cells also travel easily through blood and
the lymphoid system. The neoplasms arising from these tissues can, therefore, disseminate easily. They also harbor detectable genetic defects, more
so than with solid tumors; some translocations are actually pathognomonic
of certain types of neoplasms, such as t (9, 22) in CML and t (15, 17) in
promyelocytic leukemia.

TX Most chemotherapeutic drugs target the DNA of cycling cells and produce DNA damage. Subsequently, the cells either attempt to repair the damage or, alternatively, undergo programmed cell death (apoptosis). The exact
basis for clinical efficacy of various chemotherapy agents is unknown at
this time. The answer may come from the understanding of the probable
complex interplay between mechanisms that control drug uptake, metabolism, and detoxification on the one hand and mechanisms that determine
cell growth and susceptibility to apoptosis on the other. Mechanisms controlling growth and death, in turn, reflect the basic genetic changes
involved in cancer development. **The combination of two or more
chemotherapeutic agents may be superior to single-agent** treatment for
the following reasons:

- Drugs with different mechanisms of action may overcome single-
  drug resistance
- Synergism, in which one agent's effectiveness is augmented by
  another agent, can be achieved

- Drugs whose toxicities do not overlap can be used, thus increasing the therapeutic effect
- Some agents can reach cellular sites not accessible by others

The concept of "total cell kill" implies the complete destruction of all invading cancer cells. Antineoplastic agents follow **first-order kinetics** rather than a constant number of cells killed. Hence, if a certain drug is capable of killing 99.99% of tumor cells and clinically evident tumors are typically in excess of 10^9 cells, then even after therapy there will be about 10^5 tumor cells remaining. These remaining cells can later cause relapse. It is from this concept that the idea of combination therapy evolved. **By using several chemotherapeutic agents concurrently or in rational sequences, one attempts to achieve total cell kill.** Recently, we have witnessed the arrival of some biological agents targeting signal pathways in the cell. Newer agents are antibodies or small molecules that are expected to have a better toxicity profile than classical chemotherapy.

The cells from these neoplasms are often quite sensitive to chemotherapeutic agents. Cure can be achieved with chemotherapy with or without radiation therapy in Hodgkin's disease, intermediate- and high-grade lymphomas, and acute leukemias. Meaningful palliation can be achieved in other instances. Curative combination chemotherapy (e.g., mechlorethamine, vincristine [Oncovin], procarbazine, prednisone regimen in Hodgkin's disease) was a breakthrough. High-dose chemotherapy, taking advantage of the increased cell killing attainable mainly with alkylating agents while circumventing marrow ablation with autologous or allogenic transplant of stem cells, was also first used in these disorders. In addition, the first clinically useful antibody (rituximab [Rituxan] in low-grade lymphoma), the first clinical application of an antiangiogenic agent (thalidomide in multiple myeloma), and the first agent targeting a signal pathway (imatinib [Gleevec] in CML) were all directed at hematopoietic neoplasms.

RX Table 14–1 lists common chemotherapeutic agents and their mechanisms of action against tumor cells. Table 14–2 compares the activity of commonly used agents against certain tumor types. Table 14–3 gives examples of combination regimens used in the treatment of given cancers. Table 14–4 lists available therapeutic agents other than classic chemotherapy.

DS Dosages and protocols for different chemotherapeutic regimens are beyond the scope of the chapter.

SE The immediate side effects caused by chemotherapy are predictable, as treatment frequently affects rapidly proliferating normal tissue, such as bone marrow, gut mucosa, and hair follicles. Another major side effect is nausea and vomiting, probably caused by direct central nervous system effects. Table 14–5 describes these commonly encountered events and the treatment of choice for each. **Chemotherapy is one of the few pharmacologic treatments in which there is a narrow therapeutic index. The more tumor toxicity achieved, the more normal cells destroyed, and, accordingly, the more side effects experienced by the patient.** Hence, chemotherapeutic side effects can be used as a guide to monitor safe drug

(text continues on page 269)

Table 14-1. Established Chemotherapeutic Agents and Their Mechanisms of Action

Class	Generic (Brand) Name	Mechanism of Action
Alkylating agents	Busulfan (Busulfex, Myleran) [D] Chlorambucil (Leukeran) [D] Cyclophosphamide (Cytoxan, Neosar—U.S.; Procytox—Can.) [D] Hexamethylmelamine (Hexalen) Ifosfamide (Ifex) [D] Mechlorethamine (Mustargen) [D] Melphalan (Alkeran) [D] Temozolomide (Temodar) [D] Thiotepa (Thioplex) [D]	**Alkylates DNA; causes breaks in DNA,** interstrand and intrastrand cross-linking Hexamethylmelamine has the structure of an alkylating agent but the mechanism of action is unknown.
Alkylating agents, nonclassical	Dacarbazine (DTIC-Dome) [C] Procarbazine (Matulane—U.S.; Natulan—Can.) [D]	Methylates nucleic acids, blocks replication; procarbazine has various other effects.
Anthracenedione*	Mitoxantrone (Novantrone) [D]	**Intercalates** DNA, interstrand and intrastrand cross-linking, DNA breaks, and topoisomerase II inhibitor
Anthracyclines*	Daunorubicin (Cerubidine) [D] Doxorubicin (Adriamycin, Rubex) [D] Epirubicin (Ellence—U.S.; Pharmorubicin—Can.) [D] Idarubicin (Idamycin) [D] Liposomal daunorubicin (DaunoXome) [D] Liposomal doxorubicin (Doxil—U.S.; Caelyx—Can.) [D]	Multiple effects, including intercalates DNA, direct DNA damage, and inhibits topoisomerase I and, especially, topoisomerase II

(continued)

Table 14–1. Established Chemotherapeutic Agents and Their Mechanisms of Action *(Continued)*

Class	Generic (Brand) Name	Mechanism of Action
Antimetabolites	Capecitabine (Xeloda) [D]	Inhibits methylation of deoxyuridylate to thymidylate
	Cladribine (Leustatin) [D]	Blocks adenosine deaminase, inhibits RNA synthesis
	Cytarabine/ara-C (Cytosar-U) [D]	Inhibits DNA polymerase; ara-CTP incorporates into DNA
	Fludarabine (Fludara) [D]	Inhibits ribonucleotide reductase and DNA polymerase
	Fluorouracil (Adrucil, Carac, Efudex, Fluoroplex) [D]	See Capecitabine
	Gemcitabine (Gemzar) [D]	Di- and triphosphate metabolites inhibit DNA synthesis
	Hydroxyurea (Droxia, Hydrea, Mylocel) [D]	Inhibits ribonucleotide reductase
	Mercaptopurine (Purinethol) [D]	Inhibits purine synthesis; incorporates a metabolite into DNA
	Methotrexate (Folex, Rheumatrex, Trexall) [D]	**Folate antagonist, which interferes with thymidylate synthesis**
	Pentostatin (Nepent) [D]	Inhibits adenosine deaminase, causing toxic buildup of adenine deoxynucleotide; DNA strand breaks
	Raltitrexed (Tomudex)	Inhibits thymidylate synthase
	Thioguanine (Lanvis) [D]	Inhibits purine synthesis; incorporates into DNA and RNA

Antibiotics	Bleomycin (Blenoxane) [D]	Single and double strand breaks from a redox reaction involving oxygen and iron
	Dactinomycin (Cosmegen) [C]	**Intercalates** and cross-links DNA
	Mitomycin (Mutamycin) [D]	Acts as a bifunctional alkylator, which inhibits DNA synthesis
Camptothecin	Irinotecan (Camptosar) [D] Topotecan (Hycamtin) [D]	Topoisomerase I inhibitor
Enzyme	Asparaginase (Elspar) [C]	Depletes asparagine
Epipodophyllotoxins	Etoposide/VP16 (Toposar, Vepesid) [D] Teniposide/VM26 (Vumon) [D]	Topoisomerase II inhibitor
Nitrosoureas	Carmustine [BCNU] (BiCNU, Gliadel) [D] Lomustine [CCNU] (CeeNU) [D] Semustine [methyl-CCNU] Streptozocin (Zanosar) [D]	Chloroethylates DNA, interstrand and intrastrand cross-linking; restricts strand uncoiling and replication
Platinum compounds	Cisplatin (Platinol) [D] Carboplatin (Paraplatin) [D] Oxaliplatin	**Intercalates** and intracalates between DNA strands inhibiting their uncoiling and especially replication
Taxanes	Docetaxel (Taxotere) [D] Paclitaxel (Taxol) [D]	Prevents the depolymerization of microtubules
Vinca alkaloids	Vinblastine (Alkaban-AB, Velban—*U.S.*; Velbe—*Can.*) [D] Vincristine (Oncovin, Vincasar) [D] Vinorelbine (Navelbine) [D]	Alters the microtubular protein, producing mitotic arrest

*Anthracyclines and anthracenedione are also antitumor antibiotics.

Table 14-2. Activity of Selected Chemotherapeutic Agents in the Treatment of Common Cancers*

Agent	ALL	AML	BL	Brain	Breast	CLL	CML	Colon	CX	GC	HL	Lung NSC	Lung SC	Melanoma	Myeloma	NHL	Ovary	Pancreas	Prostate
Alkylators	+++	++	+++	+	++	+++	++	-	+	++	+++	-	++	+	+++	+++	++	-	+
Anthracyclines	+++	+++	+	-	+++	++	++	-	-	++	+++	+	+++	-	+++	+++	+	-	+
Camptothecins								++					++				++		
Cisplatin		-	+++		+			-	++	+++		+	+++	+			+++	-	-
Corticosteroids	+++	-			+	+++					+++				+++	++			-
Cytarabine	+++	+++			+	+	++				++		+	+	-	++			-
Dacarbazine										++	++			+					
Epipodophyllotoxin	+++	++			+	+				++	++		+++		+	++	+		
Fluorouracil	-	-			++	-		++	+	-		-	+					+	-
Gemcitabine			++		++					++		+	+				+	+	
Hydroxyurea	+	++				-	++							-					
Methotrexate	+	-	++		++	+				+	+	+	+	+		+	+		-
Nitrosoureas			-	++	-	++		+			++	-	+	+	+	++	-	-	-
Raltitrexed								++											
Taxanes	+++	-	++	-	+++	++				++		+	++	-	++	++	+++		-
Vincas	+++	-	+	+	++	++	++		-	++	+++	+	++	-	++	++	-	-	+

ALL = acute lymphoblastic leukemia; AML = acute myelogenous leukemia; BL = bladder; CLL = chronic lymphocytic leukemia; CML = chronic myelogenous leukemia; CX = cervix; GC = germ cell (e.g., testes); HL = Hodgkin's lymphoma; Lung NSC = non–small cell lung cancer; Lung SC = small cell lung cancer; NHL = non-Hodgkin's lymphoma; + = drug somewhat active against tumor type; ++ = drug moderately active against tumor type; +++ = drug highly active against tumor type; − = drug not active against tumor type; [blank] = activity of drug unknown in that tumor type or simply not used; bold type = more frequently used drug.

*Note: Within a drug class there may be only one or a few specific drugs that are effective against the tumor sites listed.

268

Table 14–3. Combination Chemotherapeutic Regimens

Cancer	Combination Regimen
ALL	Cytarabine + mitoxantrone Cytarabine + mitoxantrone + methylprednisolone + vincristine Vincristine + prednisone + asparaginase
AML	Daunorubicin + cytarabine
Bladder	**CMV** (cisplatin + methotrexate + vinblastine) Cisplatin + gemcitabine **M-VAC** (methotrexate + vinblastine + doxorubicin + cisplatin)
Breast	**AC** (doxorubicin + cyclophosphamide) **CMF** (cyclophosphamide + methotrexate + fluorouracil) **FAC** (fluorouracil + doxorubicin + cyclophosphamide) **FEC** (fluorouracil + epirubicin + cyclophosphamide) **TAC** (docetaxel + doxorubicin + cyclophosphamide)
Colon	Fluorouracil + leucovorin + irinotecan
Hodgkin's lymphoma	**ABVD** (doxorubicin + bleomycin + vinblastine + dacarbazine) **MOPP** (mechlorethamine + vincristine + procarbazine + prednisone) **MOPP/ABV** (MOPP + doxorubicin + bleomycin + vinblastine)
Lung, small cell	CAV (cyclophosphamide + doxorubicin + vincristine) PE (cisplatin + etoposide)
Lung, non–small cell	Carboplatin + Taxol Cisplatin + gemcitabine Cisplatin + vinorelbine
Non-Hodgkin's lymphoma	**CHOP** (cyclophosphamide + doxorubicin + vincristine + prednisone) **DHAP** (dexamethasone + cytarabine + cisplatin) **ESHAP** (etoposide + Solu-Medrol + ara-C + cisplatin)
Ovary	Cisplatin + cyclophosphamide Paclitaxel + cisplatin
Testis	**PEB** (cisplatin + etoposide + bleomycin)

ALL = acute lymphoblastic leukemia; AML = acute myelogenous leukemia.

dosing. Other side effects are more drug specific, and some can be encountered a long time after the treatment has been completed. The most important of these are included in Table 14–6. As a consequence of the myelosuppressive effects of chemotherapy, many patients experience infections during and after chemotherapy. Table 14–7 lists treatment options most commonly administered. In patients with hematologic malignancies, prophylactic antibiotics can be administered. These patients are sometimes prescribed fluoroquinolone antibiotics, which have been shown to reduce febrile morbidity but not change survival outcome.

Table 14–4. Therapeutic Agents Other Than Classic Chemotherapy

Therapeutic Agents	Mechanism of Action
Agent targeting signal pathways	
ST-571 imatinib (Gleevec) [D]	Tyrosine kinase inhibitor (active in chronic myelogenous leukemia and stromal tumors)
Antiangiogenic agent	
Thalidomide (Thalomid) [X]	Antiangiogenesis (active in multiple myeloma)
Hormonal agents	
Anastrozole (Arimidex) D]	Nonsteroidal inhibitor of aromatase (↓ estrogen)
Bicalutamide (Casodex) [D]	Competitive inhibitor at the androgen receptor level
Corticosteroids (prednisone) [B]	Cytotoxic to lymphoid cells
Exemestane (Aromasin) [D]	Steroidal inactivator of aromatase (↓ estrogen)
Flutamide (Eulexin—*U.S.*; Euflex—*Can.*) [D]	Competitive inhibitor at the androgen receptor level
Goserelin (Zoladex) [X]	LHRH agonist (analog): eventually produces castration level of androgen or estrogen
Letrozole (Femara) [D]	Nonsteroidal inhibitor of aromatase (↓ estrogen)
Leuprolide (Lupron) [X]	LHRH agonist (analog): eventually produces castration level of androgen or estrogen
Megestrol acetate (Megace) [X]	Progestin mechanism uncertain
Tamoxifen (Nolvadex—*U.S.*; Tamofen, Tamone—*Can.*) [D]	Binds to estrogen receptor and blocks estrogen effect
Immune modulators	
Interferon alfa-2B recomb (Intron A) [C]	Complex activity, including direct anti-proliferative effect, activates lymphocytes, antiangiogenic effect among others
Interleukin-2 or aldesleukin (Proleukin) [C]	Stimulates growth and activation of T cells
Monoclonal antibodies	
Rituximab (Rituxan) [C]	Causes B-cell lysis through mechanisms initiated by CD20 receptor binding
Trastuzumab (Herceptin) [B]	Inhibits tumor proliferation through binding to the HER-2 receptor when overexpressed

LHRH = luteinizing hormone–releasing hormone.

SOLID TUMORS

These tumors can arise from virtually all organs in the body. Cancer cells have to acquire different characteristics, including self-renewal and the capacity to invade surrounding tissue and eventually to metastasize. A number of gene defects usually accumulate, some we can detect, for the cells to acquire this malignant phenotype.

Table 14–5. Short-term Side Effects Associated With Chemotherapy

Side Effect	Description	Treatment or Prevention
Alopecia	Hair loss caused by direct cytotoxic effects on the hair follicle. Most commonly caused by anthracycline, cyclophosphamide, dactinomycin, etoposide, irinotecan, and taxanes.	Scalp cooling may reduce hair loss by reducing blood flow through the scalp
Myelosuppression (most problematic side effect, which can be fatal)	Bone marrow suppression (often a dose-limiting factor). Manifests as anemia, leukopenia, and thrombocytopenia.	Antibiotics for fever Blood transfusions Recombinant hematopoietic growth factors: G-CSF or filgrastim (Neupogen) [C] GM-CSF or sargramostim (Leukine) [C] Erythropoietin or epoetin alpha (Epogen, Procrit—U.S.; Eprex—Can.)
Nausea, vomiting	Commonly experienced. Highly emetogenic agents: cisplatin, dacarbazine, high-dose doxorubicin, mechlorethamine, high-dose ara-C, and streptozocin.	Benzamides: Metoclopramide* (Reglan—U.S.; Maxeran—Can.) [B] Phenothiazines: Chlorpromazine (Thorazine—U.S.; Largactil—Can.) [C] Prochlorperazine (Compazine, Compro—U.S.; Stemetil—Can.) [C] Serotoninergic antagonist: Ondansetron (Zofran) [B] Granisetron (Kytril) [B]
Stomatitis	Inflammation of the oral mucosa.	Modification of drug dose Oral antiseptic rinse Topical oral anesthetic: Viscous lidocaine (Xylocaine) [B]

G-CSF = granulocyte colony-stimulating factor; GM-CSF, granulocyte-macrophage colony-stimulating factor.

*Metoclopramide, when used in high dosages, should be administered with an antihistamine (diphenhydramine) or benzodiazepine (lorazepam) to prevent extrapyramidal side effects.

Table 14–6. Drug-Specific Side Effects

Side Effect	Drugs	Note
Cardiotoxicity	Anthracenedione Anthracyclines High-dose cyclophosphamide	Cardiotoxicity is dose related. Protective agent (iron chelator) is available for anthracyclines.
Central nervous system toxicity	High-dose ara-C Rarely, fluorouracil Ifosfamide	Cerebellar toxicity necessitates drug cessation.
Cystitis	Ifosfamide > cyclophosphamide	Hydration Mesna (Mesnex—*U.S.*; Uromitexan—*Can.*) [B]
Diarrhea	Cisplatin Fluorouracil Irinotecan	Dose reduction if not severe. Nonspecific measures.
Extravasation injury	Anthracyclines Mechlorethamine Mitomycin C Vinca alkaloids	Local measures: stopping the infusion, remove drug, apply cold (or heat in the case of vinca alkaloids).
Hypersensitivity	Bleomycin L-asparaginase Paclitaxel	Premedication using steroids with or without diphenhydramine can be useful.
Infertility and menopause	Alkylating agents Nitrosoureas	Side effects are age and dose related.
Lung toxicity	Ara-C Bleomycin Busulfan Carmustine Cyclophosphamide Gemcitabine Methotrexate Mitomycin C	Most frequently dose related, but some cases are acute (e.g., hypersensitivity) and can respond to steroids.
Malignancies (subsequent)	Alkylating agents Anthracyclines Epipodophyllotoxins Nitrosoureas	Alkylators and nitrosoureas can cause leukemia and solid tumors. Anthracyclines and epipodophyllotoxins can cause AML.
Nephrotoxicity	Cisplatin High-dose methotrexate	Vigorous hydration and diuresis prevents toxicity.
Peripheral nerve toxicity	Cisplatin Hexamethylmelamine Procarbazine Taxanes Vinca alkaloids	Drug has to be discontinued if symptoms become severe.

AML = acute myelogenous leukemia.

Early and Locally Advanced Disease

KY **Early disease** refers most of the time to cancer that has not invaded adjacent organs or lymph nodes. Local therapy is paramount at this stage, although chemotherapy or hormonal therapy may have a role. **Locally advanced disease** usually means that an adjacent structure or regional

Table 14–7. Chemotherapy-Induced Infections and Their Pharmacologic Treatment

Infection	Drugs	Doses*
Bacterial	Single-agent therapy: **Ceftazidime** (Ceftaz, Fortaz, Tazicef, Tazidime) [B]	2 g IV q8hr
	Imipenem and cilastatin (Primaxin) [C]	500 mg IV q6hr
	Meropenem (Merrem) [B] Combination therapy:	1 g IV q8hr
	Piperacillin (Pipracil) [B] or	3–4 g IV q4–6hr
	Piperacillin (pip) and **tazobactam** (taz) (Zosyn—*U.S.*; Tazocin—*Can.*) [B] and	(pip) 12–16 g + (taz) 1.5–2 g IV qd in divided doses (q6–8hr)
	Gentamicin† (Garamycin) [C] or any other aminoglycoside	3–5 mg/kg/day IV in divided doses (q8hr)
Cytomegalovirus	**Ganciclovir**† (Cytovene) [C]	Induction dose: 5 mg/kg IV q12hr, then 6 mg/kg IV q24hr
Fungal	**Amphotericin B**† (conventional) (Fungizone) [B] (lipid complex) (Abelcet) [B]	0.3–1.5 mg/kg IV q24hr
Herpes zoster	**Acyclovir**† (Zovirax) or	800 mg PO q4hr
	Famciclovir (Famvir) or	500 mg PO tid
	Valacyclovir (Valtrex) [B]	1,000 mg PO tid
Pneumocystis carinii	**Trimethoprim (TMP)** and **sulfamethoxazole (SMX)** (Bactrim, Septra, Sulfatrim) [C/D at term]	(TMP) 20 mg/kg/day + (SMX) 100 mg/kg/day PO in four divided doses

*Note that doses are approximate, assuming normal organ function (which is not always present, especially in patients with cancer).

†Amphotericin B has been associated with (increased) renal dysfunction (azotemia) when coadministered with other nephrotoxic drugs. Aminoglycosides (i.e., gentamicin), when administered with amphotericin B, can produce additive toxicity to kidneys. Blood levels of aminoglycosides should be checked after the third dose routinely.

lymph nodes are involved. In some cancers, including the most common (i.e., lung, breast, and colon), systemic therapy has become complementary to local therapy to increase survival.

TX **Adjuvant chemotherapy is used in situations in which there is a high risk of recurrence after potentially curative surgery,** for example, lymph node–positive breast or colon cancer. Chemotherapy used in an adjuvant setting may be capable of eliminating micrometastatic disease, even though it cannot eliminate clinically evident metastases. This is explained by the first-order kinetic killing (see HEMATOPOIETIC NEO-PLASMS). **Neoadjuvant chemotherapy means that systemic therapy is used before local therapy takes place.** It can reduce the bulk of tumor, thus reducing morbidity and enhancing the efficiency of local treatment (e.g., cancer of the larynx). It can also eliminate micrometastatic disease. In recent years, it has become apparent that the best way to improve survival sometimes is to use both radiotherapy and chemotherapy at the same time. This concomitant therapy, which increases both response and toxicity, has found a niche in head and neck, lung, esophageal, rectal, and anal cancer.

RX Table 14–1, Table 14–2, Table 14–3, and Table 14–4

DS Dosages and protocols for different chemotherapeutic regimens are beyond the scope of the chapter.

SE Table 14–5, Table 14–6, and Table 14–7

Metastatic Disease

KY When deposits of cancer cells are found outside of the areas of origin, the disease is metastatic.** Most of the time, the goal of treatment is palliative, except for the most responsive diseases (e.g., testicular cancer).

TX The principles supporting the use of chemotherapeutic agents are addressed in HEMATOPOIETIC NEOPLASMS. Biological agents look promising. Hormonal agents that we have used for many years in breast, prostate, and, to a lesser extent, endometrial cancer were already an application of that principle. Immune therapy has a role in a few cancers, such as melanoma and renal cell carcinoma.

RX Table 14–1, Table 14–2, Table 14–3, and Table 14–4

DS Dosages and protocols for different chemotherapeutic regimens are beyond the scope of the chapter.

SE Table 14–5, Table 14–6, and Table 14–7

15

Ophthalmology

NATHALIE LABRECQUE

This chapter focuses on the differential diagnosis of red eye (Table 15–1), with emphasis on the pharmacotherapy of each pathologic condition. Red eye refers to hyperemia, or engorgement, of the superficially visible vessels of the conjunctiva, episclera, or sclera. Hyperemia can be caused by disorders of these structures or of adjoining structures, including the cornea, iris, ciliary body, and ocular adnexa.

CONJUNCTIVITIS

Inflammation of the conjunctiva.

Acute Bacterial Conjunctivitis (Other Than Gonococcal)

KY The etiologic factors in adults include *Staphylococcus aureus* and *Staphylococcus epidermidis*. The etiology in children includes *Streptococcus pneumoniae* and *Haemophilus influenzae*, and it is often associated with upper respiratory tract infections.

TX Bacterial conjunctivitis is treated with frequent antibiotic eyedrops as well as antibiotic ointment applied at bedtime.

RX1 Antibiotic eyedrops/solution: neomycin–polymyxin B–gramicidin (Neosporin); polymyxin B–trimethoprim (Polytrim); and sulfacetamide (Ocu-Sol—*U.S.*, Sulfex—*Can.*) [C]

DS1 Instill 1–2 drops in affected eye q4–6hr for 7–10 days.

SE1 Burning on instillation, local irritation, and hypersensitivity reaction.

with or without

RX2 Antibiotic ointment: bacitracin (Baciguent—*U.S.*; Bacitin—*Can.*), bacitracin–polymyxin-B (AK-Poly-Bac, Polysporin—*U.S.*; Bacimyxin—*Can.*), erythromycin (Erye), sulfacetamide (AK-Sulf—*U.S.*; Sulfex—*Can.*) [C]

DS2 Apply to lower conjunctival sac 2–6 times/day for 7–10 days.

SE2 Local irritation and burning. Rarely, hypersensitivity reactions.

Allergic Conjunctivitis (Including Vernal and Atopic Keratoconjunctivitis)

KY Allergic conjunctivitis is inflammation of the conjunctiva in reaction to an allergin. **Seasonal allergic** conjunctivitis is usually caused by grass pollens and ragweed. **Vernal** keratoconjunctivitis occurs mostly in children

Table 15–1. Differential Diagnosis of Red Eye

Cause of Red Eye	Visual Acuity	Pain	Discharge
Conjunctivitis, acute bacterial	Normal	Mild or burning	Purulent
Conjunctivitis, allergic	Normal	Itching	Mucoid or tearing
Conjunctivitis, herpes simplex virus (with no corneal involvement)	Normal or decreased	Burning	Tearing
Glaucoma, acute	Decreased	Severe pain Nausea	Tearing
Keratitis, bacterial or herpes simplex virus	Usually decreased	Burning	Tearing
Uveitis, anterior	Decreased	Severe pain	Tearing

and young adults with a family history of atopy. **Atopic** keratoconjunctivitis is seen more commonly in the late teens.

TX The treatment of allergic conjunctivitis is directed at the **underlying allergic reaction.** Ophthalmic corticosteroid solutions can be used, but with caution, in the treatment of acute moderate and severe allergic conjunctivitis, especially in vernal and atopic keratoconjunctivitis.

RX Table 15–2

DS Table 15–2

SE Table 15–2

Herpes Simplex Virus Conjunctivitis (With No Corneal Involvement)

KY Usually caused by herpes simplex virus type 1.

TX Treatment consists of **topical antiviral agents.**

RX1 **Trifluridine 1%** (Viroptic) [C]

DS1 Instill 1 drop in eye(s) qid × 1 week.

SE1 Local irritation. Rarely, hyperemia, keratitis, increased intraocular pressure, and hypersensitivity reactions.

Preauricular Adenopathy	Hyperemia	Pupils	Photophobia
Present if gonococcal in adults	Diffuse chemosis	Normal	None
None	Diffuse chemosis	Normal	Usually none
Present	Diffuse chemosis Subconjunctival membrane/ pseudomembrane hemorrhages	Normal	None or present
None	Diffuse	Semidilated and non-reactive to light	Present
None	Ciliary or diffuse	Normal	Present
None	Ciliary or diffuse	Miosis	Present

or

RX2 **Vidarabine 3%** (Vira-A) [C]

DS2 3% ointment applied to lower conjunctival sac 2 times/day.

SE2 Local irritation, lacrimation, and photophobia.

Newborn Conjunctivitis

KY Newborn conjunctivitis can be caused by either a **chemical irritant** or by **bacterial** or **viral** etiologic factors.

TX Treatment depends on the etiology of newborn conjunctivitis.

RX Table 15–3

DS Table 15–3

SE Table 15–3

Viral Conjunctivitis

KY The etiology includes adenovirus and enterovirus 70. Can present with acute hemorrhagic conjunctivitis.

Table 15–2. Drugs Used in Allergic Conjunctivitis

Condition	Class	Generic (Brand) Name
Allergic conjunctivitis (seasonal)	Antiallergic + anti-inflammatory (mast cell stabilizer)	Nedocromil sodium (Alocril—U.S., Mireze—Can.) [B]
	Antihistamine (H₁ blocker)	Levocabastine (Livostin) [C]
	Antihistamine + vasoconstrictor	Antazoline + naphazoline (Vasocon A—U.S., Albalon A—Can.) [C]
		Pheniramine + naphazoline (Naphcon A —U.S.; Opcon A —Can.) [C]
Atopic, vernal, and seasonal kerato conjunctivitis	Mast cell stabilizers	Cromolyn sodium (Opticrom) [B]
		Lodoxamide tromethamine (Alomide) [B]
		Olopatadine (Patanol) [C]

MAO = monoamine oxidase.

TX Treatment includes **artifical tears** and **topical steroids,** such as fluorometholone or prednisolone.

RX Fluorometholone (Flarex, Fluor-Op) or prednisolone acetate [C]

DS Start with 0.125%, 4 times/day for 1 week, then slowly taper.

SE Can cause glaucoma with optic nerve damage, visual acuity and field defects, cataract formation, and secondary ocular infection. Prolonged use may attribute to the development of increased intraocular pressure.

GLAUCOMA

Glaucoma can be defined as a group of diseases that share two of the following three elements: ocular hypertension, progressive atrophy/excavation of the optic nerve, and visual field loss.

Dose	Side Effects
1–2 drops in eye(s) bid	Headache and local irritation and burning Rarely, eye redness, photophobia, asthma
1 drop in eye(s) qid for up to 2 weeks	Local irritation Rarely, headache, blurred vision, eye pain, eye redness, dyspnea
1–2 drops in eye(s) q3–4hr	Local irritation, headache, hypertension, mydriasis, increased intraocular pressure, blurred vision
1–2 drops in eye(s) q3–4hr	Pupillary dilation, increase in intraocular pressure, hypertension, hyperglycemia Increased adrenergic effects may result with concomitant MAO inhibitor administration.
1–2 drops in eye(s) q4–6hr	Local irritation
1–2 drops in eye(s) q6hr for up to 3 months	Local irritation, headache, corneal erosion/ulcer and abrasion Patients cannot wear soft contact lenses during treatment.
1–2 drops in eye(s) bid for up to 6 weeks	Headache, local irritation

Acute Glaucoma

KY **Pupillary block is responsible for closed-angle glaucoma;** this occurs when the aqueous humor flows between the posterior and the anterior chambers, causing apposition of the iris on the surface of the lens. Because elimination of the aqueous humor is impossible, the intraocular pressure increases very rapidly. **Risk factors** for acute glaucoma include age ($\geq$ 60 years), sex (women more than men), race (white), hypermetropia, and chronic uveitis.

TX Pharmacologic treatment options include **topical beta-blockers, carbonic anhydrase inhibitors,** and **osmotic agents** when the glaucoma is severe or when the pressure is unable to be controlled by other agents. **Laser iridotomy is the definitive treatment option.**

RX Table 15–4

Table 15–3. Etiology and Treatment of Newborn Conjunctivitis

Etiology	Generic (Brand) Name	Dose	Side Effects
Chemical (e.g., silver nitrate)	No treatment		
Bacteria	**Gram-negative bacteria:** Tobramycin (Tobrex) or gentamicin (Genoptic—*U.S.*, Lomicin Ophthalmic, Ocugram—*Can.*) **Gram-positive bacteria:** Bacitracin ointment (Baciguent—*U.S.*, Bacitin—*Can.*)	1–2 drops in eye(s) q4hr and reduce to less frequent intervals over 2 weeks Apply into conjunctival sac qid for 2 weeks	Local irritation
Chlamydia	Erythromycin (EryPed) Erythromycin ointment (Ilotycin)	50 mg/kg/day PO (divided into four doses) for 2–3 weeks Apply into conjunctival sac qid for 2 weeks	Cardiac arrhythmias, oral candidiasis, diarrhea, pseudomembranous colitis, eosinophilia, hepatic impairment, allergic reactions Local irritation
Herpes simplex virus	See treatment for herpes simplex corneal keratitis, Table 15–6		
*Neisseria gonorrhea**	Ceftriaxone (Rocephin) Bacitracin ointment (Baciguent—*U.S.*, Bacitin—*Can.*)	25–50 mg/kg (maximum 125 mg) IM/IV single dose Infection treatment: 25–50 mg/kg (maximum 125 mg) IM/IV q24hr for 10–14 days Apply into conjunctival sac q4hr for 2 weeks	Hypersensitivity, eosinophilia, thrombocytosis, leukopenia, elevation in liver function tests (ALT, ALP, AST) and bilirubin Local irritation

ALT = alanine transaminase; ALP = alkaline phosphatase; AST = aspartate transaminase.
*Treat also for *Chlamydia* infection.

DS Table 15–4
SE Table 15–4

Chronic Glaucoma

KY **Risk factors** for chronic open angle glaucoma include the following: ocular hypertension, age ($\geq$ 40 years), family history of glaucoma, long-term use of topical steroids, diabetes, myopia, black race, and vasospastic vascular disease. Symptoms are usually absent until late in the disease and may begin with decreased night vision.

TX **The goal of treatment is to decrease intraocular pressure** to prevent atrophy of the optic nerve and, thus, loss of visual fields. **The treatment of choice is based on the characteristics of the individual patient,** such as age, systemic diseases, cataracts, pseudophakia, and glaucoma evolution. Table 15–4 describes the various treatment options for glaucoma.

RX Table 15–4
DS Table 15–4
SE Table 15–4

KERATITIS AND KERATOCONJUNCTIVITIS

Inflammation of the cornea and conjunctiva.

Bacterial Keratitis

KY Corneal infection is usually secondary to trauma, prolonged contact lens wear, or chronic corneal disease. **Bacteria that are most often involved** in bacterial keratitis are staphylococci and streptococci; however, in contact lens wearers, *Pseudomonas aeruginosa* infection can occur.

TX **Topical medication** (Table 15–5) **is the treatment of choice** because of the efficient absorption of most of the antibiotics used and the possibility of achieving high intracorneal concentrations. In general, corneal infiltrates and ulcers of unknown etiology are **treated as bacterial until proven otherwise** by laboratory studies. Always **keep in mind the possibility of a fungal or acanthamoeba keratitis.**

RX Table 15–5
DS Table 15–5
SE Table 15–5

Herpes Simplex Corneal Keratitis

KY A common inflammation of the cornea caused by the herpes simplex virus. It is **potentially serious and can lead to corneal ulceration.**

TX Treatment is **topical** and/or systemic if there is stromal or uveitis, and depends on the degree of involvement, as outlined in Table 15–6.

RX Table 15–6

Table 15–4. Treatment Options for Glaucoma

Class	Generic (Brand) Name
Topical beta-blockers (decrease aqueous humor production)	Timolol (Timoptic, 0.25%, 0.5%) [C]
	Levobunolol (Betagan, 0.25%, 0.5%—*U.S.*; Ophtho-Bunolol—*Can.*) [C] Betaxolol (Betoptic) [C]
Parasympathomimetics (increase aqueous humor production)	Pilocarpine (Isopto Carpine, Miocarpine, 1%, 2%, 4%, 6% solution; Pilopine, 4% [gel]) [C]
	Carbachol (Carboptic, 0.75%–3%) [C]
Adrenergic agonists (β_2 agonists; increase aqueous humor outflow)	Apraclonidine (Iopidine, 0.5%) [C]
	Brimonidine (Alphagan, 0.2%) [B]
Carbonic anhydrase inhibitors (decrease aqueous humor production)	Acetazolamide Diamox—*U.S.*; Acetazolam—*Can.* [C]
	Dorzolamide (Trusopt, 2% topical) [C] Brinzolamide (Azopt, 2% topical) [C]
Prostaglandin analogs (increase uveoscleral outflow)	Latanoprost (Xalatan, 0.005%) [C] Travoprost (Travatan, 0.004%) [C]
Prostamide analogs (increase uveoscleral outflow and trabecular meshwork outflow)	Bimatoprost (Lumigan, 0.03%) [C]
Beta-blocker and carbonic anhydrase inhibitor	Dorzolamide, 2% + timolol, 0.5% (Cosopt)

DS Table 15–6
SE Table 15–6

UVEITIS

The uvea is composed of three ocular structures: the iris, the ciliary body, and the choroid. Although the uvea is often the site of ocular inflammation, the primary site of inflammation may come from another ocular structure (e.g., cornea, retina, or sclera).

Dose	Side Effects
Instill 1 drop in eye(s) bid	Chronic pulmonary obstructive disease, cardiac arrhythmias, cardiac insufficiency
Instill 1 drop in eye(s) qd–bid	
Instill 1 drop in eye(s) bid	
Instill 1–2 drops in eye(s) up to 6 times/day as needed to control intraocular pressure	Local irritation, headache, hypotension, hypersensitivity reactions. Parasympathomimetics must be discontinued 6 weeks if needs general anesthesia that contains succinylcholine
Instill 1–2 drops in eye(s) up to tid	
Instill 1 drop in eye(s) bid	
Instill 1–2 drops in eye(s) tid	Hypertension, tachycardia, cystoid macular edema, allergic conjunctivitis
Instill 1 drop in eye(s) q8hr	Blurred vision, local irritation, allergic conjunctivitis
	Headache, conjunctival hyperemia, allergic conjunctivitis
Acute: 250–500 mg IM/IV and repeat in 2–4 hours (maximum 1 g/day)	Renal or hepatic insufficiency, electrolytic disorders, allergic reactions, aplastic anemia
Chronic: 250 mg PO qd–qid	
Instill 1 drop in eye(s) tid	
Instill 1 drop in eye(s) tid	
Instill 1 drop in eye(s) qhs	Increased iris pigmentation, hypertrichosis, iritis, cystoid macular edema, and conjunctival hyperemia.
Instill 1 drop in eye(s) qhs	
Instill 1 drop in eye(s) qhs	Increased iris pigmentation, hypertrichosis, and conjunctival hyperemia.
Instill 1 drop q12hr	See beta-blockers and carbonic anhydrase.

Anterior Uveitis (Noninfectious)

KY Anterior uveitis (iritis, iridocyclitis) can be caused by idiopathic noninfectious and infectious etiologies. **Noninfectious:** Ankylosing spondylitis, Behçet disease, corneal graft rejection, Fuchs heterochromia, HLA-B$_{27}$, inflammatory bowel disease, juvenile arthritis, lens induced, psoriatic arthritis, Reiter's syndrome/reactive arthritis, sarcoidosis, secondary to posterior inflammation, and trauma. **Infectious:** Exogenous or endogenous endophthalmitis, herpes simplex virus, herpes zoster virus, other retinitis or choroiditis of infectious etiology, syphilis, and toxoplasmosis.

Table 15-5. Treatment Options for Bacterial Keratitis

Generic (Brand) Name	Dose	Effective Against	Side Effects
Bacitracin (Baciguent—*U.S.*; Bacitin—*Can.*) [C]	Ointment: Apply into conjunctival sac q3–4hr for 7–10 days	Gram positive mostly (staphylococci)	Hypersensitivity, local irritation
Polymyxin B + trimethoprim (Polytrim) [C]	Solution: Instill 1–2 drops in eye(s) q4–6hr for 7–10 days	Broad spectrum	Local irritation, pruritus, hypersensitivity
Aminoglycosides:			
Gentamicin (Garamycin, Genoptic) [C]	Ointment: Apply into conjunctival sac 2–6 times/day	Gram negative mostly	Local irritation, corneal toxicity
Tobramycin (AKTob, Tobrex)	Solution: Instill 1–2 drops in eye(s) q2–4hr		
Quinolones:			
Norfloxacin (Chibroxin) [C]	Solution: Instill 1–2 drops in eye(s) qid for up to 7 days	Gram positive mostly (staphylococci)	Local irritation, photophobia, pruritus
Ciprofloxacin (Ciloxan, Cipro) [C]		Broad spectrum	
Ofloxacin (Floxin, Ocuflox) [C]		Broad spectrum	

Table 15–6. Treatment of Herpes Simplex Corneal Keratitis

Treatment	Corneal Epithelial Disease	Corneal Stromal Disease	Side Effects
Trifluridine 1% drops (Viroptic) [C]	9 times/day	4 times/day	Local irritation, superficial keratitis
Vidarabine 3% (Vira-A) ointment [C]	5 times/day	Not used	Local irritation, keratitis, photophobia, and uveitis.
Prednisolone acetate (Pred Forte) 1% drops [C]	**Contraindicated**	4 times/day, if condition is severe or central	Herpes simplex epithelial keratitis, cataract, glaucoma, ptosis, mydriasis
Cycloplegics (Homatropine 5%) drops [C]	If iritis present, bid	2 times/day	Loss of accommodation, mydriasis, photophobia
Valacyclovir (Valtrex) [B]	—	5 mg PO qd × 3–6 months	Headache, nausea, and GI irritation
Acyclovir (Zovirax—U.S.; Aviran—Can.)	—	400 mg PO qd	Headache, nausea, and GI irritation

TX Treatment depends on the etiology, severity, and response to initial treatment. Topical steroids and cycloplegics are first-line treatment options for noninfectious uveitis. If there is no favorable response to this, the use of subconjunctival steroids is warranted. If treatment is still unsuccessful, consider the use of systemic steroids, immunosuppressive agents, or both.

RX1 Topical steroids: Prednisolone acetate, dexamethasone.

DS1 Topical application qid and up to q30min as needed.

SE1 Local irritation and aggravation and masking of infection.

RX2 Homatropine (Isopto-Homatropine) [C]: Anticholinergic agent.

DS2 Topical application bid–qid.

SE2 Local irritation.

RX3 Triamcinolone acetonide (Kenalog): Only used if no response to topical treatment.

DS3 Inject 1 cc subconjunctival of a 40 mg/cc solution.

SE3 Glaucoma, anaphylactoid reaction, and aggravation and masking of infection. With long-term use, headache, hypopigmentation, and cataracts.

16

Otolaryngology

ADRIAN L. JAMES, BLAKE C. PAPSIN

Otolaryngology encompasses the wide variety of pathology that affects the **ear, nose, and throat**. This chapter focuses on those conditions that respond to pharmacologic treatment. Many conditions are best managed by surgical intervention, but these are beyond the scope of this text.

THE EAR

Acute Otitis Media

KY An **acute infection of the middle ear,** more common in children, that usually resolves spontaneously, through rupture of the eardrum. It is followed by an effusion. Rarely, there are serious local or intracranial complications. *Streptococcus pneumoniae, Moraxella catarrhalis,* and *Haemophilus influenzae* are the most common pathogens.

TX **Analgesics and antipyretics** are required. Antibiotic use, although common, is controversial; it reduces risks of rare complications and leads to a more rapid diminution of pain but has been implicated in increasing antibiotic resistance. **Surgery** is required when significant antibiotic resistance is encountered or when complications occur (e.g., facial paralysis).

RX1 **Acetaminophen** (Tylenol) [B]: This drug is a prostaglandin synthesis inhibitor in the central nervous system.

DS1 0.5–1 g PO qid (**PEDS:** — *15 mg/kg PO qid*)

SE1 There is a **risk of hepatic impairment.** In situations of **overdose** (> 150 μg/mL at 4 hours), acetaminophen causes hepatotoxicity.

ANTIDOTE

Antidote for acetaminophen intoxication is acetylcysteine (Mucomyst, Mucosil—*U.S.*; Parvolex—*Can.*) 140 mg/kg PO loading dose followed by 70 mg/kg PO q4hr for 72 hours (total dose 1,330 mg/kg). In Canada, acetylcysteine 300 mg/kg is given by continuous IV infusion over 20 hours.

or

RX2 **Ibuprofen** (Advil, Motrin) [B/D depending on trimester]: This is a nonsteroidal anti-inflammatory.

DS2 400–600 mg PO tid (**PEDS:** — *5–10 mg/kg PO tid–qid*)

SE2 Risk of peptic ulceration, exacerbation of asthma, and bleeding if surgery is required.

or

RX3 **Amoxicillin** (Amoxil) [B]: This is a semisynthetic penicillin of the aminopenicillin group. It acts by inhibiting the mucopeptide synthesis in the bacterial cell wall (Table 16–1).

DS3 Recommended regular dosing is 20–50 mg/kg/day PO divided tid. High dose is 80–90 mg/kg/day PO divided tid and may be used in patients for whom regular-dose amoxicillin was not effective.

SE3 Urticaria, diarrhea, and anaphylaxis. **Amoxicillin should be avoided in the setting of infectious mononucleosis** owing to an increased incidence of maculopapular rash. Dosage is decreased in renal impairment.

Chronic Suppurative Otitis Media

KY Chronic purulent otorrhea through a defect in the tympanic membrane, which is associated with inflammation of the middle ear mucosa or cholesteatoma. Pseudomonas, *Staphylococcus aureus,* and anaerobic bacteria are commonly associated pathogens. **Serious local and intracranial complications can follow.**

TX Inflammation and discharge can virtually always be controlled by **topical preparations** (Table 16–2). **Aminoglycoside drops, although effective, should be used with caution because of ototoxicity.** Short courses are recommended. **Surgery** is necessary to remove cholesteatoma.

RX Table 16–2

DS Table 16–2

SE Table 16–2

Ménière's Disease

KY This **triad of vertigo, sensorineural hearing loss, and tinnitus** is associated with **endolymphatic hydrops** (raised pressure in the inner ear), but the pathophysiology is uncertain.

TX **Antivertiginous drugs** are useful in symptom control (see Table 16–3). **Betahistine** and **diuretics** are used to try to prevent further attacks (although no good evidence of efficacy is shown). **When vertigo is debilitating it can be abolished by the vestibulotoxic effect of instilling high-dose aminoglycosides into the middle ear. Surgery is occasionally required for refractory cases.**

RX1 **Betahistine:** This drug probably works by improving blood flow through the cochlea or by inhibiting the vestibular nuclei via histamine receptors.

DS1 8–16 mg PO tid

SE1 Peptic ulceration and exacerbation of pheochromocytoma.

(text continues on page 292)

Table 16–1. Oral Antibiotics for Otolaryngologic Infections

Generic (Brand) Name	Adult Dose PO (Pediatric Dose PO)	Indications	Side Effects
Amoxicillin (Amoxil) [B]*	500 mg tid (6–15 mg/kg tid)	Acute otitis media (first line)	Anaphylaxis, diarrhea, urticaria
Amoxicillin-clavulanate (Augmentin—U.S., Clavulin—Can.) [B]	500/125 mg tid (13 mg/kg tid)	Acute otitis media Neck space infections Sinusitis	Anaphylaxis, diarrhea, hepatic impairment, urticaria
Cefaclor (Ceclor) [B]	250–500 mg tid (7–13 mg/kg tid)	Acute otitis media Sinusitis	Anaphylaxis, GI upset, urticaria
Cefixime (Suprax) [B]	200 mg bid (8 mg/kg daily)	Acute otitis media Sinusitis	Anaphylaxis, GI upset, urticaria
Ciprofloxacin (Ciloxan, Cipro) [C]	500 mg bid (not applicable in children)	Acute otitis media	GI upset, hepatic or renal failure, growth impairment (questionable)

Clarithromycin (Biaxin)† [C]	250–500 mg bid (7.5 mg/kg bid)	Acute otitis media Sinusitis	GI upset
Clindamycin (Cleocin—*U.S.*; Dalacin—*Can.*) [B]	150–300 mg qid (2.5–7.5 mg/kg qid)	Neck space infections Tonsillitis (second line)	Jaundice, pseudomembranous colitis, rash
Erythromycin (Eryc, EryPed, Erythrocin—*U.S.*; Diomycin, Erybid—*Can.*) [B]	250–500 mg qid (10 mg/kg qid)	Acute otitis media Tonsillitis (second line)	GI upset, urticaria
Penicillin V potassium (Suspen, Truxcillin, Veetids—*U.S.*; Nadopen—*Can.*) [B]	500 mg qid (6–15 mg/kg tid–qid)	Tonsillitis	Anaphylaxis, diarrhea, urticaria
Trimethoprim/sulfamethoxazole (Septra)	Not generally used in adults with this infection (4/20 mg/kg bid)	Acute otitis media	GI upset, hypersensitivity reactions

GI = gastrointestinal.

*Avoid amoxicillin in the presence of infectious mononucleosis because of increased incidence of maculopapular rash.

†Clarithromycin is principally excreted by the kidney and liver, so for patients with both liver and renal impairment, or severe renal impairment, decreased dosage or a prolonged dosing interval must be used.

Table 16–2. Topical Preparations for Ear Disease

Brand Name	Contents	Dose	Indications
Auralgan [C]	Antipyrine (analgesic) and benzocaine	Insert saturated cotton plug into ear canal; change 5–6 times/day for 3 days	Acute otitis media Otitis externa
Chloromycetin [C]	Chloramphenicol	2–3 drops tid–qid for 7 days	Otitis externa
Cipro-HC Otic	Ciprofloxacin Hydrocortisone	1–2 drops bid for 7 days	CSOM
Garamycin* [C]	Gentamicin	3–4 drops tid for 7 days	CSOM* Otitis externa
Vioform—U.S.; Clioquinol—Can. [C]	Flumethasone pivalate Clioquinol	2–3 drops bid for 7 days	CSOM Fungal otitis externa
NeoDecadron [C]	Neomycin Dexamethasone	3–4 drops bid–tid for 7 days	CSOM* Dermatitis Eczema Otitis externa
Neosporin [C]	Neomycin Polymyxin B	3–4 drops bid–qid for 7 days	CSOM* Otitis externa

CSOM = chronic suppurative otitis media.

*Aminoglycoside-containing drops should be **used with caution and for short periods only in the presence of a perforated eardrum** because of the **risk of ototoxicity**.

Table 16-3. Antivertiginous Drugs

Class	Generic (Brand) Name	Dose	Mechanism of Action	Side Effects	Contraindications
Anticholinergics	Scopolamine (Scopace, Transderm Scop—*U.S.*; Buscopan, Transderm-V—*Can.*) [C]	300 µg PO tid, or 1 skin patch (1.5 mg/patch) q3d	Muscarinic antagonists: central vestibular suppression	Drowsiness, blurred vision, urinary retention	Closed angle glaucoma Prostatic hypertrophy
Antihistamines	Cyclizine (Marzine—*U.S.*) [B]	50 mg PO, PR, or IM tid	Histaminergic and muscarinic antagonists: central vestibular suppression	Sedation, dry mouth, extrapyramidal symptoms	Caution when using dimenhydrinate in the presence of closed angle glaucoma, stenotic peptic ulcer, urinary tract obstruction, cardiovascular disease
	Dimenhydrinate (Calm-X, Dramamine, Dymenate, Hydrate—*U.S.*; Gravol—*Can.*) [B]	50–100 mg PO, PR, or IM tid			
Benzodiazepines	Diazepam (Valium) [D]	2 mg PO tid (1 mg in elderly patients)	GABA receptor modification: sedative and anxiolytic	Prolonged drowsiness, confusion, dependence	Respiratory depression
Phenothiazines	Prochlorperazine (Compazine, Compro—*U.S.*; Prorazin, Stemetil—*Can.*) [C]	5 mg PO or SL tid, or 12.5 mg IM	Central vestibular suppression	Extrapyramidal symptoms, drowsiness, hypotension	Pheochromocytoma

291

or

RX2 **Hydrochlorothiazide** (HydroDIURIL) [B]: This diuretic and antihypertensive drug interferes with the renal tubular mechanism of electrolyte reabsorption, increasing the excretion of sodium and chloride.

DS2 25 mg PO qd

SE2 Electrolyte disturbances (e.g., hypokalemia) and postural hypotension.

Otitis

See Acute Otitis Media, Chronic Suppurative Otitis Media, and Otitis Externa (OE).

Otitis Externa (OE)

KY **Infection of the skin of the ear canal** is facilitated by entry of water and trauma by scratching. *Pseudomonas aeruginosa,* streptococci, and fungi are commonly involved. Progression to skull base osteomyelitis in people with diabetes and the immunocompromised patient is known as **necrotizing OE.**

TX **Aural toilet** (using suction and an otologic microscope) and **keeping the ear dry** are important treatments. Numerous **antiseptic** and **antibiotic** preparations are used (for examples, see Table 16–2). **Necrotizing OE requires systemic antibiotics** (Table 16–4) **and surgical debridement.**

RX Table 16–2 and Table 16–4

DS Table 16–2 and Table 16–4

SE Table 16–2 and Table 16–4

Otitis Media

See Acute Otitis Media and Chronic Suppurative Otitis Media.

Vertigo

KY Vertigo is an illusion of movement in which the sufferer classically feels everything rotating around him. It arises from disturbances of the inner ear or central vestibular system.

TX **Identification of the cause** of vertigo should be the first part of management to allow definitive treatment. For **symptomatic relief** of vertigo, see Table 16–3.

RX Table 16–3

DS Table 16–3

SE Table 16–3

Table 16-4. Intravenous Antibiotics for Severe Otolaryngologic Infections

Generic (Brand) Name	Adult Dose PO (Pediatric Dose PO)	Indications	Side Effects
Amoxicillin-clavulanate	1.2 g tid (25 mg/kg tid) Infuse slowly	Neck space infections Otitis media Sialadenitis Sinusitis	Table 16-1
Ceftazidime (Ceptaz, Fortaz, Tazicef, Tazidime) [B]	1-2 g bid-tid (25-50 mg/kg tid)	Otitis externa	Anaphylaxis, GI disturbance, urticaria
Cefuroxime (Ceftin, Kefurox, Zinacef) [B]	0.75-1.5 g tid (25 mg/kg tid)	Epiglottitis Neck space infections (use with metronidazole) Otitis media	Same as for ceftazidime
Clindamycin	300-600 mg tid (4-10 mg/kg tid-qid)	Neck space infections	Table 16-1
Gentamicin (Garamycin, Gentacidin—*U.S.*; Cidomycin—*Can.*) [C]*	1-2.5 mg/kg bid (1-2.5 mg/kg bid)	Necrotizing otitis externa	Ototoxicity and vestibular toxicity, nephrotoxicity, hypersensitivity reactions
Metronidazole (Flagyl) [B]	500 mg tid (10 mg/kg tid)	With penicillin or cefuroxime in tonsillitis and neck space infections	GI upset, headache, seizure, disulfiram-type reaction with alcohol, pancreatitis
Penicillin G (Pfizerpen) [B]	0.6-1.2 g qid (15-60 mg/kg qid)	Tonsillitis (use with metronidazole)	Anaphylaxis, urticaria

GI = gastrointestinal.
*Decreased doses required in the presence of renal impairment; monitoring of levels is essential.

THE NOSE

Acute Sinusitis

KY Acute infection localized to one or more sinuses is usually bacterial (*S. pneumoniae, M. catarrhalis,* and *H. influenzae*). It is associated with rhinitis (see below). Although usually self-limiting, it may persist (chronic sinusitis is defined as > 3 months of symptoms). **Serious intraorbital and intracranial complications can occur from acute and chronic sinusitis.**

TX Treatment of acute sinusitis is with **analgesia, topical decongestants,** and **antibiotics.** Topical decongestants relieve blockage but should be used for short periods only to avoid the rebound phenomenon of rhinitis medicamentosa. For chronic sinusitis, see Rhinosinusitis. **Surgical intervention** is indicated in severe or complicated acute sinusitis and chronic disease.

RX1 **Xylometazoline** (Otrivin) [C]: This is a sympathomimetic decongestant.

DS1 2–3 drops in each nostril bid (for a maximum of 7 days).

SE1 When used for > 7 days, there is increased risk of developing rhinitis medicamentosa.

or

RX2 **Amoxicillin-clavulanate** (*Augmentin—U.S.; Clavulin—Can.*) [B]

DS2 Table 16–1 and Table 16–4

SE2 Table 16–1 and Table 16–4

or

RX3 **Clarithromycin** (Biaxin) [C]

DS3 Table 16–1

SE3 Table 16–1

Epistaxis

KY Rupture of blood vessels in the anterior nasal mucosa is often secondary to trauma from nose picking. Spontaneous bleeding also occurs posteriorly.

TX **Application of pressure or packing** stops most bleeding. **Topical decongestants** (see Acute Sinusitis) may help. **Cauterization** (with heat or silver nitrate) is effective. **Antibiotic ointment** can reduce further episodes.

RX **Bacitracin, neomycin, polymyxin B, and hydrocortisone** (Cortisporin) [C]: Bacitracin, neomycin, and polymyxin B reduce bacterial activity; hydrocortisone reduces inflammation; and the ointment prevents drying of the mucosa.

DS Smear inside nostril bid for 10 days.

SE No significant side effects.

Rhinosinusitis

KY Rhinitis, inflammation of the nasal mucosa, is **caused by allergy** (seasonal, e.g., hayfever, and perennial, e.g., to house dust mite) or **infection** (viral, e.g., the common cold, or bacterial), or **it may be vasomotor** (i.e., sympathetic underactivity). Because these processes may affect the sinus mucosa along with the nasal mucosa, rhinosinusitis is a better term.

TX Most forms of rhinosinusitis improve with **topical corticosteroids.** Benefit typically occurs after 2–3 weeks of regular use and requires good compliance to be maintained. **Antihistamines** are effective in allergic disease.

RX1 **Mometasone furoate** (Elocon, Nasonex) or fluticasone (Flonase) [C]: **Corticosteroid agents** that reduce mucosal inflammation.

DS1 Two sprays in each side of the nose daily (**PEDS:** *[4–11 years]—one spray in each side*).

SE1 Prolonged use in children has a theoretical risk of growth impairment. Can cause mild epistaxis.

or

RX2 **Loratadine** (Claritin) [B]: This is an H_1 receptor antagonist.

DS2 10 mg PO qd (**PEDS:** *[2–5 years]—5 mg PO qd*)

SE2 **Contraindicated in the presence of glaucoma and hepatic disease.** Can rarely cause sedation.

Sinusitis

See Acute Sinusitis and Rhinosinusitis.

THE THROAT

Epiglottitis

KY In children, *H. influenzae* was previously a common cause, but the disease has become rare since introduction of the *H. influenzae* type b vaccine. Other upper aerodigestive tract organisms can cause infection and inflammation of the supraglottic area in children and adults. **Fatal airway obstruction occurs readily without adequate treatment.**

TX The priority is airway protection: this may require **intubation** (which is difficult and requires experienced hands) or **tracheotomy.** Inhalation of **nebulized epinephrine** (adrenaline) and **intravenous steroids** reduce airway inflammation. **Intravenous antibiotics are essential. Medical therapy of epiglottitis requires administration of the three drugs described next.**

RX **Epinephrine or adrenaline (racemic)** [C]: This agent causes mucosal vasoconstriction.

DS 0.5 mL of 2.25% in 3 mL of normal saline q15min via nebulizer.

SE **Caution in ischemic heart disease.** Can cause tachycardia, tremor, and restlessness.

with

RX **Hydrocortisone [C]:** This is a corticosteroid that reduces inflammation.

DS 100 mg IV qid (**PEDS:** — *5 mg/kg IV qid*)

SE Aggravation of diabetes, gastrointestinal upset, and avascular osteonecrosis of the femoral head.

with

RX **Cefuroxime** (Ceftin, Kefurox, Zinacef) [B]

DS Table 16–4

SE Table 16–4

Neck Space Infections

KY Infection can spread from tonsillitis, dental infection, lymphadenopathy, or trauma to anatomical spaces within the neck (e.g., parapharyngeal and submandibular spaces). Without treatment, an abscess forms and swelling can cause airway obstruction. Oral anaerobes are often the cause. Atypical mycobacteria and tuberculosis are rarer causes.

TX Initial management is similar to that for epiglottitis (see Epiglottitis), with **airway protection being the main priority.** Surgical drainage is necessary for abscesses.

RX **Amoxicillin-clavulanate**

DS Table 16–4

SE Table 16–4

Pharyngitis

See Tonsillitis and Pharyngitis.

Sialadenitis (Salivary Gland Enlargement)

KY **Acute parotitis and submandibular gland infections** are usually from oral bacteria. A calculus may be present. Viruses (e.g., mumps) can cause bilateral parotitis.

TX **Good hydration** and **sialogogues** (substances such as lemon drops that encourage salivation) aid resolution. **Antibiotics,** if required, must often be given intravenously.

RX **Amoxicillin-clavulanate**

DS Table 16–4

SE Table 16–4

Tonsillitis and Pharyngitis

KY Infection of the tonsils is commonly **viral** and is usually self-limiting. **Epstein-Barr virus causes a severe form (infectious mononucleosis).** Streptococci and other **bacteria** are also commonly involved.

TX **Analgesia is the most important treatment.** Soluble formulations and local anesthetic gargles are useful when pain prevents swallowing. **Adequate hydration must be maintained.** Antibiotics are often prescribed, but with little benefit because of the frequently viral etiology and spontaneous resolution. Widespread use probably contributes to increasing antibiotic resistance. **Ampicillin is contraindicated in patients with infectious mononucleosis.**

RX1 **Ibuprofen** (Advil, Motrin): See Acute Otitis Media.

DS1 See Acute Otitis Media.

SE1 See Acute Otitis Media.

or

RX2 **Acetaminophen** (Tylenol): See Acute Otitis Media.

DS2 See Acute Otitis Media.

SE2 See Acute Otitis Media.

with or without

RX3 **Antibiotics**

DS3 Table 16–1 and Table 16–4

SE3 Table 16–1 and Table 16–4

17

Pain Management

ALINE BOULANGER, M. JANE POULSON

The International Association for Study of Pain defines pain as "an unpleasant sensory and emotional experience associated with actual or potential tissue damage or described in terms of such damage." It is a complex phenomenon with physical, psychological, social, and spiritual elements. The contribution of each of these elements varies depending on the patient and the underlying pathophysiology.

GENERAL PRINCIPLES OF PAIN MANAGEMENT

Pain is almost invariably a sign of an underlying process (e.g., ischemia or inflammation). Analgesic medications treat the symptom of pain without altering the underlying pathologic process. Appropriate concurrent investigations of underlying pathology are always indicated—never treat pain without addressing the underlying pathophysiologic process.

In general, the physician should accept patients' assessment of pain severity. Pain is a subjective symptom, and no objective observer can rate someone else's pain. Pain control and side effects need to be evaluated during the treatment.

In the presence of constant pain, administration on a prn basis is certainly the worst way to give an analgesic. A **regular administration of the analgesic** prevents the important fluctuation in blood concentration of the drug.

DEFINITIONS

Addiction

Compulsive drug use and a **continued craving** for an opioid despite its harm to the health of the user characterize addiction. **Addiction is extremely rare in patients with pain.** It is, however, a major cause of concern for patients and families, who must be repeatedly reassured.

Breakthrough Analgesics

This is analgesic made available to the patient as **a rescue dose if regular analgesic provides insufficient relief.** If the patient requires breakthrough doses frequently, these are no longer breakthrough doses, and regular medications should be increased. Breakthrough analgesia is **also useful to administer prophylactically if a painful event is anticipated** (e.g., physiotherapy, physical care, or a procedure).

Table 17–1. Equianalgesic Doses

Generic (Brand) Name	Equianalgesic Dose	
	SC	PO
Codeine [C/D depending on dose and duration of use]	120	200
Hydromorphone (Dilaudid) [B/D depending on dose and duration of use]	1.5	7.5
Morphine [B/D depending on dose and duration of use]	10	20–30
Oxycodone (Endocodone, OxyContin, Percolone, Roxicodone—*U.S.*; Supendol—*Can.*) [B/D depending on dose and duration of use]	n/a	15

Dependence

There is an important distinction between physical and psychological dependence on drugs. Persons receiving opioids develop **physical dependence,** manifested by the development of **acute abstinence syndrome** if opioid antagonists are administered or drug delivery is discontinued. Acute abstinence syndrome includes diaphoresis, tachycardia, diarrhea, lacrimation, salivation, and piloerection. This syndrome can be avoided by gradually *tapering* the opioid dosage rather than abrupt cessation. **Psychological dependence** includes craving and drug-seeking behavior. **It has no relationship to physical dependence and is extremely rare in patients treated for pain.**

Equianalgesic Dose

This is an important clinical concept that facilitates substituting different drugs (e.g., morphine to hydromorphone) or routes of administration (PO to SC). Equianalgesic dose charts do not provide information about usual doses or recommended starting doses (Tables 17–1 and Table 17–2).

Neuropathic Pain

This is pain resulting from activation of damaged nerves. Neuropathic pain is described as a burning or a lancinating sensation and is associated with altered perceptions (e.g., light touch is perceived as painful).

Table 17–2. Dose Conversion of Oral Morphine to Fentanyl-TTS*

Daily Dose PO Morphine (mg)	Fentanyl Equivalent Dose (µg/hr)
45–134	25
135–224	50
225–314	75
315–404	100

*Transdermal patch.

Nociceptive Pain

Nociceptive pain results from the activation by noxious stimuli of peripheral pain receptors, which transduce the information to the a-delta fibers and smaller unmyelinated c-fibers. Then information is transmitted by way of the ascending spinothalamic tracts to the brain, where the perception of pain occurs. **Nociceptive pain includes somatic and visceral pain. Somatic** pain results from the activation of nociceptors in musculoskeletal tissues (bone or soft tissue) and is usually sharp, well localized, and exacerbated by movement. **Visceral** pain results from the involvement of visceral organs, stretching of the liver capsule, or obstruction of hollow viscera (e.g., bowel, bladder). It is usually poorly localized and is often associated with autonomic symptoms such as nausea and vomiting.

Tolerance

Tolerance is a pharmacologic principle relating to the need for an increased drug dose to achieve the same effect. Tolerance to the analgesic effect of opioids is rarely problematic. **Opioids should not be withheld to prevent tolerance.** Disease progression rather than tolerance should be suspected in patients who develop increased pain subsequent to management with stable doses of opioids.

Total Pain

This is a concept whereby **the patient expresses global despairs—** including psychological, emotional, and existential—using the word "pain." It is important to recognize this concept because the use of analgesic medications is unlikely to relieve the patient's suffering. A **multidisciplinary approach is required** to manage a total pain picture. It should be noted that a patient's suffering is not proportional to physical pain.

CLASSIFICATION AND MANAGEMENT OF PAIN

Pain might be classified into **acute** and **chronic** pain. Acute pain includes acute pain syndromes, obstetric pain, postoperative and procedural pain, exacerbation of cancer or chronic pain, tissue ischemia, inflammation, and obstruction and dilatation of hollow viscus. Pain will be qualified as chronic when it persists for more than the normal time of cure. Chronic pain includes malignant (nociceptive and neuropathic) and nonmalignant.

Acute Pain Syndromes

Management of acute pain syndromes is generally targeted at the underlying pathology rather than simply administering analgesic medications. For example, myocardial ischemia is managed with revascularization and vasodilating medications (e.g., nitrates). Small doses of morphine may be required for analgesia, but primary treatment is directed toward reducing tissue ischemia. Similarly, the pain of inflammatory arthropathies is best managed by anti-inflammatory and immunologic therapies. It is beyond the scope of this chapter to deal with specific management of acute pain syndromes, and the reader is referred to appropriate sources elsewhere.

Obstetric Pain

See Ch 13 Obstetrics and Ch 2 Anesthesiology for discussions of pain management in obstetrics.

Postoperative Pain

KY Postoperative pain is acute and generally of the nociceptive type. Postoperative pain should improve quite quickly. If your patient has persistent or worsening pain, consider complications such as wound infection or deep venous thrombosis.

TX **Good pain management is necessary** to ensure postoperative recuperation and to prevent complications.

RX1 **Continuous epidural infusion** represents an effective way to treat postoperative pain.

DS1 Many types of epidural solutions are possible. In general, it consists of a combination of an opioid (e.g., fentanyl 2–5 μg/mL, meperidine 1–2.5 mg/mL), and a local anesthetic drug (e.g., bupivacaine 0.0625%–0.25%). Also see Table 17–3 and Table 17–4 for factors that affect doses.

SE1 Low blood pressure may occur secondary to the sympathetic block induced by the local anesthetic solution. This side effect occurs mainly in the hypovolemic patient. Correction of the hypovolemia or administration of a vasopressor (e.g., phenylephrine hydrochloride 100 μg IV) is recommended.

Table 17–3. Factors Influencing Dose of Opioids

Factor	Influence
Age of patient	Elderly patients are very susceptible to opioid effects. Halve the doses for geriatric patients.
Renal and hepatic failure	All opioids metabolized by the liver are excreted in urine. For patients with renal or hepatic failure or those who have a reduced oral intake or dehydration, the dose should be reduced, the interval of administration should be lengthened, or both.
Previous exposure to opioids	Patients who are on chronic opioid use will have a lower effect from initial opioid therapy; initial doses should be increased.

Table 17–4. Side Effects of Opioids

Side Effect	Frequency	Management
Cognitive impairment	Variable	Eliminate other causes. If no cause elucidated then opioid should be changed if cognitive state does not improve within 48 hours.
Constipation	Universal	All patients receiving opioids should receive concurrent stool softeners (e.g., docusate) and laxatives (e.g., Senna).
Dry mouth	Frequent	Mouth irrigation. Chewing gum and sour candies to stimulate saliva.
Nausea	Frequent	Antiemetics should be administered, particularly in early phases of opioid therapy. See Ch 14 Oncology.
Pruritus	Infrequent	Opioids release histamine from mast cells. Concurrent treatment with antihistamines is sometimes required. True allergy to opioids is extremely rare.
Respiratory depression	Variable and dose dependent	**Naloxone should be administered immediately as described in Table 17–5.** The patient requires close monitoring for 4 hours after the respiratory depression event as this can recur and repeated doses of naloxone may be required.
Sedation	Variable, tolerance quickly develops	Eliminate other causes. If no causes elucidated the dose should be reduced. If sedation remains problematic, a different opioid should be used. The addition of methylphenidate (Ritalin) 5–10 mg bid may allow analgesia without sedation.
Urinary retention	Infrequent	Always consider other possible etiologic factors (e.g., cord compression).

ANTIDOTE

In situations of opioid overdose, an opioid antagonist, naloxone (Narcan), can be used (Table 17–5). The action of naloxone is via competitive antagonism at the opioid receptor. Competition between agonist and antagonist may persist for 3–4 hours. **Patients must be carefully monitored because repeated naloxone injections may be required.** It is also important to try to administer the minimum required dose to reverse life-threatening respiratory depression without reversing all desirable opioid effects, which could lead to the precipitation of acute abstinence syndrome.

RX2 **Patient-controlled analgesia:** These pumps allow the patient to self-administer a fixed amount of analgesic. A typical setting might be 1–2 mg every 6–10 minutes. Maximum doses can be predetermined. Alternatively, the pumps can be set to administer a continuous infusion alone or a combination of patient-controlled analgesia and infusion.

Table 17–5. Opioid Antagonist

Generic (Brand) Name	Recommended Dose	Peak Effect	Duration	Side Effects
Naloxone (Narcan) [B]	0.2–0.4 mg IV q2–3min prn	Immediate	Variable*	Symptoms of opiate withdrawal, in patients addicted to opiates (e.g., pain, hypertension, irritability, seizure, and violent behavior)

*Action is via competitive antagonism at the opioid receptor. Competition between agonist and antagonist may persist for 3–4 hours. Patients must be carefully monitored because repeated naloxone injections may be required.

DS2 **Morphine** up to 1–2 mg q6–10min (maximum: 40 mg/4 hr)

SE2 **In opioid overdose, an opioid antagonist, naloxone (Narcan), can be used.** See the epidural section and Table 17–5.

RX3 **Parenteral analgesia:** If postoperative pain is not being managed by epidural or patient-controlled analgesia pumps, patients who cannot take the medication by mouth should receive regular subcutaneous or intravenous doses of opioids. The amount each patient will require will vary widely, and the patient must be reassessed regularly to ensure sufficient analgesia.

DS3 Morphine 5–10 mg q4hr SC, with 5 mg q2hr as a breakthrough dose (morphine may be administered via an indwelling SC butterfly to avoid repeated injections; morphine does not need to be administered IM), or

Morphine 1–2 mg/hr by continuous IV infusion, or

Morphine 1–2 mg/hr by continuous SC infusion.

When the patient can tolerate medications by mouth, he or she might be switched to: Acetaminophen with codeine 1–2 tablets q4hr, or

Acetaminophen with oxycodone 1–2 tablets q4hr.

SE3 Table 17–4 and Table 17–5

Procedural Pain

Many medical procedures are painful and require analgesic management. Some procedures can be executed with **local anesthetic administered at the time of the procedure.** For other painful procedures (e.g., radiologic biopsies or orthopedic maneuvers), **patients may be premedicated with an opioid.** A reasonable approach: morphine 5 mg SC 20 minutes before the procedure. Concurrent administration of **sublingual benzodiazepines may help if anxiety is a key feature.**

Chronic Nonmalignant Pain

Chronic nonmalignant pain is a complex process with psychosocial, economic, and societal consequences. Patients with chronic pain are **best managed by an interdisciplinary team,** which can help address the various aspects of this syndrome. **Multimodality therapy is required** (e.g., phys-

Table 17–6. Guidelines for the Utilization of Opioids

Generic (Brand) Name	Dose	Peak Effect (hours)	Duration (hours)	Side Effects*
Weak Opioids				
Codeine 15–30 mg and acetaminophen [C]	1–2 tablets PO q4hr	1–2	4–6	Constipation, nausea, and vomiting are common.
Codeine [D]	30–60 mg PO q4hr	0.5	4–6	Table 17–4
Codeine parenteral	30–60 mg SC q4hr			
Codeine SR	50–100 mg PO q12 hr			
Oxycodone 5 mg and acetaminophen (Percocet) [C]	1–2 tablets PO q4hr	1–2	4–6	
Oxycodone (Endocodone, OxyContin, Percolone, Roxicodone—*U.S.*; Supendol—*Can.*) [B/D depending on dose and duration of use]	5–10 mg PO q4hr SR: 10–20 mg PO q12hr	n/a	12	
Strong Opioids				
Morphine elixir [B/D depending on dose and duration of use]	5–10 mg PO q4hr	1–2	4–6	Sweet taste may cause nausea with this preparation.
Morphine tablet	5–10 mg PO q4hr	1–2	4–6	Table 17–4
Morphine SR	10–30 mg PO q8–12hr–24 hr	n/a	8–12	
Morphine parenteral†	5–10 mg SC q4hr see Table 17–6	0.25–0.5	4–6	

Strong Opioids				
Hydromorphone [B/D depending on dose and duration of use]	1–2 mg PO q4hr SR: 3 mg PO q12hr	1–2	4–6	
Hydromorphone parenteral	0.5–1.0 SC q4hr	0.5	4–6	Generally less effective when given by mouth. Table 17–4.
Meperidine (Demerol)‡ [B/D depending on dose and duration of use]	75–150 PO q4hr	1–2	4	
Meperidine parenteral	50–75 mg IM q4hr	0.5–1.0	3–4	Seizure inducing with repeated use. Table 17–4.
Fentanyl-TTS [B/D depending on dose and duration of use]	Recommended for initial therapy§ Dermal patch□ Change patch q3d	n/a	n/a	Table 17–4. Prolonged duration of both effects and side effects is the result of subdermal pooling of medication.

n/a = not available; SR = sustained release.

*Common side effects and their management are listed in Table 17–4.

†Subcutaneous and intravenous doses are equivalent. The onset of action and side effects is more rapid with intravenous injection. If given intravenously, low initial dose with gradual dose augmentation is recommended.

‡Demerol is not recommended for chronic pain.

§Starting dose depends on previous dose of morphine or hydromorphone.

□Oral preparation is currently not available.

iotherapy and rehabilitation services, medical and psychological support, vocational counseling). The use of opioids in chronic nonmalignant pain is controversial. However, properly used, opioid therapy can be helpful, and acceptance and use are increasing. See Table 17–6 on pages 304–305 for guidelines for the use of opioids. The following steps must be taken when initiating opioid therapy: assessment for etiology of pain syndrome; evaluation of the efficacy of opioid therapy with respect to symptom relief and side effects (Table 17–4), and assessment for development of addictive behaviors (e.g., lost prescriptions or alterations in drug use).

Cancer Pain

Cancer pain is generally grossly undertreated and is a major cause of suffering and reduced productivity. Careful history and physical examination are required to determine nociceptive (somatic and visceral) and neuro-

Table 17–7. Adjuvant Analgesics for Neuropathic Pain

Generic (Brand) Name	Dose
*Tricyclic antidepressants** Amitriptyline (Elavil, Vanatrip) [D] Nortriptyline (Aventyl, Pamelor) [D]	Initial dose: 10–25 mg PO qhs; gradually increase to 150–200 mg PO qhs
Anticonvulsants† Carbamazepine (Tegretol) [D] Valproic acid (Depacon, Depakene—*U.S.*; Epival—*Can.*) [D] Gabapentin (Neurontin) [C]	Initial dose 100 mg PO tid; increase to 800 mg PO daily dose Initial dose 250 mg PO bid; increase to 1 g PO daily dose Initial dose 100 mg PO tid; increase to 3,600 mg PO daily dose
Antiarrhythmics Mexiletine (Mexitil) [C]	Start with 100 mg PO bid; increase as required to a maximum of 600–900 mg PO daily dose
Steroids Dexamethasone (Decadron) [C]	2–4 mg PO qid
NMDA receptor blockers Ketamine (Ketalar) [D]	Continuous SC infusion with anesthesia supervision, PO, SC bolus

CNS = central nervous system; GI = gastrointestinal; NMDA, N-methyl-D-aspartate.

*Also see Ch 19 Pyschiatry.

†Also see Ch 12 Neurology.

pathic components of pain. Neuropathic pain classically requires addition of adjuvant analgesics for sufficient pain control. **Cancer pain management requires multimodality therapy,** often including chemotherapy, radiation, surgery, and multiple analgesics and adjuvant medications.

The World Health Organization recommends a stepwise approach to cancer pain. Mild pain is managed with **nonopioid medications** (e.g., aspirin, nonsteroidal anti-inflammatory drugs [NSAIDs], and acetaminophen). More severe pain is an indication for the addition of **weak opioids** (e.g., codeine, oxycodone). If regular use of maximum doses is insufficient, weak opioids are discontinued and **strong opioids** (e.g., morphine, hydromorphone) are initiated. Appropriate **adjuvant analgesics** are concurrently administered with opioid analgesics.

Like chronic pain, cancer pain is a complex phenomenon of physical, psychological, social, and spiritual concerns, and support from an interdisciplinary team is helpful.

Mechanism of Action	Side Effects
Enhanced catecholamine-neurotransmitters for analgesic pathways	Weight gain, dry mouth, dry eyes, blurred vision, urinary retention, sedation, hypotension, cardiac arrhythmias, sexual dysfunction, mania, withdrawal syndrome
Membrane stabilization	Drowsiness, pruritus, hypertension, tachycardia, edema, bone marrow suppression, hepatotoxicity, blurred vision, ototoxicity, allergic reactions
Membrane stabilization	Dizziness, nervousness, ataxia, GI upset, cardiac arrhythmias, insomnia, headache, blurred vision, tinnitus, dyspnea, bone marrow suppression, allergic reactions
Not well defined	Ulcer disease, glucose intolerance, hypertension, osteoporosis, osteonecrosis cataract, skin fragility, increased susceptibility to infections, gastric ulcer, cushingoid features, avascular necrosis, myopathy, cataract, glaucoma, mood changes
NMDA receptor blockade interrupts aberrant pain pathways at level of CNS	Hypotension, confusion, disorientation, aggression

Table 17–8. Adjuvant Analgesics for Bone Pain

Generic (Brand) Name	Dose	Mechanism of Action	Side Effects
NSAIDs	Table 17–9		
Bisphosphonates			
Pamidronate (Aredia) [C]	60 mg IV over 6 hours	Decreased osteoclastic activity	Monitor serum calcium and phosphate. May require repeated administration to control pain.
Steroids			
Dexamethasone (Decadron) [C]	2–4 mg PO bid-qid	Anti-inflammatory (in part) but incompletely understood	Peptic ulcer disease, glucose intolerance, hypertension, osteoporosis, osteonecrosis, cataract, skin fragility, increased susceptibility to infections, gastric ulcer, cushingoid features, avascular necrosis, myopathy, cataract, glaucoma, mood changes

NSAIDs = nonsteroidal anti-inflammatory drugs.

MEDICATIONS

Adjuvant Analgesics

Adjuvant analgesics are medications that are not primarily analgesics but that act synergistically when used with them. For example, tricyclic antidepressants and anticonvulsants are very useful in treating neuropathic pain, and bisphosphates and steroid drugs are helpful in treating bone pain (See Table 17–7 on pages 306–307 and Table 17–8).

Nonsteroidal Anti-Inflammatory Drugs (NSAIDs)

NSAIDS are very effective analgesics (Table 17–9). **They act via interruption of prostaglandin synthesis.** They are effective when used as single agents in mild to moderate pain and are synergistic when administered with opioids in moderate to severe pain. They are particularly effective in nociceptive pain. **Major side effects** include peptic ulcer disease with significant gastrointestinal bleeding, renal failure in elderly or volume-depleted patients, confusion, and headache. **NSAIDs impair platelet activity and must be used with caution in patients with impaired marrow function or bleeding diathesis. Extreme caution must be used in prescribing NSAIDs in patients receiving anticoagulation.** Prophylaxis against peptic ulcer disease with misoprostol (Cytotec) is generally recommended for patients at high risk of peptic ulcer disease or who would tolerate gastrointestinal bleeding poorly. The **new selective COX-2 inhibitor molecules** (Table 17–9) are less disruptive on the gastric mucosa and do not impair platelet activity. They are indicated for at-risk patients. However, there has

Table 17–9. Recommended Dose of Commonly Used Nonsteroidal Anti-inflammatory Drugs

Generic (Brand) Name	Route	Dose
Diclofenac (Voltaren)*	PO or PR	100 mg qd
Ketorolac (Toradol)*	PO IM	10 mg q5hr prn 30 mg q6hr prn
Indomethacin (Indocin, Indocid)*	PO PR	25 mg tid 50 mg tid
Ibuprofen (Advil, Motrin)	PO	400 mg tid
Naproxen*	PR	100 mg qd
Naproxen (Naprosyn)*	PO	375 mg bid
Celecoxib†	PO	100–200 mg bid
Rofecoxib†	PO	1.25–25 mg qd

*Pregnancy risk category B in first and second trimester and D in third trimester.

†Selective COX-2 inhibitors have been associated with increased cardiovascular risk (e.g., myocardial infarction, ischemic stroke); pregnancy risk category C in first and second trimester and D in third trimester.

been an association between selective COX-2 inhibitors and increased cardiovascular risk, including myocardial infarctions and ischemic stroke.

Opioids

Opioids produce analgesia by a **specific action on opioid receptors.** They are **the cornerstone of pain management.** Opioids are particularly effective for nociceptive pain (somatic and visceral). Their action on neuropathic pain is more limited but useful in some patients. **Common side effects** are listed in Table 17–4. When opioids are titrated properly for the individual patient, side effects may be mild but will persist and require preventive treatment (e.g., prophylactic laxatives for the treatment of constipation side effect).

18

Pediatrics

DAT J. TRAN

Informed use of medications and therapeutic agents is essential, especially in pediatrics, where drug therapy presents with unique challenges. Complicating factors include (1) developmental changes in body composition and organ function that affect both pharmacokinetic and pharmacodynamic characteristics; (2) availability of appropriate dosage forms that have an impact on adherence; (3) limited prescribing information; and (4) concomitant disease states. This chapter attempts to provide an overview of the salient pharmacokinetic considerations in pediatric therapy and to focus on the common conditions encountered in pediatrics that are amenable to pharmacologic therapy. The reader will note that infectious diseases form a significant proportion of pediatric practice, and, for the purpose of this discussion, the focus will be on bacterial infections. However, given that active immunization is an integral part of pediatric practice, the chapter begins with a brief review of the recommended routine vaccinations before proceeding to a discussion of drug therapy. Throughout this chapter, the terminology used for the various age groups will be defined as follows: **neonate,** first month of postnatal life; **infant,** 1–12 months of age; **child,** 1–12 years of age; and **adolescent,** 12–18 years of age.

IMMUNIZATIONS

Immunization is key to preventing disease among the general population, and it is children who receive most of the vaccinations.

KY Active immunization involves administration of all or part of a microorganism or modified product of that microorganism (e.g., toxoid, purified antigen, genetically engineered antigen) to elicit a protective, immunologic response without producing significant illness. Vaccines incorporating an intact microorganism may be either **live (attenuated)** or **killed (inactivated).** Although live vaccines are more likely to induce long-lasting immunity without the need for booster injections, they carry with them the risk of causing vaccine-induced disease in recipients or spreading the vaccine strain to secondary hosts. They may also be inadvertently inactivated if improperly stored. Refer to the footnotes of Table 18-1 for the type of vaccine for each of the routine vaccines.

TX **Some general guidelines for vaccine administration are as follows:** (1) written informed consent is required; (2) the schedule for premature infants should be based on postnatal age; (3) there is no need to restart when schedule interruptions occur; (4) children with unknown/undocumented immunization status should receive all appropriate vaccinations; (5) simultaneous administration of routine immunizations at different sites is safe and effective; (6) injection pain may be managed with topical anesthetic agents such as EMLA cream or vapo-coolant spray; (7) acetaminophen 15 mg/kg at 0 and 4

Table 18-1. Immunization Schedule for Infants and Children*

											Age		
Vaccine	Birth	1 mo	2 mo	4 mo	6 mo	12 mo	15 mo	18 mo	24 mo	4–6 yr	11–12 yr	14–16 yr
Hep B		X										
			X				X				(X)†	
DTaP			X	X	X		X			X		
Td												X
IPV			X	X		X				X		
Hib			X	X	X	X						
PCV7			X	X	X	X						
MMR						X				X	(X)†	
Var						X					(X)†	
Hep A										X—in selected areas		

*Based on recommendations of the Advisory Committee on Immunization Practices, the American Academy of Pediatrics, and the American Academy of Family Physicians.

†Vaccine to be given if previously recommended doses were missed or given earlier than the recommended minimum age.

Vaccine [Type of Vaccine]:

Hep B = hepatitis B vaccine [inactivated viral antigen]: Infants born to hepatitis B surface antigen (HBsAg)–negative mothers should receive the first dose by 2 months of age. The second dose should be administered at least 1 month after the first dose; the third dose should be given at least 4 months after the first dose and 2 months after the second dose but not before 6 months of age. Infants born to HBsAg-positive mothers should receive the first dose of vaccine and 0.5 mL of hepatitis B immune globulin (HBIG) within 12 hours of birth (at separate sites). Infants born to mothers with unknown HBsAg status should receive the first dose of vaccine within 12 hours of birth. If the HBsAg test (drawn during labor and delivery) is positive, HBIG should be given as soon as possible (no later than 1 week of age).

DTaP = diphtheria, tetanus, and acellular pertussis vaccine [toxoids and inactivated bacterial components]: The fourth dose may be given as early as 12 months of age, provided 6 months have elapsed since the third dose and the child is unlikely to return at 15–18 months of age.

Td = tetanus and diphtheria "adult-type" vaccine [toxoids]: Contains less diphtheria toxoid and is less likely to cause reactions; for use in persons ≥ 7 years of age. It can be given at age 11–12 years if at least 5 years have elapsed since the last dose of DTP, DTaP, or DT. Subsequent routine Td boosters are recommended every 10 years.

IPV = inactivated polio vaccine [inactivated virus]: A schedule using only IPV is recommended to eliminate the risk of vaccine-associated paralytic polio. Oral polio vaccine may be used for special circumstances.

Hib = *Haemophilus influenzae* type b vaccine [polysaccharide-protein conjugate]: Schedule shown is for PRP-T or HbOC vaccine. If PRP-OMP (PedvaxHIB or COMVAX) is used, the 6-month dose is not required. DTaP/Hib combination products should not be used for the primary immunization series (2, 4, 6 months).

PCV7 = heptavalent conjugate pneumococcal vaccine [polysaccharide]: Recommended for all children 2–23 months of age. It is also recommended for children 24–59 months with sickle cell hemoglobinopathies, chronic illnesses, human immunodeficiency virus infection, and other immunocompromised states. Not recommended in children ≥ 5 years of age.

MMR = measles, mumps, and rubella vaccine [live]: The second dose may be administered during any visit provided that at least 4 weeks have elapsed since the first dose and both doses are given at ≥ 12 months of age.

Var = varicella vaccine [live]: Recommended for susceptible children. Susceptible persons ≥ 13 years of age should receive two doses given at least 4 weeks apart.

Hep A = hepatitis A vaccine [inactivated viral antigen]: Indicated for use in communities with approximately twice the national average. Two doses should be administered 6–12 months apart.

hours after vaccination and then q4hr prn to decrease fever and irritability; (8) preferred sites for injection are the anterolateral aspect of the upper thigh for infants (children < 1 year of age) and the deltoid area of the upper arm for all other age groups; (9) monitor recipients for 15 minutes after vaccination and have epinephrine immediately available for possible anaphylaxis.

RX Recommended routine childhood immunization schedule: Table 18-1.

DS For all those younger than 18 years, the dose of each of the recommended routine vaccinations is 0.5 mL. IPV, MMR vaccine, and varicella vaccine are administered SC. Pneumococcal conjugate virus can be administered via IM or SC route. The remainder of the routine vaccines are given IM.

SE Table 18-2

PHARMACOKINETIC CHARACTERISTICS IN PEDIATRICS

There are a variety of age-related physiologic changes that may have an impact on drug absorption, distribution, and elimination. These maturational changes, as summarized in Table 18-3, have various clinical implications. Although beyond the scope of this chapter, it should also be noted that there is increasing evidence that developmental differences in drug receptor sensitivity and binding characteristics may have important implications for response to specific drugs in pediatric patients, especially neonates. Last, like in adults, underlying disease states such as hepatic disease, renal disease, and cardiac disorders have been shown to result in altered pharmacokinetics. More specific to pediatric practice, cystic fibrosis is an important disorder that is associated with alterations in drug disposition. In these patients, volume of distribution, hepatic metabolism, and renal clearance of many medications, particularly broad-spectrum antibiotics, are increased; as a result, increased doses may be required for effective treatment.

DOSING PRINCIPLES IN PEDIATRICS

Dosing in pediatrics is often based on weight (occasionally on body surface area). Table 18-4 provides a rough guideline to dosing in pediatrics.

DRUGS TO AVOID IN PEDIATRICS

Not surprisingly, natural maturational changes also lead to pharmacodynamic differences and place the pediatric patient at risk for drug toxicity not seen in adults. **It is therefore important to be aware of medications that are contraindicated or must be used with extreme caution in specific age groups. Aspirin** is associated with Reye syndrome (characterized by acute encephalopathy and fatty degeneration of the liver), particularly in patients with varicella or influenza infection. **Fluoroquinolones** can potentially damage growing cartilage. **Sulfonamides** are associated with kernicterus (bilirubin encephalopathy) in icteric neonates by displacing bilirubin from albumin binding sites. **Tetracyclines** and **doxycycline** cause dental enamel dysplasia and discoloration; **contraindicated** under 9 years of age.

314 NMS Clinical Manual of Medical Drug Therapy

Table 18–2. Side Effects, Contraindications, and Precautions to Immunizations*

Vaccine	Side Effects
All vaccines	See below
DTaP	Fever in 5%. Local discomfort or inflammation in 20%. Transient nodule may develop at injection site lasting a few weeks. Redness and swelling in up to 70% at the 4–6 year booster.
Hep B	Local pain in 3%–29%. Fever in 1%–6%.
Hib	Minimal local reactions in up to 25%.
IPV	Local discomfort or inflammation in 5%.
Influenza‡	Local reactions in 10% of children ≥ 13 years of age. Associated with GBS in 1/1,000,000.
MMR	**Measles:** Discomfort, local inflammation, or fever with or without a noninfectious rash in 5%–10%. Encephalitis in 1/1,000,000. Transient thrombocytopenia in 1/24,000. **Mumps:** Fever and mild rash occasionally. Parotitis in 1%. Aseptic meningitis in 1/3 million. **Rubella:** Discomfort, local inflammation, or fever in 10%. Swollen glands, stiff neck, or joint pain in 5%. Noninfectious rash in 1%. Transient arthralgias or arthritis may occur, more in postpubertal females.
PCV7	Local reaction rate similar to Hib. Fever more often than with Hib.
Varicella	Minor local reactions in 20%. Localized rash in 3%–5%. Generalized varicella-like rash 5–26 days after immunization in 3%–5%. Fever in 10% of adolescents and adults.

GBS = group B streptococcal infection; DTaP, Hep B, Hib, IPV, MMR, and PCV7 are defined in Table 18–1.

*Based on recommendations of the Advisory Committee on Immunization Practices, the American Academy of Pediatrics, and the American Academy of Family Physicians.

†The vaccine should be given if the benefits are believed to outweigh the risks. Whether and when to administer DTaP to children with proven or suspected underlying neurologic disorders should be decided on an individual basis.

Absolute Contraindications	Precautions†
Anaphylactic reaction to a previous dose or to a constituent of the vaccine.	Moderate or severe illness with or without fever.
Encephalopathy within 7 days of a previous dose.	Temperature of 40.5°C (104.8°F) or a hypotonic-hyporesponsive episode or persistent inconsolable crying lasting 3 hours within 48 hours of a previous dose. Seizures within 3 days of a previous dose. Guillain-Barré syndrome within 6 weeks after a previous dose.
Anaphylactic reaction to baker's yeast.	None
None	None
Anaphylactic reaction to neomycin or streptomycin.	Pregnancy
Anaphylactic reaction to chicken or egg protein.	None
Anaphylactic reaction to neomycin or gelatin. Pregnancy or immunocompromised state.	Recent§ administration of immunoglobulin. Thrombocytopenia or history of thrombocytopenic purpura
None	Pregnancy: Vaccination should be deferred during pregnancy, given limited data available regarding effects on fetus (although other inactivated or killed and polysaccharide vaccines have been used safely in pregnancy).
Anaphylactic reaction to neomycin or gelatin. Pregnancy or immunodeficient state.	Recent§ administration of immunoglobulin. Family history of immunodeficiency.‖

‡Can be administered annually to those > 6 months of age; recommended for high-risk patients (e.g., cystic fibrosis), close contacts of high-risk patients, and foreign travelers to areas where influenza outbreaks are or may be occurring.

§Definition of recent varies from 3 to 11 months, depending on dose.

‖Immune status of other children in the family should be documented before administration.

Table 18–3. Effect of Age-Dependent Physiologic Factors on Pharmacokinetic Variables and Drug Disposition Compared With Adults

Pharmacokinetic Variable	Physiologic Factor	Age Group	Drug Disposition
Absorption	Increased gastric pH	Neonates to children aged 5–12 years	Bioavailability of basic drugs increases (e.g., semisynthetic penicillins) Bioavailability of acidic drugs decreases (e.g., acetaminophen, phenobarbital, phenytoin)
	Reduced or irregular gastric emptying and intestinal motility	Neonates and infants	Unpredictable bioavailability (e.g., digoxin, sulfonamides)
	Reduced bile acids and pancreatic enzymes; increased β-glucuronidase (a gastrointestinal enzyme) activity	Neonates	Reduced bioavailability (e.g., vitamin E)
Distribution	Increased total body water and extracellular water	Neonates and infants	Increased volume of distribution of water-soluble drugs (e.g., aminoglycosides)
	Reduced body fat	Neonates and infants	Decreased volume of distribution of lipophilic drugs (e.g., diazepam)
	Reduced plasma protein binding (caused by lower concentrations of proteins, reduced affinity of proteins for many drugs, and competition* for binding sites by endogenous substances such as bilirubin and free fatty acids)	Neonates and infants	Increased volume of distribution and free drug concentration (e.g., phenytoin, phenobarbital, sulfonamides, propranolol)

Elimination[†] Metabolism	Reduced hepatic enzymatic activity	Neonates and infants	Increased half-life of drug (e.g., phenobarbital)
	Increased hepatic enzymatic activity	Older infants and young children	Decreased half-life of drug (e.g., carbamazepine, phenytoin, quinidine)
Excretion	Reduced glomerular filtration rate	Neonates and infants	Increased half-life of drug (e.g., aminoglycosides)
	Reduced tubular secretion rate	Neonates and infants	Increased half-life of drug (e.g., penicillins, cephalosporins)

*Conversely, highly protein-bound drugs (e.g., sulfonamides), at therapeutic concentrations, are capable of displacing unconjugated bilirubin from albumin, thereby placing neonates with hyperbilirubinemia at risk for kernicterus.

[†]In general, drug elimination expressed as a percentage of body weight is low in neonates, peaks in infants and young children, and thereafter gradually approaches adult levels.

Table 18–4. A Rough Guide to Pediatric Doses

Weight (kg)	Age	Percentage of Adult Dose
4	1 month	10
10	1 year	25
20	6 years	50
40	12 years	75
65	>18 years	100

ACUTE LARYNGOTRACHEOBRONCHITIS OR CROUP

KY **A common infection of the upper respiratory tract with potential for airway obstruction** caused by marked inflammation of the larynx and subglottic area that gives rise to the characteristic hoarseness, barking cough, and stridor. Attack rates are highest in children 6–36 months of age and in boys, with peaks in late fall and early winter. Croup is caused mainly by viruses, with parainfluenza virus type 1 accounting for most cases as well as being responsible for winter epidemics.

TX Most cases can be managed at home; the decision to admit depends on the severity of upper airway obstruction, the degree of toxicity, and the likelihood of a more serious diagnosis such as bacterial tracheitis or epiglottitis. Systemic or inhaled **steroid administration should be considered in children with mild to moderate croup.**

RX1 **Dexamethasone** (Decadron): **a systemic steroidal anti-inflammatory agent.** This is **the drug of choice** owing to wider availability, easier administration (especially in distressed young children), and lower cost.

DS1 0.6 mg/kg PO/IM for 1 dose

SE1 No side effects documented with 1 dose.

or

RX2 **Budesonide** (Pulmicort): an inhaled **steroidal anti-inflammatory agent.**

DS2 2 mg via nebulizer for 1 dose

SE2 No side effects documented with 1 dose.

RX3 **Racemic epinephrine** (2.25%) or **epinephrine** (1:1000 solution) (Adrenalin): **an alpha-adrenergic agent that causes mucosal vasoconstriction, reducing subglottic edema. It does not affect the natural history of the disease but may prevent the need for intubation or tracheotomy.** It should be given to those with marked stridor at rest with tracheal tug.

DS3 **Racemic epinephrine:** 0.25 mL SC 1hr prn (< 6 months); 0.5 mL SC 1hr prn (≥ 6 mo)
   Epinephrine (1:1000): 0.5 mL/kg SC 1hr prn (> 5 kg); 2.5–5 mL SC 1hr prn (≥ 5 kg).

SE3 Tremor, tachycardia, hypertension, pallor, emesis, and rebound edema (patient should be observed for at least 2 hours after administration). **Contraindicated in patients with obstructive right, left, or cyanotic cardiac lesions.**

ASTHMA

Management of asthma in adults is discussed in Ch 20 Pulmonology.

🔑 Asthma is characterized by paroxysmal or persistent symptoms of airway hyperresponsiveness and airflow limitation such as wheezing, shortness of breath, chest tightness, and cough with or without sputum production. Although **endogenous and exogenous triggers** such as emotional stress, exercise, viral infections, tobacco smoke, allergens, and weather/humidity changes exaggerate symptoms of bronchoconstriction, it is **chronic inflammation and the resulting pathologic effects on airway morphology** (edema, bronchial epithelial injury, goblet cell hyperplasia leading to increased mucus secretion, collagen deposition beneath the basement membrane, and smooth muscle thickening) that are responsible for the development and maintenance of asthma. This inflammatory process and its effects involve both **inflammatory cell infiltration** and **release of mediators** via mast cell activation. Moreover, the **morphologic changes from chronic inflammation may not be completely reversible and may contribute to airway remodeling.**

Acute Exacerbation of Asthma

🅃🅇 Emergent management includes supplemental oxygen (to maintain oxygen saturation > 92%), IV hydration (to avoid fluid overload), and specific pharmacologic therapy.

🆁🆇 The general approach to pharmacotherapy in such cases includes **concurrent use of systemic corticosteroids and bronchodilators,** starting with aggressive treatments and then weaning as the patient improves and stabilizes (Table 18-5).

🅳🆂 Table 18-5
🆂🅴 Table 18-5

Chronic Asthma

🅃🅇 **The goal in asthma management is to maintain control** (Table 18-6) **of symptoms with the least amount of medication.** This can best be achieved with a multifaceted strategy that includes (1) regular individualized assessment and monitoring, (2) environmental measures to limit exposure to triggering factors, (3) asthma education including an action plan for exacerbations, and (4) pharmacologic therapy.

🆁🆇 Medications available for the treatment of asthma may be divided into two major categories: **controllers** and **relievers** (Table 18-7). Relievers are used to treat acute intercurrent symptoms on demand. Controllers include agents that are taken regularly to maintain control and prevent exacerbations. Whether one uses the stepped care approach endorsed by the American Academy of Allergy, Asthma & Immunology, Inc (Table 18-8) or the asthma treatment continuum concept adopted by the Canadian Asthma Consensus Group (Figure 18-1), **the choice of drug therapy is dictated by illness severity and the degree of control.**

(Text continues on page 327)

Table 18–5. Pharmacologic Management of an Acute Exacerbation of Asthma

Generic (Brand) Name	Dose	Note
Albuterol (Proventil, Ventolin)	Nebulizer: 0.15 mg/kg q20min for three doses, then q2hr prn (if improving) MDI*: 0.2 puffs/kg q20min for three doses, then q1–2hr prn (if improving) (maximum 8 puffs/dose)	If not improving after first three doses, may continue the q20min dosing (essentially continuous†) until the patient can be weaned to q1hr schedule (maximum: 15 mg/hr).
Corticosteroids Prednisone or Prednisolone	2 mg/kg PO for one dose, then 1–2 mg/kg PO qd for 4–6 days (starting the day after initial dosing)	Corticosteroids should be given to all except those with mild disease. Although IV corticosteroids are often used in very severe exacerbations, evidence suggests that PO and IV administration are equally effective. Its main utility is for those who are unable to tolerate oral corticosteroids.‡
Hydrocortisone (Solu-Cortef)	4–6 mg/kg IV q4–6hr	
Methylprednisolone (Solu-Medrol)	0.5–2 mg/kg IV q6hr	
Ipratropium (Atrovent)	Nebulizer: 250 µg q20min for three doses, then q2–4hr prn (depending on severity)	Should be reserved for moderate to severe disease in the ED,§ although there is controversy over its use in patients with signs of severe airflow obstruction.

ED = emergency department.

*Delivery of inhaled albuterol by metered-dose inhaler with spacer is equally as effective as nebulization in children as young as 2 years; however, nebulization is generally recommended for those younger than 6 years or those with severe asthma or poor air movement.

†Continuous administration may reduce the need for endotracheal intubation in status asthmaticus.

‡Dexamethasone (Decadron) 0.3 mg/kg IM/IV for one dose at initial presentation is an option for patients who are unable to tolerate prednisone or prednisolone.

§Its use in inpatients is not generally recommended.

Table 18–6. Criteria for Asthma Control

Parameter	Acceptable Control
Daytime symptoms	< 4 days/week
Nighttime symptoms	< 1 night/week
Physical activity	Normal
Exacerbations	Mild, infrequent
Absence from work or school	None
Need for short-acting β_2-agonist	< 4 doses/week*
FEV_1 or PEF	> 85% of personal best, ideally 90%
PEF diurnal variation	< 15% of diurnal variation

FEV_1 = forced expiratory volume in 1 second; PEF = peak expiratory flow using a portable peak flow meter; PEF diurnal variation = [(highest PEF − lowest PEF)/highest PEF] × 100.

*Excludes 1 dose/day for prevention of exercise-induced symptoms.

Adapted from Canadian Asthma Consensus Group. Boulet LP, et al. *Summary of Recommendations from the Canadian Asthma Consensus Report, 1999.* CMAJ 1999;161(11 Suppl):S2.

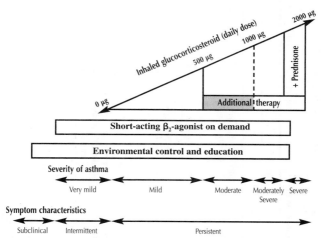

FIGURE 18-1. Continuum of Asthma Management. Note the dynamic approach, starting with environmental control and education and short-acting β_2-agonist on an as-needed basis. Gradually increasing requirements for inhaled corticosteroid therapy should prompt consideration of additional therapy (e.g., long-acting β_2-agonists, leukotriene antagonists) and, last, systemic corticosteroids in severe asthma.

Adapted from Canadian Asthma Consensus Group. Boulet LP, et al. *Summary of Recommendations from the Canadian Asthma Consensus Report, 1999.* CMAJ 1999;161(11 Suppl):S2.

Table 18–7. Selected Medications in the Maintenance Therapy of Children With Asthma

Class and Generic (Brand) Name	Dose	Side Effects
Relievers		
SHORT-ACTING β_2-AGONISTS* Albuterol (Proventil, Ventolin) MDI: 90 µg/puff Nebulizer: 5 mg/mL	MDI: 1–2 puffs q4hr prn Nebulizer: 0.15 mg/kg q4hr prn (minimum 1 mg/dose) (maximum 5 mg/dose) Oral: 0.3 mg/kg/day PO divided tid–qid	Tremor, tachycardia, and hypokalemia may occur with frequent dosing.
ANTICHOLINERGICS Ipratropium (Atrovent) MDI: 20 µg/puff Nebulizer: 250 µg/mL	MDI: 1–2 puffs q4hr prn Nebulizer: 250 µg/dose q4hr prn	This drug is poorly absorbed from the lung, so systemic effects are not common. Rarely, urinary retention and glaucoma have been reported.
Controllers		
STEROIDAL ANTI-INFLAMMATORY AGENTS **Inhaled glucocorticosteroids** Beclomethasone (Beclovent) MDI: 50 µg/puff Fluticasone (Flovent) MDI: 25, 50, 125, or 250 µg/puff Budesonide (Pulmicort) Nebulizer: 0.125, 0.25, or 0.5 mg/mL	Initial dose depends on severity of symptoms and degree of control (Fig 18–1). Dose (µg/day) Low Medium High MDI <400 400–1000 >1000 Nebulizer <1000 1000–2000 >2000 Dosing frequency should be bid.	Oral candidiasis, hoarseness, sore throat, cough (with MDI). Potential increase in risk of systemic side effects at high doses, although children receiving more than "low" doses should be monitored for impaired growth and osteoporosis.

Oral glucocorticosteroids Prednisolone (Pediapred) Prednisone (Deltasone)	For both prednisolone and prednisone: 0.25–2 mg/kg/day (maximum 60 mg/day)	Need to monitor for systemic side effects of corticosteroids; hyperglycemia, edema, osteonecrosis, osteoporosis, peptic ulcer disease, cushingoid appearance, growth suppression, myopathy, and susceptibility to infections.
NONSTEROIDAL ANTI-INFLAMMATORY AGENTS **Leukotriene-receptor antagonists** Zileuton (Zyflo) Zafirlukast (Accolate)	 >12 years: 600 mg PO qid 7–11 years: 10 mg PO bid >12 years: 20 mg PO bid	**Zileuton:** headache, elevation of liver enzymes, GI upset, leukopenia, myalgia, arthralgia, conjunctivitis **Zafirlukast:** headache, GI upset, hepatitis, hepatic failure, hyperbilirubinemia, agranulocytosis, hypersensitivity reactions
Montelukast (Singulair)	6–14 years: 5 mg PO qhs ≥ 15 years: 10 mg PO qhs	**Montelukast:** headache, GI upset, vasculitis, hypersensitivity reactions
Antiallergic agents Cromolyn sodium (Intal) MDI: 1 mg/puff Nebulizer: 10 mg/mL Nedocromil (Alocril, Tilade—*U.S.*; Mireze—*Can.*) MDI: 2 mg/puff	 MDI: 2 puffs tid–qid Nebulizer: 20 mg bid–qid >6 years: 2 puffs bid–qid	**Cromolyn sodium:** unpleasant taste, headache, diarrhea, myalgia, hypersensitivity reactions **Nedocromil:** unpleasant taste, dizziness, fatigue, headache, GI upset, chest pain, arthralgia, pharyngitis, bronchitis, broncho- spasm, upper respiratory tract infection, and increased sputum production

(continued)

Table 18-7. Selected Medications in the Maintenance Therapy of Children With Asthma *(Continued)*

Class and Generic (Brand) Name	Dose	Side Effects
BRONCHODILATORS		
Long-acting β₂-agonists		Headache, tremor, GI upset, cardiac arrhythmias, broncho-spasm, hypersensitivity reactions
Salmeterol (Serevent)	> 12 years: 2 puffs bid	
MDI: 25 μg/puff		
Formoterol (Foradil)	> 12 years: 1 capsule bid	
Aerolizer inhaler: 12 μg/capsule		
Methylxanthines	Maximum maintenance dose before	Nausea, vomiting, tremor
Theophylline (Aminophylline, Uniphyl)	TDM‡:	Risk of seizures and arrhythmias with high doses. Note that
	[0.2 (age in weeks) + 5]mg/kg/day PO divided tid–qid	theophylline has many drug interactions and is also affected by changes in diet and concomitant illness.
	1–12 years: 20 mg/kg/day PO divided bid–tid	
	12–16 years: 18 mg/kg/day PO divided bid	
	> 12 years: 14 mg/kg/day PO divided bid (maximum 900 mg/day)	

GI, gastrointestinal; MDI = metered-dose inhaler; TDM = therapeutic drug monitoring.

*Dosing schedule for inhaled β₂-agonists is q4hr prn, but regular use implies poor control and other agent(s) should be added.

†A short course may be used in the treatment of moderately severe acute asthmatic exacerbations and in this way is considered by some as also a reliever.

‡TDM is crucial as theophylline has a narrow therapeutic index; titrate according to clinical response and serum levels (optimal range, 10–20 μg/mL); start at 50% of recommended doses.

Table 18–8. Stepwise Approach for Managing Asthma*

(Symptom Severity and Control)	Long-Term Control	Quick Relief†
Step 4 (severe persistent)	Daily medications: Anti-inflammatory: high-dose inhaled corticosteroid. and If needed, add systemic corticosteroids; make repeated attempts to reduce to lowest daily or alternate dose that controls symptoms. and Long-acting inhaled β₂-agonist or theophylline (if age >5 years)	Short-acting inhaled‡ β₂-agonist as needed for symptoms.
Step 3 (moderate persistent)	Daily medication: Anti-inflammatory: medium-dose inhaled corticosteroid. or Low- to medium-dose inhaled corticosteroid. and If age ≤ 5 years: nedocromil or theophylline. If age > 5 years: long-acting inhaled β₂-agonist or theophylline. If needed, medium- to high-dose inhaled corticosteroid plus long-acting inhaled β₂-agonist or theophylline, especially for nighttime symptoms.	Short-acting inhaled‡ β₂-agonist as needed for symptoms.

(continued)

Table 18–8. Stepwise Approach for Managing Asthma* (Continued)

(Symptom Severity and Control)	Long-Term Control	Quick Relief†
Step 2 (mild persistent)	One daily medication: Anti-inflammatory: low-dose inhaled corticosteroid **or** Cromolyn sodium or nedocromil (infants and young children usually begin with a trial of cromolyn or nedocromil) Theophylline is an alternative to anti-inflammatory agents, but not preferred (if age > 5 years). Leukotriene-receptor antagonist may be considered if age > 5 years.	Short-acting inhaled‡ β₂-agonist as needed for symptoms.
Step 1 (mild intermittent)	No daily medication needed.	Short-acting inhaled‡ β₂-agonist as needed for symptoms.
Step Up		**Step Up**
Step Down		
Review treatment every 1–6 months, and step down gradually if possible.	If control is not maintained (after reviewing medication technique, adherence, environmental control), consider stepping up.	

*Based on recommendations from the American Academy of Allergy, Asthma & Immunology, Inc.

†Daily or increasing use of quick-relief medication may indicate a need for additional long-term control therapy.

‡Oral β₂-agonist also an option for children ≤ 5 years of age.

DS Table 18-7
SE Table 18-7

BACTEREMIA AND SEPSIS

KY **Bacteremia is defined as the presence of a positive blood culture indicating viable bacteria in the blood.** The bacteremia may be occult, and the patient presents with only fever. The term *sepsis* is used when there is an infection or clinical suspicion of an infection that is accompanied by a systemic inflammatory response syndrome—manifested by two or more of the following: (1) fever or hypothermia, (2) tachycardia, (3) tachypnea, (4) significant leukocytosis or leukopenia or increased band counts. The etiology of bacteremia and sepsis varies according to age and other determining factors (Table 18-9). **The pathogenesis of bacteremia is highly variable and depends on the etiologic agent, the host's immunologic status, and other predisposing factors.**

TX **Empiric antibiotic selection is based on age and presence of risk factors for unusual pathogens. Supportive care** (including pharmacologic inotropic support) is critical, particularly when hypotension or shock ensues. The role of corticosteroids in sepsis remains debated; at this time,

Table 18–9. Bacteremia/Septicemia (Without Meningitis): Microbiology and Initial Empiric Antibiotic Therapy

Age/Immune Status	Common Etiologic Agents	Antibiotic*
Neonate†	Same as for pneumonia (Table 18–11)	Same as for pneumonia (Table 18–11)
1–3 months	Organisms commonly seen in neonates and older children	Ampicillin + cefotaxime
3 months–18 years	*Haemophilus influenzae, Neisseria meningitidis, Staphylococcus aureus, Streptococcus pneumoniae*	Cefuroxime + aminoglycoside‡
Immunocompromised state		
Terminal complement deficiencies	*N. meningitidis*	Third-generation cephalosporin
Asplenia (anatomic or functional) (e.g., sickle cell disease)	*H. influenzae, Salmonella* species, *S. pneumoniae*	Third-generation cephalosporin + vancomycin§

*See Table 18–10 for dosing information.
†The list of pathogens does not include those that infect long-term residents in the neonatal intensive care unit.
‡If suspected urinary or abdominal source.
§If the patient is seriously ill.

the **evidence does not justify recommendation of large doses of steroids as adjunctive therapy.** The role of other adjunctive measures, such as anticoagulation and other immunomodulating agents, remains unclear.

RX Table 18-9

DS Table 18-10

SE Table 18-10

BRONCHIOLITIS

KY Patients with bronchiolitis present with **signs and symptoms of upper respiratory tract infection and obstructive airways disease.** Bronchiolitis **occurs during the first 2 years of life,** although it is primarily a disease of infants, with a peak incidence at 2–6 months of age, and is more common in boys. Its incidence steadily increases as survival rates of premature infants and those with cardiopulmonary disorders increase. **Respiratory syncytial virus (RSV) is the major cause of bronchiolitis in infants.** Bronchiolitis is characterized by submucosal inflammation, epithelial necrosis, mucus plugging, and atelectasis of small airways. Young infants are especially predisposed to severe clinical illness not only because of the diminutive caliber of their small airways but also because of the relatively large contribution of their small airways to total airway resistance (up to sevenfold more compared with adults). In addition, there is evidence that airways of infants are intrinsically more reactive to irritative stimuli than airways of older children, especially in those with a family history of asthma. It also seems that cell-mediated hypersensitivity to RSV may play an important role in the pathogenesis of bronchiolitis. Last, **environmental factors, such as crowding and passive smoking, have been associated with increased risk of severe clinical illness.**

TX **Infants with disease severe enough to require hospitalization often need supplemental oxygen and IV fluids.** However, **care should be taken not to overhydrate** as edema is an important component of the pathophysiologic process. The efficacy of **bronchodilator therapy is of questionable benefit,** but because these medications are frequently used in clinical practice and seem to be the standard of care, they are listed here as potential therapeutic agents. Drugs and doses are generally the same as those for asthma. However, because deteriorations including oxygen desaturations have been associated with nebulized treatments, **if the patient shows no clinical improvement after a trial of bronchodilator therapy, it is recommended that inhalation therapy be discontinued. Corticosteroids are not recommended.** Perhaps the best approach to RSV management is prevention of infection in at-risk patients (mainly those with chronic lung disease or those born before 32 weeks' gestation) younger than 2 years with either **RSV immune globulin intravenous (RSV-IGIV)** or the newer product, **palivizumab (the preferred product because of its advantages**—see below). Both have been shown to reduce hospitalization rates, duration of hospital stay, and duration of oxygen requirement.

RX1 **Albuterol or salbutamol** (Table 18-7).

DS1 Table 18-7

SE1 Table 18-7

or

RX2 **Ipratropium** (Table 18-7)

DS2 Table 18-7

SE2 Table 18-7

or

RX3 **Racemic epinephrine** (2.25%) or epinephrine (1:1,000 solution). Studies comparing epinephrine to β_2-agonists have been mixed; perhaps epinephrine use should be deferred until a trial of a β_2-agonist proves ineffective.

DS3 **Racemic epinephrine:** 0.25 mL q1hr prn SC (< 6 months); 0.5 mL SC q1hr prn (≥ 6 months)
   Epinephrine (1:1,000): 0.5 mL/kg SC q1hr prn (< 5 kg); 2.5–5 mL SC q1hr prn (≥ 5 kg).

SE3 See ACUTE LARYNGOTRACHEOBRONCHITIS OR CROUP.

or

RX4 **RSV-IGIV:** Immune globulin from donors with high serum titers of RSV neutralizing antibody, or **Palivizumab:** Humanized mouse monoclonal antibody against F protein of RSV.

DS4 **RSV-IGIV:** 750 mg/kg/dose (15 mL/kg/dose) IV.
   Palivizumab: 15 mg/kg/dose IM
   Both are given monthly at onset of and throughout the RSV season.

SE4 **RSV-IGIV:** Fluid overload from infusions, small risk of anaphylaxis, requires deferral of live vaccines for 9 months.
   Palivizumab: Well tolerated with only local reactions, and does not have the disadvantages of RSV-IGIV.

CROUP

See ACUTE LARYNGOTRACHEOBRONCHITIS OR CROUP.

HERPES SIMPLEX ENCEPHALITIS

KY The term **encephalitis refers to inflammation of the brain without significant involvement of the meninges or spinal cord.** Discussion is limited to encephalitis caused by herpes simplex virus (HSV), as it is the leading cause of severe encephalitis at all ages and where **specific antiviral therapy results in a significant reduction in mortality (28% compared with 70% if untreated). Beyond the neonatal period, HSV encephalitis is almost always caused by HSV-1.** The virus enters the central nervous system (CNS) by retrograde neurotropic spread as a result of reactivation or primary infection, where hematogenous spread may also play a role. In contrast, **most neonatal HSV encephalitis is caused by HSV-2** and results from perinatal exposure to infectious maternal genital secretions. Hematogenous dissemination to the CNS is important in such

Table 18–10. Recommended Dosing and Side Effects of Antibiotics Recommended in Empiric Management of Pneumonia and Bacteremia/Septicemia

Class and Generic (Brand) Name	Dose
PENICILLINS	
Penicillin G (parenteral) (Pfizerpen)	Mild-moderate infections: 25,000–50,000 U/kg/day IV/IM divided q6hr Severe infections: 100,000–400,000 U/kg/day IV/IM divided q4–6hr
Ampicillin (Omnipen, Principen, Marcillin—U.S.; Ampicin—Can.)	Meningitis: Neonate: < 2 kg: 0–7 days: 100 mg/kg/day IV divided q12hr > 7 days: 150 mg/kg/day IV divided q8hr ≥ 2 kg: 0–7 days: 150 mg/kg/day IV divided q8hr > 7 days: 200 mg/kg/day IV divided q6hr GBS: 0–7 days: 200 mg/kg/day IV divided q8hr > 7 days: 300 mg/kg/day IV divided q6hr Beyond neonatal period: 200–300 mg/kg/day IV divided q6hr Other: Neonate: < 2 kg: 0–7 days: 50 mg/kg/day IV divided q12hr > 7 days: 75 mg/kg/day IV divided q8hr ≥ 2 kg: 0–7 days: 75 mg/kg/day IV divided q8hr > 7 days: 100 mg/kg/day IV divided q6hr Beyond neonatal period: 50–100 mg/kg/day IV divided q6hr
Amoxicillin (Amoxil, Trimox)	20–50 mg/kg/day PO divided tid 80–90 mg/kg/day PO divided tid (high-dose therapy*)
Cloxacillin (Cloxapen—U.S.; Orbenin—Can.)	Neonate: > 2 kg: 0–7 days: 50–100 mg/kg/day IV divided q12hr > 7 days: 75–150 mg/kg/day IV divided q8hr ≥ 2 kg: 0–7 days: 75–150 mg/kg/day IV divided q8hr > 7 days: 100–200 mg/kg/day IV divided q6hr Beyond the neonatal period: 50–200 mg/kg/day IV divided q6hr (depending on severity)
CEPHALOSPORINS	
Cefuroxime (Ceftin, Kefurox, Zinacef)	75–150 mg/kg/day IV divided q8hr
Cefotaxime (Claforan)	Neonate: 0–7 days: 100–150 mg/kg/day IV/IM divided q8–12hr > 7 days: 150–200 mg/kg/day IV/IM divided q6–8hr Beyond neonatal period: Meningitis and sickle cell disease: 200 mg/kg/day IV/IM divided q6hr Other: Mild-moderate infections: 75–100 mg/kg/day IV/IM divided q8hr Severe infections: 150–200 mg/kg/day IV/IM divided q6–8hr

Dose Limit	Side Effects
20 MIU/day	**Frequent:** Diarrhea (especially with ampicillin and amoxicillin) Hypersensitivity reactions (1%–4%) Rash (especially with ampicillin and amoxicillin); increased incidence of rash in patients with infectious mononucleosis taking amoxicillin.
10 g/day	Ampicillin should be injected slowly over 10–15 minutes as more rapid administration could cause convulsive seizures. **Occasional:** Fever, phlebitis at infusion site (especially with cloxacillin) **Rare but important:** Anemia, *Clostridium difficile* colitis (especially with ampicillin), convulsions (with high dose in renal failure), hepatic damage, leucopenia, thrombocytopenia
4 g/day	
12 g/day	
4.5 g/day	**Frequent:** Phlebitis at infusion site
8 g/day	**Occasional:** Cholelithiasis (ceftriaxone), diarrhea, hypersensitivity reactions **Rare but important:** Convulsions (with high dose in renal failure), hemolytic anemia, hepatic dysfunction, intersitial nephritis, neutropenia, thrombocytopenia

(continued)

Table 18–10. Recommended Dosing and Side Effects of Antibiotics Recommended in Empiric Management of Pneumonia and Bacteremia/Septicemia *(Continued)*

Class and Generic (Brand) Name	Dose
Ceftriaxone (Rocephin)	Meningitis: 80 mg/kg/dose at 0, 12, 24 hours, then 80 mg/kg/dose IV/IM q24hr Other: 80 mg/kg/dose IV/IM q24hr
Ceftazidime (Ceptaz, Fortaz, Tazicef, Tazidime)	Neonate: 0–7 days: 100 mg/kg/day IV/IM divided q8–12hr > 7 days: 150 mg/kg/day IV/IM divided q8hr Beyond neonatal period: Mild-moderate infections: 75–100 mg/kg/day IV/IM divided q8hr Severe infections: 125–150 mg/kg/day IV/IM divided q8hr
AMINOGLYCOSIDES	
Gentamicin (Garamycin—*U.S.*; Cidomycin—*Can.*) Tobramycin (Nebrex, Tobrex)	Neonate: 0–7 days: < 34 weeks†: 3 mg/kg/dose IV q24hr ≥34 weeks: 3 mg/kg/dose IV q18hr > 7 days: ≤ 1 kg: 3.5 mg/kg/dose IV q24hr > 1 kg: < 37 weeks: 2.5 mg/kg/dose IV q12hr ≥ 37 weeks: 2.5 mg/kg/dose IV q8hr Beyond neonatal period: 7.5 mg/kg/day divided q8hr
AZALIDE-MACROLIDES	
Erythromycin	20–50 mg/kg/day IV divided q6hr 20–40 mg/kg/day PO divided qid–bid
Clarithromycin (Biaxin)	15 mg/kg/day PO divided q12hr
Azithromycin (Zithromax)	10 mg/kg on day 1, then 5 mg/kg daily on days 2–5
OTHER	
Clindamycin (Cleocin—*U.S.*; Dalacin—*Can.*)	Mild-moderate infections: 15–25 mg/kg/day IV/IM divided q6–8hr Severe infections: 25–40 mg/kg/day IV/IM divided q6–8hr
Vancomycin (Vancocin)	Meningitis: 60 mg/kg/day IV divided q6hr Other: 40–60 mg/kg/day IV divided q6hr

GBS = group B streptococcal infection.

*Useful for otitis media unresponsive to regular-dose amoxicillin.

†Postconceptional age (i.e., corrected gestational age).

‡Red man syndrome is erythematous rash on the face and upper body.

Dose Limit	Side Effects
2 g/dose 4 g/day	
6 g/day	
	Hearing loss (related more to duration or cumulative dose) Nephrotoxicity, usually reversible **Ototoxicity is irreversible.** Renal failure (related to dose, duration, previous renal function, concurrent nephrotoxic drugs, hydration status)

2 g/day PO
4 g/day IV
1 g/day
	Cholestatic hepatitis
	Gastrointestinal intolerance (most with erythromycin, least
	    with azithromycin)
	Interaction with many important drugs (e.g., elevate serum
	    levels of theophylline and digoxin)
	Phlebitis (IV erythromycin)

2.7 g/day	C. *difficile* colitis

4 g/day	Bitter taste, nausea, vomiting, drug fever, hematologic
	    dyscrasias, vasculitis, hypotension, red man syndrome‡
	    (infusion rate related), renal failure, hypersensitivity reac-
	    tions

cases. Infection may be limited to the skin, eye, and mouth or to the CNS, or it may be disseminated. Once in the CNS, virus-induced cell death can lead to perivascular and parenchymal inflammation intense enough to cause localized vasculitis, resulting in hemorrhage and necrosis.

TX **Supportive care, seizure control,** and, particularly, **early antiviral (acyclovir) treatment are crucial** in reducing mortality and morbidity. **Slow rate of infusion of acyclovir and good hydration are important in avoiding transient renal insufficiency associated with the drug.** Recommended total duration of therapy is 21 days.

RX **Acyclovir** (Zovirax): an acyclic nucleoside analog that, once phosphorylated by HSV-specified thymidine kinase and incorporated into the growing DNA chain of the virus, causes chain termination.

DS **Neonatal HSV encephalitis:** 60 mg/kg/day IV divided q8hr
HSV encephalitis beyond the neonatal period: 30–45 mg/kg/day IV divided q8hr

SE Transient renal insufficiency caused by crystallization of the drug in the renal parenchyma.

MENINGITIS

See Ch 10 Infectious Diseases.

OTITIS MEDIA

See Ch 16 Otolaryngology.

PHARYNGITIS AND TONSILITIS

See Ch 16 Otolaryngology.

PNEUMONIA

Management of pneumonia in adults is discussed in Ch 10 Infectious Diseases.

KY Pneumonia, an **inflammation of the lung,** can be caused by a wide array of microorganisms, including bacteria, viruses, fungi, rickettsiae, and parasites; its incidence is highest in infants. Although the focus here is **bacterial pneumonia,** the reader should be cognizant of the significant role of **respiratory viruses** (e.g., RSV, parainfluenza, influenza, adenoviruses), particularly in pneumonia beyond the neonatal period. This is especially important given that there are **specific antiviral agents** (e.g., ribavirin for RSV; amantadine, rimantadine, and the newer neuraminidase inhibitors for influenza) that may be helpful in select cases. In pediatrics, age is the most important factor in determining microbiologic etiology and in guiding initial therapy in bacterial pneumonia (Table 18-11), although clinical and radiographic patterns of infection may also be helpful. Aspiration of nasopharyngeal flora and inhalation of infected aerosols are the usual routes of infection, with hematogenous seeding being less common. In newborns, infection may also develop through transplacental spread or aspiration of infected amniotic fluid or infected genital secretions during the birthing process.

TX **Once diagnosis is made, empiric therapy should be started promptly.** Criteria for hospitalization include severe disease, toxic appearance, significant pulmonary dysfunction, and inability to cope by the family. Hospitalization should also be considered for infants, especially those younger than 3 months. Treatment duration is 7–14 days depending on age, circumstance, and likely causative agent(s), with longer duration in neonates, young infants, hospital-acquired aspiration pneumonia, and *Staphylococcus aureus* infections. **Supportive and symptomatic treatment,** such as antipyretics, fluid hydration, supplemental oxygen, physiotherapy, and treatment of secondary reactive airways disease, should also be given as needed.

RX Table 18-11

DS Table 18-10

SE Table 18-10

SEPSIS

See BACTEREMIA AND SEPSIS

URINARY TRACT INFECTION (UTI)

KY UTI is more common (5–8 times) in boys during the first 3 months of life and thereafter occurs more often (10–20 times) in girls. Most offending organisms originate from the fecal flora. *Escherichia coli* accounts for most cases; the remainder are caused by other gram-negative enteric bacilli (*Proteus, Klebsiella, Enterobacter,* and *Pseudomonas* species) and gram-positive cocci (enterococci, *Staphylococcus epidermidis* [primarily seen in adolescents]). Vesicoureteral reflux (usually caused by a congenital abnormality of the ureterovesical junction) increases the risk of UTI including pyelonephritis and should be ruled out in girls < 5 years of age and all boys irrespective of age.

TX **Empiric therapy should be targeted at the likely infective organism** based on age and on previous culture and sensitivity result(s) in the case of recurrent UTIs, and **then adjusted as necessary using culture and susceptibility results.** In general, UTIs in children are considered "complicated" and should generally be treated as such (i.e., 7–10 days of treatment). The choice between IV and oral therapy depends on the severity of symptoms, likelihood of pyelonephritis, and age (neonates should be given parenteral therapy). Management should also include appropriate use of antipyretics as needed, good fluid hydration to increase urine flow, correction of any anatomical or functional abnormalities, and measures to prevent recurrences (e.g., vaginal/vulvar hygiene, avoidance of irritants such as perfumed soaps and bubble baths, encouragement of normal patterns of

Table 18–11. Acute Uncomplicated Bacterial Pneumonia: Microbiology and Initial Empiric Antibiotic Therapy

Age Group or Circumstance	Common Etiologic Agents*	Antibiotic†		Note
		Inpatient	Outpatient	
Neonate‡	GBS, *Escherichia coli*, other gram-negative bacilli, *Listeria monocytogenes*, *Staphylococcus aureus*	Ampicillin + aminoglycoside ± cloxacillin	Not recommended and generally not feasible	Cloxacillin if suspected *S. aureus* infection.
1–3 months	*Streptococcus pneumoniae*, *Chlamydia trachomatis*, *Bordetella pertussis*, *S. aureus*, *Haemophilus influenzae*	Cefuroxime ± azalide-macrolide	Not recommended as initial therapy	Azalide-macrolide if suspected *C. trachomatis* or *B. pertussis* infection.
3 months– 5 years	*S. pneumoniae*, *Mycoplasma pneumoniae*, *S. aureus*	Ampicillin ± cloxacillin (or cefuroxime alone) ± azalide-macrolide	Amoxicillin	Cefuroxime alone if suspected *S. aureus* infection. Azalide-macrolide if suspected *M. pneumoniae* infection.

5–18 years	M. pneumoniae, C. pneumoniae, S. pneumoniae, S. aureus	Ampicillin or cefuroxime + azalide-macrolide	Azalide-macrolide or amoxicillin	Ampicillin or cefuroxime if suspected bacterial pneumonia in ill inpatient.
Aspiration pneumonia§ Community acquired	Oral anaerobes or mixed oropharyngeal flora ± gram-negative enteric bacilli, S. aureus in ill patients.	Penicillin	Not recommended if severe enough for treatment	Penicillin or clindamycin if suspected penicillin-resistant organisms or life threatening.
Hospital acquired		Penicillin or clindamycin ± aminoglycoside		Aminoglycoside use depends on severity, previous use of antibiotics, or respiratory flora.

GBS = group B streptococcal infection.

*Mycobacterium tuberculosis (TB) should be considered in all children (especially adolescents) in highly endemic areas, with a history of possible contact. Group A β-hemolytic streptococci are an uncommon but important cause of severe necrotizing pneumonia and often occur as a complication of varicella infection. For S. pneumoniae pulmonary infections, it seems that penicillins and other β-lactam antibiotics remain effective for most penicillin-intermediate and penicillin-resistant strains.

†See Table 18–10 for dosing information.

‡The list of pathogens does not include those that infect long-term residents in the neonatal intensive care unit.

§No treatment needed unless severe.

Table 18–12. Commonly Used Antibiotics for Empiric* Therapy and Prophylaxis in UTIs

Generic (Brand) Name	Dose	Side Effects
Empiric Therapy		
Ampicillin + gentamicin† (or another aminoglycoside)	Ampicillin: 50–100 mg/kg IV/PO divided q6hr (max 2–3 g/day)	See Table 18–10 for side effects.
	Gentamicin: 1.5–2.5 mg/kg IV divided q8hr	Gentamicin active against *Pseudomonas.*
TMP-SMX† (Bactrim, Septra)	8 mg TMP/kg PO divided q12hr	Fever, GI intolerance, hemolytic anemia with G-6-PD deficiency, hepatitis with cholestatic jaundice, rash (especially in HIV patients), risk of kernicterus in hyperbilirubinemic newborns
Sulfisoxazole (Gantrisin, Truxazole—*U.S.*; Sulfizole—*Can.*)	120–150 mg/kg PO divided q4–6hr (max 6 g/day)	Not active against *Pseudomonas.*
Nitrofurantoin (Furadantin, Macrobid, Macrodantin—*U.S.*; Nephronex—*Can.*)	5–7 mg/kg PO divided q6hr (maximum 400 mg/day)	Acute pneumonitis, GI intolerance, hemolytic anemia with G-6-PD deficiency, peripheral neuropathy
		Active against *Klebsiella-Enterobacter* species.

Amoxicillin (Amoxil, Trimox)	20–50 mg/kg PO divided q8hr	See Table 18–10 for side effects. Increasing resistance in *Escherichia coli* to amoxicillin limits its use.
Prophylactic Therapy		
TMP-SMX‡	2 mg TMP/kg PO qd	See above.
Nitrofurantoin	1–2 mg/kg PO divided q6hr (max 100 mg/day)	See above.
Sulfisoxazole	100 mg/kg PO divided q6hr (max 6 g/day)	See above.

GI = gastrointestinal; G-6-PD, glucose-6-phosphate dehydrogenase; HIV = human immunodeficiency virus; TMP-SMX = trimethoprim and sulfamethoxazole; UTI = urinary tract infection.

*Patients with recurrent UTIs may require a more individualized regimen based on past culture results.

†May be considered as first-line therapy for treatment.

‡May be considered as first-line therapy for prophylaxis.

voiding and defecation). **Follow-up cultures should be obtained at 1 week after completion of treatment and then periodically for 12 months** thereafter (even if asymptomatic) to identify patients with recurrent UTIs. Patients at risk for recurrent UTIs (e.g., vesicoureteral reflux) or with a history of recurrent UTIs should receive **prophylactic therapy** for at least 6–12 months. If no infection occurs during this period, prophylaxis may be discontinued, with subsequent monitoring.

RX **Empiric treatment and prophylactic options** (Table 18-12)

DS Table 18-12

SE Table 18-12

19

Psychiatry

ADAM WAESE, ROGER S. MCINTYRE

ADDICTIVE SUBSTANCE WITHDRAWAL

Substance withdrawal is characterized by a substance-specific syndrome occurring on cessation of heavy and prolonged use of the substance.

Alcohol Withdrawal

KY This is the most common withdrawal syndrome posing significant health risks. It is usually characterized early by symptoms of autonomic arousal (e.g., sweating, tachycardia, tremor, insomnia), and later-onset symptoms may include disorientation, altered level of consciousness, hallucinations, seizures, or death. The pathophysiology is accounted for by changes in neurotransmitter systems, including gamma-aminobutyric acid (GABA), that accompany sustained, heavy alcohol use. It is acutely triggered by the abrupt cessation of alcohol use.

TX Alcohol withdrawal is treated with **benzodiazepines** (Table 19–1). Diazepam (Valium) is used with most patients and can be given 10–20 mg q1hr until symptoms subside without further dosing. **Caution** should be used in prescribing the drug when excessive drowsiness, ataxia, or respiratory depression is present. **In patients with hepatic impairment,** use lorazepam (Ativan), oxazepam (Serax—*U.S.*; Zaprex—*Can.*), or temazepam (Restoril), and taper the daily dose over 3–4 days.

RX **Anxiolytic agents:** Table 19–1

DS Table 19–1

SE Table 19–1

Opioid Withdrawal

KY Occurs with abrupt cessation of opioid use, or administration of an opioid antagonist, after chronic use. Consists of symptoms such as dysphoric mood, nausea and vomiting, diarrhea, lacrimation, muscle aches, pupillary dilation, sweating, fever, yawning, and insomnia that last several days, based on the duration of action of the opioid that was used. Changes in opioid receptor number and sensitivity, in addition to probable changes to other neurotransmitter systems, associated with chronic opioid use result in withdrawal symptoms on abrupt cessation.

TX The syndrome may not require treatment, as it is generally not physically dangerous. **Methadone** or **pentazocine** (the latter only for pentazocine dependence) may be used for detoxification, tapered gradually over

Table 19–1. Anxiolytic Agents

Generic (Brand) Name	Average Dose (PO)
Benzodiazepines	
Lorazepam (Ativan) [D]	0.5–2 mg tid
Clonazepam (Klonopin—*U.S.*; Rivotril—*Can.*) [D]	0.5–2 mg bid
Diazepam (Valium) [D]	2–10 mg qd or bid
Alprazolam (Xanax) [D]	0.25–1 mg tid
Temazepam (Restoril) [X]	15–30 mg qhs
Oxazepam (Serax—*U.S.*; Zaprex—*Can.*)	15–30 mg qhs
Other agents	
Buspirone (BuSpar) [B]	5–30 mg/day
Gabapentin (Neurontin) [C]	600–2,400 mg/day divided bid–tid

CNS = central nervous system; GI, gastrointestinal; MAOIs = monoamine oxidase inhibitors; OCPs = oral contraceptive pills; SSRIs = specific serotonin reuptake inhibitors.

*There are many possible drug interactions, but it is beyond the scope of this book to list them all.

†Serotonin syndrome includes hyperpyrexia, hypertension, tachycardia, confusion, seizures, and death.

several days. **Clonidine** (Catapres—*U.S.*; Dixarit—*Can.*) may help relieve nausea, vomiting, and diarrhea.

RX Table 19–2

DS Table 19–2

SE Table 19–2

ANXIETY DISORDERS

Generalized Anxiety Disorder

KY Characterized by excessive uncontrollable and pervasive anxiety and worry, associated with symptoms of chronic arousal (e.g., muscle

Side Effects	Drug Interactions*
Drowsiness, fatigue, confusion, amnesia, cognitive impairment, incoordination, ataxia, disinhibition, dizziness, blood dyscrasias, dependence, withdrawal syndrome **With liver impairment or for elderly patients: oxazepam, lorazepam, or temazepam should be used.**	Concomitant use with CNS depressants can have additive effects. OCPs, P-450 inhibitors may increase the serum levels of benzodiazepines. Disulfiram can increase the serum levels of clonazepam. Concomitant use of valproic acid and clonazepam is associated with absence seizures.
Headaches, dizziness, activation, mania, hyperprolactinemia, serotonin syndrome,† blurred vision, allergic reactions	Increases the risk of extrapyramidal side effects with concomitant use of antipsychotics. Calcium channel blockers can increase the serum levels of buspirone. Concomitant use with MAOIs is contraindicated because it can cause hypertension. Concomitant use with SSRIs can cause serotonin syndrome.† P-450 inhibitors can increase serum levels of buspirone.
Somnolence, ataxia, edema, amnesia, depression, dysarthria, GI upset, weight gain, tremor, hypotension, blood dyscrasias, allergic reactions, alopecia, hyperlipidemia, withdrawal syndrome	Antacids can reduce the bioavailability of gabapentin and should be avoided 2 hours before and after gabapentin administration. Phenytoin may increase serum levels of gabapentin.

tension, sleep disturbance). Substances (e.g., caffeine), medical conditions (e.g., hyperthyroidism), and primary mood disturbances can account for similar symptoms. The pathophysiology is not fully understood. GABA and serotonin neurotransmitter systems are thought to be involved.

TX **First-line treatment:** Selective **serotonin norepinephrine reuptake inhibitor** (SNRI) venlafaxine (Effexor) and the **specific serotonin reuptake inhibitors** (SSRIs). **Nonselective cyclic antidepressants** and **irreversible monoamine oxidase inhibitors** (MAOIs) are also effective (Table 19–3). Treatment may need to be initiated at lower doses than for depression.

Table 19–2. Agents Used for Substance Withdrawal

Generic (Brand) Name	Dose (PO)
Clonidine (Catapres—*U.S.*; Dixarit—*Can.*)	0.1–0.2 mg q3hr, up to 0.8 mg/day Taper over 2 weeks
Methadone (Dolophine, Methadose) [B/D depending on dose and duration of use]	Initially 10 mg q6hr until withdrawal effects are controlled; after 24–48 hours, can be lengthened to q12–24hr. Taper by 5 mg per day.
Pentazocine (Talwin) [B/D depending on dose and duration of use]	Dose often varies. Average is 50 mg q3–4hr, and it can be increased to 100 mg q3–4hr if needed. Maximum is 600 mg/day. Taper gradually.

CNS = central nervous system.

*There are many possible drug interactions, but it is beyond the scope of this book to list them all.

Second-line treatment: Benzodiazepines, for example, clonazepam (Klonopin—*U.S.*; Rivotril—*Can.*) and lorazepam (Ativan) are also effective agents but are not considered primary treatments. They are often used in combination with an antidepressant for initial short-term control of symptoms while the antidepressant takes effect. Evidence suggests that they address only some symptoms of anxiety (somatic symptoms and not psychic symptoms) as opposed to antidepressants, which have demonstrated efficacy for both classes of symptoms of anxiety. **Other agents** with reported efficacy include buspirone (Buspar), particularly in patients who have not previously received benzodiazepine therapy. See Table 19–1 for selected benzodiazepines and other anxiolytic agents.

RX Table 19–1 and Table 19–3

DS Table 19–1 and Table 19–3

SE Table 19–1 and Table 19–3

Side Effects	Drug Interactions*
Drowsiness, hypotension, dry mouth, bradycardia, hepatitis, withdrawal syndrome	Concomitant use with antipsychotics, narcotic analgesics, and nitroprusside may produce additive hypotensive effects. Beta-blockers may potentiate bradycardia and can increase rebound hypertension of withdrawal. Concomitant use with CNS depressants can cause additive sedative effects. Concurrent administration of verapamil and clonidine is associated with hypotension and atrioventricular block.
Drowsiness, constipation, respiratory depression, hallucinations, physical and psychological dependence	P-450 inhibitors and zidovudine may increase serum levels of methadone. Barbiturates, carbamazepine, phenytoin, primidone, rifampin, and somatostatin can decrease the therapeutic effect of methadone. Avoid concurrent use with MAOIs, selegiline, and furazolidone.
Drowsiness, dizziness, euphoria, nausea, vomiting, constipation, respiratory depression, hypertension, anxiety, physical and psychological dependence Can cause withdrawal symptoms in opioid addicts owing to its agonist/antagonist properties.	CNS depressants can cause additive sedative effects. Pentazocine can precipitate withdrawal in those addicted to narcotic analgesics.

Obsessive-Compulsive Disorder

KV Characterized by obsessions (recurrent and intrusive thoughts, impulses, or images), which cause anxiety or distress, and compulsions (repetitive and unwanted behaviors), which are performed to alleviate anxiety or to prevent an unrealistic dreaded situation. Dysregulation of the serotonergic neurotransmitter system has been hypothesized as the cause for this disorder. Structural and blood perfusion abnormalities have been noted with brain imaging studies.

TX **SSRIs** at higher doses than for depression are generally required. An adequate trial consists of 6–8 weeks at the maximum recommended dose. Clomipramine (Anafranil) is the most effective agent, used in refractory cases, owing to its increased side effect burden. The **SNRI**, serotonin-2 antagonists/reuptake inhibitors (**SARIs**), and **MAOIs** can also be used (Table 19–3). **Lithium** (Table 19–4) and **L-tryptophan** (Table 19–5) can be used as **adjunctive agents** for partial responders.

RX **Antidepressants:** Table 19–3, with or without lithium (Table 19–4) or L-tryptophan (Table 19.5)

DS Table 19–3, Table 19–4, Table 19–5

SE Table 19–3, Table 19–4, Table 19–5

Table 19–3. Antidepressants

Generic (Brand) Name	Daily Dose (PO)	Maximum Dose (PO)
Selective Serotonin Reuptake Inhibitors		
Citalopram (Celexa) [C]	20–40 mg	60 mg
Proxetine (Paxil) [C]	20–40 mg	60 mg
Sertraline (Zoloft) [C]	50–150 mg	200 mg
Fluoxetine (Prozac) [C]	20–40 mg	80 mg
Fluvoxamine (Luvox) [C]	100–200 mg	300 mg
Selective Serotonin Norepinephrine Reuptake Inhibitor		
Venlafaxine (Effexor) [C]	75–225 mg	375 mg
Norepinephrine Dopamine Reuptake Inhibitor		
Bupropion (Wellbutrin, Zyban) [B]	150–300 mg	300 mg
SARIs (Serotonin-2 Antagonist/Reuptake Inhibitors)		
Nefazodone (Serzone) [C]	200–400 mg	600 mg
Trazodone (Desyrel) [C]	200–400 mg	600 mg
Reversible Inhibitor of MAO-A		
Moclobemide (Manerix)	450–600 mg	900 mg

Panic Disorder With or Without Agoraphobia

KY Characterized by recurrent unexpected panic attacks, followed by at least 1 month of persistent concern about having additional attacks or worrying about the possible consequences of the attacks. Agoraphobia is diag-

Side Effects	Drug Interactions*
GI upset, nausea, headaches, sexual dysfunction, tremor, anxiety, akathisia, asthenia, insomnia, mania, sedation, dry mouth, constipation, withdrawal syndrome	Ergotamine, MAOIs, and tryptophan; concomitant use can cause serotonin syndrome.† Can potentiate the effects of P-450 inhibitors. Can increase the level of some beta-blockers.
Hypertension, insomnia, headache, dry mouth, GI upset, sexual dysfunction, mania, withdrawal syndrome	Avoid concomitant use with MAOIs, as this can cause serotonin syndrome.† Can potentiate the effects of P-450 inhibitors.
Seizures, tremor, headache, agitation, insomnia, mania	Avoid concomitant use with MAOIs, as this can cause serotonin syndrome.† Levodopa increases the toxicity of bupropion.
Risk of life-threatening hepatic failure, and it is **contraindicated** in patients with active liver disease or elevated transaminase levels. Sedation, hypotension, lowers seizure threshold, headache, mania, impotence, urinary frequency and retention, vision impairment and visual field defect, and hypersensitivity reactions. Use with caution in patients with cardiovascular disease.	Serum concentrations of amiodarone, lidocaine, propaterone, and quinidine could be increased with concomitant use. Can potentiate the effects of P-450 inhibitors.
Priapism, sedation, hypotension, hypertension, tremor, blurred vision, extrapyramidal effects, cardiac arrhythmias, urinary retention	Concomitant use with other antipsychotic agents can have additive hypotension effects. Can potentiate the effects of P-450 inhibitors. Avoid concomitant use with MAOIs, as this can cause serotonin syndrome.† Use caution with tyramine-rich foods (e.g., ethanol, cheese), particularly > 600 mg.
Insomnia, agitation, headache, GI upset, dry mouth, blurred vision, mania	Avoid concurrent use with sympathomimetic drugs and meperidine. *(continued)*

Table 19–3. Antidepressants *(Continued)*

Generic (Brand) Name	Daily Dose (PO)	Maximum Dose (PO)
Noradrenergic/Specific Serotonergic Antidepressants		
Mirtazapine (Remeron) [C]	30 mg	45 mg
Nonselective Cyclic Antidepressants		
Amitriptyline‡ (Elavil, Vanatrip— U.S.; Levate—Can.) [D]	100–250 mg	300 mg
Clomipramine (Anafranil) [C]	100–250 mg	300 mg
Desipramine (Norpramin) [C]	100–250 mg	300 mg
Imipramine (Tofranil) [D]	100–250 mg	300 mg
Nortriptyline (Aventyl, Pamelor) [D]	75–150 mg	200 mg
Irreversible MAOIs		
Phenelzine (Nardil) [C]	30–75 mg	90 mg
Tranylcypromine (Parnate) [C]	20–60 mg	80 mg

GI = gastrointestinal; MAOIs = monoamine oxidase inhibitors.

*There are many possible drug interactions, but it is beyond the scope of this book to list them all.

†Serotonin syndrome includes hyperpyrexia, hypertension, tachycardia, confusion, seizures, and death.

‡Symptoms of overdose include hallucinations, hypothermia, hypotension, cardiac arrhythmias, and seizures. Alkalinization by sodium bicarbonate or hyperventilation may limit cardiac toxicity. Conventional treatment of overdose is symptomatic and supportive.

nosed in addition if there is persistent anxiety about and avoidance of places or situations in which escape might be difficult or help might not be available if an attack were to occur. Panic attacks can also be substance induced (e.g., alcohol), caused by a medical condition (e.g., hyperthyroidism), or in the context of a primary mood disorder (e.g., major depression). Dysregulation of the norepinephrine and serotonin neurotransmitter systems and heightened sensitivity to panic-inducing substances have been reported.

TX **Antidepressants for long-term control of symptoms** (Table 19–3); classes used include the SSRIs, the SNRI, the nonselective cyclic antidepressants, and MAOIs. Initiate at very low doses. Often, **benzodiazepines can be added adjunctively,** for example, clonazepam (Table 19–1) for short-term control of symptoms, while awaiting the effect of the antidepressant. They can be considered for long-term use if required.

RX **Antidepressants:** Table 19–3, with or without **benzodiazepines** (Table 19–1)

Side Effects	Drug Interactions*
Drowsiness, weight gain, dry mouth, increased cholesterol, withdrawal syndrome	Avoid concomitant use with MAOIs, as this can cause serotonin syndrome.†
Weight gain, dry mouth, dry eyes, blurred vision, urinary retention, sedation, hypotension, cardiac arrhythmias, sexual dysfunction, mania, withdrawal syndrome	Interactions have been documented with antiarrhythmics, MAOIs, P-450 inhibitors, other serotonergic agents, and warfarin
Insomnia, weight gain, mania, hypotension, edema, leukopenia, sexual dysfunction, tremor, glaucoma, withdrawal syndrome	Avoid tyramine-rich foods (e.g., cheese, ethanol). Concomitant use with amphetamines or levodopa can cause hypertension. Delirium has been reported with concomitant disulfiram. Concomitant use with serotonergic agents can result in serotonin syndrome.†

DS Table 19–1 and Table 19–3

SE Table 19–1 and Table 19–3

Posttraumatic Stress Disorder

KY Characterized by the exposure to a traumatic event generating an intense reaction (e.g., fear, helplessness, or horror) that is later reexperienced (e.g., with nightmares or flashbacks), leading to a pattern of avoidance, emotional restriction, and chronic arousal. Chronic changes and abnormal reactivity have been noted in the autonomic nervous system and in other neurologic and neurochemical systems involved in arousal.

TX **Antidepressants,** in particular **SSRIs,** can assist in modulating symptoms (Table 19–3). **Nonselective cyclic antidepressants** have been shown to be efficacious as well. **Benzodiazepines** (Table 19–1) can be considered,

Table 19-4. Mood Stabilizers

Generic (Brand) Name	Daily Dose (PO)	Blood Level	Side Effects	Drug Interactions*
Carbamazepine (Carbatrol, Epitol, Tegretol) [D]	Start 100 mg bid and then increase to 300–1,600 mg qd	4–12 µg/mL and also titrate to SE **Toxic > 12 µg/mL**	Drowsiness, ataxia, tremors, rash, blood dyscrasias, blurred vision, hepatitis, cardiac arrhythmias, hypersensitivity reactions	Anticonvulsants, antidepressants, oral contraceptive pills, some antibiotics, warfarin, and P-450 inhibitors.
Valproic acid (Depacon, Depakene, Depakote—*U.S.*; Epival—*Can.*) [D]	Start 250 mg tid and then increase to 750–3,000 mg qd	50–115 µg/mL **Toxic > 150 µg/mL**	GI symptoms, weight gain, tremor, sedation, alopecia, hepatotoxicity, thrombocytopenia, and pancreatitis	Anticonvulsants, antidepressants, diazepam, alcohol, acetylsalicylic acid, P-450 inhibitors.
Lamotrigine (Lamictal) [C]	Start 25 mg bid and then increase to 200–400 mg qd	Not required	Insomnia, activation, cognitive blunting, rash, Stevens-Johnson syndrome	Anticonvulsants affect lamotrigine levels and can increase the risk of Stevens-Johnson syndrome.
Lithium (Eskalith, Lithobid—*U.S.*; Carbolith, Duralith, Lithize—*Can.*) [D]	900–1,200 mg qd	0.8–1.2 mEq/L **Toxic > 1.5 mEq/L**	Tremor, weakness, polydipsia, polyuria, tremor, nausea, and hypothyroidism Avoid use in renal or cardiac impairment.	Sodium salts, theophylline, NSAIDs, and acetazolamide.
Topiramate (Topamax) [C]	Start with 50 mg qid and then increase to 50–500 mg qd	Not required	Weight loss, sweating, cognitive changes, dizziness, nephrolithiasis, paresthesias	Anticonvulsants

GI = gastrointestinal; NSAIDs = nonsteroidal anti-inflammatory drugs.
*There are many possible drug interactions, but it is beyond the scope of this book to list them all.

Table 19–5. Hypnotic Agents

Generic (Brand) Name	Daily Dose (PO)	Side Effects
Lorazepam (Ativan) [D]	0.5–2 mg	Table 19–1
Oxazepam (Serax—*U.S.*; Zaprex—*Can.*) [D]	15–30 mg	Table 19–1
Temazepam (Restoril) [X] Zopiclone (Imovane)	15–30 mg 7.5–15 mg	Table 19–1 Taste alteration, sedation, impaired coordination, agitation, tremor, palpitations, GI upset, dyspnea, weight loss, rebound insomnia Concomitant use with CNS depressants can cause additive sedation.
Zolpidem (Ambien) [B] L-tryptophan (Tryptan)	5–20 mg 1–3 g	Sleep disturbance, palpitations, GI upset, sedation Dry mouth, drowsiness, GI upset, headache, sexual dysfunction, emotional disorders Concomitant use with lithium can increase lithium side effects. Caution when using in combination with other serotonergic agents.
Chloral hydrate (Aquachloral, Supprettes—*U.S.*; Noctec—*Can.*) [C]	500–1000 mg	GI upset, sedation, paradoxical excitation, headache, hallucinations, rash, blood dyscrasias, physical and psychological dependence Can increase the effect of warfarin and decrease the effect of phenytoin. Concomitant use with CNS depressants can cause additive sedation. Avoid use in patients with hepatic or renal disease, GI inflammation, or porphyria.

CNS = central nervous system; GI = gastrointestinal.

for example, clonazepam, for short-term control of insomnia and anxiety. **Comorbid disorders such as major depression should be identified and treated.**

RX **Antidepressants:** Table 19–3, with or without benzodiazepines (Table 19–1)

DS Table 19–1 and Table 19–3

SE Table 19–1 and Table 19–3

Social Phobia

KY Characterized by a persistent fear of single or multiple social or performance situations, in addition to significant avoidance of the situations, or suffering intense anxiety or distress during them. The pathophysiology is similar to that of panic disorder.

TX **First-line treatment:** Treatment for generalized social phobia is with **SSRIs** (Table 19–3).

Second-line treatment: There is some evidence for nefazodone (Serzone) and venlafaxine (Effexor) (Table 19–3) and the anticonvulsant gabapentin (Neurontin) (Table 19–1).

  Third-line treatment: MAOIs should be considered only as third-line treatment owing to the decreased safety profile. **Beta-blockers,** for example, atenolol (Tenormin), **or low doses of short-duration benzodiazepines** (Table 19–1), for example, lorazepam (Ativan) or alprazolam (Xanax), can be used for anxiety related to specific performance situations 30–60 minutes before the event.

RX SSRIs (Table 19–3), SARIs (Table 19–3), venlafaxine (Table 19–3), and gabapentin (Table 19–1); or atenolol (Table 19–6) or benzodiazepines (Table 19–1)

DS Table 19–1, Table 19–3, and Table 19–6

SE Table 19–1, Table 19–3, and Table 19–6

BIPOLAR MOOD DISORDERS

Bipolar I Disorder

KY Characterized by at least one manic episode, which includes at least a week of abnormally elevated or irritable mood along with sufficient manic symptoms. An episode of major depression is not required to make this diagnosis. The pathophysiology is thought to be the same as for major depressive disorder.

TX **First-line treatment:** Treatment for bipolar mania, depression, and prophylaxis of episodes consists of **mood stabilizers** (Table 19–4), including lithium, and the anticonvulsants valproic acid (Depacon, Depakene, Depakote—*U.S.*; Epival—*Can.*) and carbamazepine (Carbatrol, Epitol, Tegretol). Blood monitoring is recommended with these medications every 6 months with chronic use.

Table 19–6. Agents for Effective Management of Medication Side Effects

Side Effect	Generic (Brand) Name of Adjunctive Medication	Average Dose
Acute extrapyramidal symptoms (antipsychotics)	Benzodiazepines	See Table 19–1
	Benztropine (Cogentin) [C]	1–2 mg PO/IM bid
	Diphenhydramine (Benadryl) [B]	25–50 mg PO/IM qd
Akathisia (antipsychotics)	Atenolol (Tenormin—*U.S.*; Tenolin—*Can.*) [D]	25–100 mg/day PO in 1–2 doses
	Benzodiazepines	See Table 19–1
	Propranolol (Inderal—*U.S.*; Detensol—*Can.*)	10–40 mg PO tid
Neuroleptic malignant syndrome (antipsychotics)	Bromocriptine (Parlodel) [B]	2.5–5 mg by NG tid
	Dantrolene (Dantrium) [C]	1 mg/kg IV prn up to 5 doses
Sexual side effects (antidepressants, some agents can be used with antipsychotics)	Amantadine (Symadine, Symmetrel—*U.S.*; Endantadine—*Can.*) [C]	100–200 mg PO qd **Avoid in cases of psychosis.**
	Bethanechol (Urecholine—*U.S.*; Duvoid—*Can.*)	10–25 mg PO prn
	Bupropion (Wellbutrin, Zyban) [B]	100–300 mg PO qd **Avoid in cases of psychosis.**
	Cyproheptadine (Periactin) [B]	4–12 mg PO prn
	Sildenafil (Viagra) [B]	50–100 mg PO prn
Sialorrhea (antipsychotics)	Amitriptyline (Elavil, Vanatrip—*U.S.*; Levate—*Can.*)	25–100 mg PO qd
	Benztropine (Cogentin) [C]	2–4 mg PO qd

NG = nasogastric tube.

Second-line treatment: Second-line mood stabilizers such as lamotrigine (Lamictal) or topiramate (Topamax) may be added in refractory cases. Lamotrigine seems promising for bipolar depression and rapid cycling bipolar disorder. **Antipsychotics** may be added in acute mania to accelerate response (Table 19–7). **Adjunctive antidepressants** (Table 19–3) may be considered for the bipolar depressed patient. Antidepressants may induce mania in some vulnerable persons. Antidepressant use is discouraged in individuals with rapid cycling bipolar I and II disorder.

RX Lithium, valproic acid, and carbamazepine (Table 19–4); lamotrigine, topiramate (Table 19–4), with or without antipsychotics (Table 19–7), with or without adjunctive antidepressants in the bipolar depressed patient (Table 19–3).

DS Table 19–3, Table 19–4, and Table 19–7

SE Table 19–3, Table 19–4, and Table 19–7

Bipolar II Disorder

KY Characterized by one or more episodes of major depression and at least one hypomanic episode. Hypomania is distinguished from mania based on severity (e.g., need for hospitalization, psychosis). The pathophysiology is thought to be the same as that for bipolar I disorder.

TX Same as for bipolar I disorder.

RX See Bipolar I Disorder.

DS See Bipolar I Disorder.

SE See Bipolar I Disorder.

BODY DYSMORPHIC DISORDER

KY Characterized by a preoccupation with an imagined or minor defect in appearance. The exact etiology is unknown.

TX SSRIs or the nonselective cyclic antidepressant clomipramine (Anafranil) at standard doses are effective for about half of the patients (Table 19–3). Management otherwise consists of minimizing harmful interventions and minimizing functional impairment.

RX SSRIs or the nonselective cyclic antidepressant clomipramine: Table 19–3

DS Table 19–3

SE Table 19–3

DELIRIUM

KY Characterized by a disturbance in consciousness (e.g., inability to focus) and changes in cognition (e.g., disorientation) that develops over a short period and fluctuates throughout the day. It is often precipitated by a general medical condition (e.g., heart attack) or substance (e.g., benzodiazepine use

Table 19-7. Antipsychotics

Generic (Brand) Name	Average Dose (PO)	High Dose (PO)	Side Effects
Novel Antipsychotics			
Risperidone (Risperdal) [C]	1–4 mg	6 mg	Agitation, akathisia, sexual dysfunction, weight gain, extrapyramidal side effects, SIADH, hyperprolactinemia, agranulocytosis, neuroleptic malignant syndrome
Olanzapine (Zyprexa, Zydis) [C]	10–15 mg	20 mg	Sedation, agitation, sexual dysfunction, weight gain, hyperglycemia, hyperuricemia, hypertriglyceridemia, SIADH, agranulocytosis, increase transaminases, neuroleptic malignant syndrome
Quetiapine (Seroquel) [C]	300–600 mg	800+ mg	Headache, sedation, sexual dysfunction, hypotension, hypothyroidism, SIADH, hypercholesterolemia, agranulocytosis, neuroleptic malignant syndrome
Clozapine (Clozaril) [B]	300–450 mg	900 mg	Sedation, delirium, sexual dysfunction, seizures, sialorrhea, cataplexy, urinary retention, blurred vision, hypotension, ECG changes, weight gain, hyperglycemia, SIADH, agranulocytosis, hypercholesterolemia, withdrawal syndrome, neuroleptic malignant syndrome.

(continued)

Table 19–7. Antipsychotics *(Continued)*

Generic (Brand) Name	Average Dose (PO)	High Dose (PO)	Side Effects
Conventional Antipsychotics			
High potency			
Haloperidol (Haldol—*U.S.*; Peridol—*Can.*) [C]	2–6 mg	10 mg	Hypotension, sedation, extrapyramidal side effects, decreased seizure threshold, urinary retention, priapism, cardiac arrhythmias, neuroleptic malignant syndrome. Use with caution in patients with prolactin-dependent tumors, renal or respiratory disease, and hemodynamic instability. Avoid use in thyrotoxicosis.
Trifluoperazine (Stelazine) [C]	5–10 mg	20 mg	Similar side effect profile as haloperidol, plus blood dyscrasias, including agranulocytosis, leukocytosis, pancytopenia, thrombocytopenic purpura, eosinophilia, hemolytic anemia, and aplastic anemia.
Medium potency			
Loxapine (Loxitane—*U.S.*; Loxapec—*Can.*) [C]	15–30 mg	50 mg	Similar to those for trifluoperazine.
Perphenazine (Trilafon) [C]	4–8 mg	16 mg	Similar to those for haloperidol.
Low potency			
Chlorpromazine (Thorazine—*U.S.*; Chlorprom, Chlorpromanyl, Largactil—*Can.*) [C]	100–200 mg	300 mg	Similar to those for trifluoperazine.

ECG = electrocardiogram; SIADH = syndrome of inappropriate secretion of antidiuretic hormone.

or alcohol withdrawal). The etiology depends on the underlying cause. Decreased acetylcholine activity in the brain is generally noted in delirium.

TX Reversible causes of delirium (e.g., dehydration/hypernatremia, infections, hypoglycemia, hypercalcemia, uremia, liver failure, heart failure, shock, hypoxia, alcohol withdrawal, and overdose) should be addressed with specific treatment. **Symptomatic treatment** is accomplished with benzodiazepines to control agitation and insomnia (Table 19–1) and high-potency antipsychotics (Table 19–7) to remediate fluctuating cognitive impairments and reality distortion. Haloperidol (Haldol, Decanoate—*U.S.*; Peridol—*Can.*) is often used, PO or IM at doses of 1–5 mg bid–qid, and can be given IV continuously in refractory cases. **Cardiac monitoring is advisable with IV haloperidol.** Risperidone (Risperdal) in low doses can also be used, but is only available in oral formulations.

RX Benzodiazepines (Table 19–1), antipsychotics (Table 19–7)

DS Table 19–1 and Table 19–7

SE Table 19–1 and Table 19–7

DEMENTIA

KY Characterized by persistent cognitive and neurologic deficits and may include behavioral, psychiatric, or functional disturbances. There are multiple etiologies, of which Alzheimer's Type, a degenerative dementia, is the most common. Exclude reversible etiologies (e.g., brain tumors). The exact cause of Alzheimer's Type dementia is unknown, but it is associated with neuropathologic changes (e.g., amyloid deposition and atrophy) and degeneration of neurotransmitter systems (e.g., acetylcholine).

TX Ten percent of etiologies are reversible. The primary treatment for vascular dementia is to prevent further vascular events. Cholinesterase inhibitors have recently been shown to have a modest effect in ameliorating and slowing cognitive deterioration and improving functional ability in mild to moderate Alzheimer's Type dementia and diffuse Lewy Body disease.

RX **Cholinesterase inhibitors:** Table 19–8

DS Table 19–8

SE Table 19–8

DEPRESSION

See Nonbipolar Mood Disorders (Major Depressive Disorder).

EATING DISORDERS

Anorexia Nervosa

KY Characterized by a refusal to keep one's body weight within 85% of the normal range, which is accompanied by amenorrhea, an intense fear of becoming fat, and a distortion of body image. The etiology is unknown, but the effects of starvation include changes in multiple body systems (e.g., bradycardia, hypokalemia) and cognitions (e.g., depressive symptoms).

Table 19–8. Cholinesterase Inhibitors

Generic (Brand) Name	Average Dose (PO)	Side Effects	Drug Interactions*
Donepezil (Aricept) [C]	5–10 mg qd	Nausea, gastrointestinal upset, diarrhea, constipation, insomnia, nightmares, dizziness, nasal congestion, flushing, muscle cramps, allergic reactions	Concomitant use with digoxin, beta-blockers, and calcium channel blockers can increase the risk of bradycardia. Anticholinergics can reduce the effects of cholinesterase inhibitors.
Rivastigmine (Exelon) [B]	6–12 mg divided bid	Drug lowers seizure threshold. **Overdose can lead to life-threatening cholinergic crisis.†**	

*There are many possible drug interactions, but it is beyond the scope of this book to list them all.

†Cholinergic crisis is caused by significant acetylcholinesterase inhibition and presents with severe nausea, vomiting, salivation, sweating, bradycardia, hypotension, respiratory depression, and convulsions. It is treated with supportive and symptomatic measures.

TX Medications have not proven consistently effective in treating the disorder, although **prokinetic agents** such as metoclopramide at 5–20 mg before meals can assist with symptoms of bloating and feelings of fullness. **Antidepressants,** in particular SSRIs (Table 19–3), can assist in treating comorbid depression. **Nutritional restoration** remains the most important immediate objective in treating depressed anorexic persons. **There are complications (e.g., hypophosphatemia) associated with rapid refeeding,** initially, after prolonged starvation.

RX SSRIs: Table 19–3

DS Table 19–3

SE Table 19–3

with or without

RX Metoclopramide (Reglan—*U.S.*; Maxeran—*Can.*) [B]: Dopamine-receptor blocker, which enhances gastrointestinal motility and accelerated gastric emptying.

DS 5–20 mg PO before meals

SE Extrapyramidal reactions, drowsiness, diarrhea, muscle weakness, insomnia, depression, and prolactin stimulation. Rarely, tachycardia, hypertension, hypotension, and methemoglobinemia.

Bulimia Nervosa

KY Characterized by episodes of binge eating, accompanied by a sense of a lack of control, and compensatory behavior (e.g., vomiting, laxative use) to prevent weight gain. The etiology is unknown. Dangerous electrolyte imbalances (e.g., hypokalemia) can occur with this disorder owing to excessive vomiting and laxative abuse.

TX SSRIs: Table 19–3. Can assist in impulse control, and reducing binging and purging behaviors and may assist with comorbid depressive symptoms.

RX SSRIs: Table 19–3

DS Table 19–3

SE Table 19–3

INSOMNIA

See PRIMARY INSOMNIA.

NONBIPOLAR MOOD DISORDERS

Depression (Major Depressive Disorder)

KY Major depressive disorder is a recurrent, often chronic disorder, characterized by at least 2 weeks of depressed mood or anhedonia with associated symptoms. The pathophysiology of depression remains to be further elucidated. Dysregulation of the norepinephrine and serotonin neurotransmitter systems, alterations in blood flow in various brain areas, and neuroendocrine changes (e.g., hypercortisolemia, thyroid axis) are often observed in depressed patients.

TX **First-line treatment:** Includes **SSRIs,** such as citalopram (Celexa) or paroxetine (Paxil); the **SNRI** venlafaxine (Effexor); the norepinephrine dopamine reuptake inhibitor (**NDRI**) bupropion (Wellbutrin, Zyban); **SARIs** such as nefazodone (Serzone); the reversible inhibitor of MAO-A (**RIMA**) moclobemide (Manerix); and the noradrenergic/specific serotonergic antidepressant (**NaSSA**) mirtazapine (Remeron).

Second-line treatment: Includes medications with proven efficacy but a less desirable safety and side effect profile, including nonselective cyclic antidepressants such as desipramine (Norpramin) or amitriptyline (Elavil, Vanatrip—*U.S.*; Levate—*Can.*) and irreversible MAOIs such as phenelzine (Nardil) or tranylcypromine (Parnate).

Adjunctive medication: Benzodiazepines (Table 19–1) can be used initially for insomnia or concurrent anxiety. **Other agents** can be added to augment antidepressant response: lithium (e.g., Eskalith: 600–900 mg PO qd), pindolol (2.5 mg PO tid), or L-tryptophan (1–3 g PO qhs). Alternatively, **antidepressants from different classes can be combined,** for example, an SSRI plus bupropion (Wellbutrin, Zyban). Some combinations can increase the risk for adverse events, for example, serotonin syndrome or hypertensive crisis. Table 19–6 lists medications used for managing **sexual side effects of antidepressants.** Lowering the antidepressant dose, if feasible, can also reduce sexual side effects.

RX SSRIs, SNRI, NDRI, SARI, RIMA, and NaSSA (Table 19–3); nonselective cyclic antidepressants; MAOIs (Table 19–3); benzodiazepines (Table 19–1); agents for effective management of medication side effects (Table 19–6).

DS In general **antidepressants should be titrated as necessary to the maximum tolerated dose.** Four to 6 weeks constitutes a minimum duration to assess efficacy at a given therapeutic dose. The maximum recommended dose should be reached if possible before switching treatments. In special populations, for example, the elderly or the developmentally delayed, initiating treatment at lower doses is generally recommended (Table 19–1, Table 19–3, and Table 19–6).

SE Table 19–1, Table 19–3, and Table 19–6

Dysthymic Disorder

KY This disorder is characterized by the presence of depressed mood for more days than not for at least 2 years, in addition to other depressive symptoms not meeting criteria for major depression. The pathophysiology is thought to be the same as that for major depressive disorder.

TX The same medication is used for dysthymic disorder as for major depressive disorder. Partial remission is often observed in patients treated with medication alone.

RX See Depression (Major Depressive Disorder).

DS See Depression (Major Depressive Disorder).

SE See Depression (Major Depressive Disorder).

PRIMARY INSOMNIA

KY Characterized by disrupted sleep for at least 1 month, including difficulty either initiating or maintaining sleep not caused by a known physical or psychiatric condition. Carefully exclude other causes, including sleep disorders (e.g., narcolepsy, sleep apnea), psychiatric conditions (e.g., depression), and substance use (e.g., alcohol). The initial cause is not fully known, but after prolonged insomnia, anxiety about being unable to sleep often aggravates the condition.

TX **Counseling** on sleep hygiene and substances that can aggravate the condition is essential. **Short-term use of hypnotic agents** can be helpful: **Benzodiazepines,** for example, lorazepam (Ativan), oxazepam (Serax), and temazepam (Restoril), or **nonbenzodiazepine agents** such as zopiclone (Imovane), zolpidem (Ambien), or trazodone (Desyrel).

RX **Hypnotic agents:** Table 19–5

DS Table 19–5

SE Table 19–5

PSYCHOTIC DISORDERS

Brief Psychotic Disorder

KY Characterized by psychotic symptoms similar to those in schizophrenia of 1 day to 1 month in duration, generally in response to a significant stressor (e.g., trauma).

TX **Benzodiazepines** (Table 19–1) help reduce anxiety initially. If psychotic symptoms persist, the addition of **short-term use of antipsychotics** (Table 19–7) can be helpful.

RX Benzodiazepines: Table 19–1, with or without antipsychotics (Table 19–7)

DS Table 19–1 and Table 19–7

SE Table 19–1 and Table 19–7

Delusional Disorder

KY Characterized by the presence of delusions of at least 1 month in duration, without the presence of other symptoms of schizophrenia (e.g., hallucinations, disorganized speech or behavior). They are classified by content: erotic, grandiose, jealous, persecutory, somatic, mixed, or unspecified type. Global functioning is more often intact than in schizophrenia, with impairments generally direct consequences of the specific delusions. The pathophysiology is not fully known, although medical conditions (e.g., brain tumors) affecting the limbic system or basal ganglia can replicate symptoms of a delusional disorder.

TX Attempt **novel antipsychotics first** (Table 19–7). See Table 19–9 for **selected depot antipsychotic agents.** Also see Schizophrenia.

RX See Table 19–7 and Table 19–9 for antipsychotic drugs and depot agents and Table 19–6 for management of medication side effects.

DS Table 19–6, Table 19–7, and Table 19–9

SE Table 19–6, Table 19–7, and Table 19–9

Schizoaffective Disorder

KY Characterized by the same features as schizophrenia, with the additional presence of manic or depressive episodes. The symptoms of schizophrenia must not occur exclusively during periods of mood disturbance. It is unclear whether the pathophysiology is closer to schizophrenia or bipolar disorder or is distinct.

TX The initial treatment consists of **antipsychotics** (Table 19–7). Mood symptoms that persist with antipsychotic treatment can be treated with a **mood stabilizer** (Table 19–4) **or an antidepressant** (Table 19–3) as appropriate.

RX Antipsychotics: Table 19–7, with or without a mood stabilizer (Table 19–4) or antidepressant (Table 19–3)

DS Table 19–3, Table 19–4, and Table 19–7

SE Table 19–3, Table 19–4, and Table 19–7

Schizophrenia

KY A disorder characterized by disturbances in thought, perceptions, language, affect, and behavior. The diagnosis is made at least 6 months after the onset of symptoms. It is often accompanied by significant social and occupational impairment, which often persists after resolution of other symptoms. In terms of pathophysiology, a myriad of neuroanatomic and neurochemical abnormalities have been observed. Dopamine dysregulation is consistently related to symptomatology.

Table 19–9. Depot Antipsychotics

Generic (Brand) Name	Average Dose Range IM
Flupenthixol (Fluanxol Depot) not available in the United States	20–60 mg q3wk
Fluphenazine (Prolixin Decanoate, Prolixin Enanthate—*U.S.*; Modecate Concentrate, Moditen Enanthate—*Can.*) [C]	12.5–37.5 mg q4wk
Haloperidol (Haldol Decanoate) [C]	50–150 mg q4wk
Zuclopenthixol (Clopixol Depot)	150–300 mg q2wk

TX **All effective agents antagonize the dopamine-2 receptor,** for example, risperidone (Risperdal) and olanzapine (Zyprexa). These **novel antipsychotics** have a lower risk of extrapyramidal symptoms (EPS) than the older conventional agents, for example, haloperidol and perphenazine (Trilafon). **Table 19–7 lists selected antipsychotic agents. Conventional agents** have the shared side effects noted in Table 19–7 and in addition have an increased rate of extrapyramidal side effects compared with novel agents. **High-potency agents** have increased rates of acute EPS and lower rates of side effects not mediated by the dopamine receptors (e.g., sedation, blurred vision, constipation, urinary retention, hypotension, dizziness, sexual dysfunction). **Medium-potency agents** have medium risks of both classes of side effects, whereas **low-potency agents** cause lower rates of acute EPS and greater rates of the other side effects mentioned. At least 4–6 weeks at a therapeutic dose is required to assess the efficacy of an antipsychotic agent. Using the lowest effective dose minimizes side effects. **If side effects persist, see Table 19–6 for adjunctive medications** that can be used to treat side effects. **Note that amantadine and bupropion should not be used in patients with psychosis for managing sexual side effects.** After a single psychotic episode, treatment is generally reassessed after 1 year of therapy. **Depot antipsychotic agents** are used for patients in whom less frequent dosing or monitored administration will assist with compliance. See Table 19–9 for selected depot agents.

RX Antipsychotics (Table 19–7) and depot antipsychotic agents (Table 19–9). Agents for effective management of side effects are listed in Table 19–6.

DS Table 19–6, Table 19–7, and Table 19–9

SE Table 19–6, Table 19–7, and Table 19–9

Schizophreniform Disorder

KY Schizophreniform disorder is characterized by the same features as schizophrenia, but its duration is 1–6 months. The pathophysiology is the same as that for schizophrenia.

TX **Same as that for schizophrenia.** With a single episode of psychosis, discontinuation of antipsychotic therapy can be considered in the stable patient after approximately 1 year.

RX See Schizophrenia.

DS See Schizophrenia.

SE See Schizophrenia.

20

Pulmonology

PATRICK BELLEMARE

BRONCHIECTASIS

KY Bronchiectasis is defined as abnormal dilatation of medium-sized bronchi by destruction of their muscular and elastic components. It is **usually associated with bacterial infection** and production of large amounts of foul-smelling purulent sputum. Several disease processes can lead to formation of bronchiectasis, but for the needs of this discussion, we only mention recurrent bacterial infections, which are the most common cause. A single acute infection can lead to bronchiectasis formation, as seen in the case of bacterial or mycobacterial pneumonia. Mucus stasis and bronchial obstruction with bacteria accumulation can also be contributive, as in cases of cystic fibrosis.

TX Treatment is largely supportive, with antibiotic therapy aimed at chronic colonizing agents such as *Pseudomonas aeruginosa, Staphylococcus aureus,* and *Burkholderia cepacia.* Other aspects of therapy aim at improving clearance of secretions and slowing the appearance of cor pulmonale.

RX1 Bronchodilators

DS1 Table 20–1

SE1 Table 20–1

with

RX2 Inhaled DNAse or dornase alpha (Pulmozyme [B]): Nucleic acid lytic enzyme that selectively cleaves DNA, thus reducing mucous viscosity; as a result, airflow in the lung is improved and the risk of bacterial infection may be decreased.

DS2 2.5 mg inhaled qd–bid

SE2 Pharyngitis, dysphonia, chest pain, dyspnea, and hemoptysis.

CHRONIC ASTHMA

The pediatric presentation of this disease and its treatment is discussed in Ch 18 Pediatrics. In the adult, chronic asthma therapy is mostly encountered. Treatment in the case of acute asthma is outlined in detail in Ch 18 Pediatrics.

KY The definition is evolving but there is general agreement that asthma is an inflammatory disease involving a **reversible** airway obstruction that can be associated with an immune response to allergen stimulation or not. The underlying mechanism for the obstruction is thought to be an inflammatory reaction thickening bronchial wall, surrounding smooth muscle spasm, and

Table 20–1. Chronic Asthma Treatment

Class	Generic (Brand) Name	Dose	Side Effects
Bronchodilator Therapy			
Short-acting beta-agonists	Albuterol (Ventolin) [C]	100–400 µg inhaled q4–6hr regularly or prn	Anxiety, insomnia, tachycardia
Long-acting beta-agonists	Formoterol (Foradil, Oxeze—Can.) [C]	12 µg PO q12hr	
	Salmeterol (Serevent) [C]	12–50 µg inhaled q12 hr	
Theophylline		200–600 mg PO qd (single or divided doses)	Diarrhea, nausea, tachycardia
Anti-Inflammatory Therapy			
Inhaled corticosteroids	Beclomethasone (Beclovent) [C]	250–1,000 mg bid	Dysphonia, thrush
Antileukotriene agents	Montelukast (Singulair) [B]	5–10 mg PO qd	Abdominal pain, flulike symptoms, headache
	Zafirlukast (Accolate) [B]	20 mg PO bid	

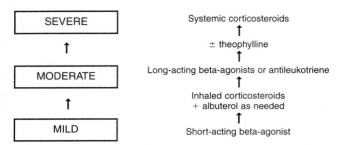

FIGURE 20-1 The treatment of chronic asthma based on severity.

secretion accumulation. That reaction can be idiopathic or triggered by a specific or nonspecific immune mechanism.

TX Treatment is titrated based on clinical and physiologic severity of illness; both the spastic and inflammatory components of the disease should be addressed (Figure 20-1).

RX Table 20–1

DS Table 20–1

SE Table 20–1

CHRONIC OBSTRUCTIVE PULMONARY DISEASE (COPD)

KY COPD is characterized by the presence of airflow obstruction caused by chronic bronchitis or emphysema. Chronic bronchitis is diagnosed by the presence of chronic productive cough for 3 months in each of 2 consecutive years in a patient with no other causes of chronic cough. Emphysema is the irreversible enlargement and destruction of the airspaces distal to the terminal bronchioles. One of five smokers will develop COPD. COPD is distinguished from asthma based on partial irreversibility of airflow obstruction. Severity criteria are based on spirometric measurements. The main parameter is forced expiratory volume in 1 second (FEV_1) (from maximal inspiration) measurement, and its proportion of forced vital capacity (FVC) (the total volume exhaled from maximal inspiration).

TX Treatment intensity is titrated based on severity of illness. Table 20–2 lists criteria for COPD severity.

RX Table 20–2 and Table 20–3

DS Table 20–3

SE Table 20–3

HYPERSENSITIVITY PNEUMONITIS

KY This group of diseases represents an **aberration of the immune response of the lung to known allergens.** The different disease names

Table 20–2. Criteria for Chronic Obstructive Pulmonary Disease Severity

Severity	Criteria	Suggested Treatment
Mild	$FEV_1/FVC > 70\%$ $FEV_1 > 80\%$	Short-acting beta-agonists as needed
Moderate	$FEV_1/FVC < 70\%$ $FEV_1 > 30\%$ and $< 80\%$	Regular bronchodilators (single or combined) + inhaled corticosteroids (if reversible component established)
Severe	$FEV_1/FVC < 70\%$ $FEV_1 < 30\%$	Moderate-severity regimen + supplemental oxygen therapy + prophylactic immunization

FEV_1 = forced expiratory volume in 1 second; FVC = forced vital capacity.

reflect the allergens involved (e.g., Farmer's lung, bird fancier's lung, flour lung), which can be microbial agents, animal proteins, and low-molecular-weight chemicals. Repeated exposure of lung lymphocytes to a defined allergen causes immune modulator release and local inflammatory response leading to alveolar damage. Intensity of exposure is directly proportional to symptoms. Diagnostic criteria include recurrent febrile episodes, infiltrates on chest x-ray, precipitating antibodies to suspected allergen, granuloma on lung biopsy, and improvement with avoidance of suspected allergen.

TX **Hallmark of therapy is withdrawal from exposure** to the suspected allergen. There is an added benefit from **corticosteroid administration.**

RX **Prednisone** [B]: A synthetic steroid that decreases inflammation.

DS 1 mg/kg/day for 4–12 weeks; taper slowly.

SE Insomnia, nervousness, hirsutism, hyperglycemia, cataracts, glaucoma, cushingoid appearance, hypertension, seizures, hypokalemia, peptic ulcer, osteoporosis, and hypersensitivity reactions. **Caution** with use in patients with hypothyroidism, cirrhosis, hypertension, congestive heart failure, ulcerative colitis, thromboembolic disorders, and in cases of increased risk for peptic ulcer disease.

INTERSTITIAL PULMONARY FIBROSIS (IPF)

KY IPF can represent a cluster of pathological processes involving fibroinflammatory infiltrates of the interstitium of the lung and ultimately leading to "stiffening" of the lung parenchyma and impairment of gas exchange. The best known of this cluster is now designated as usual interstitial pneumonia. The origin of IPF remains idiopathic, but part of the mechanism involves stimulation of cytokines with leukocyte activation and consecutive collagen deposition and scarring in the lung.

TX Generally accepted regimens involve **immune-modulating drugs.**

RX1 **Prednisone**

Table 20-3. Pharmacologic Treatment Options for Chronic Obstructive Pulmonary Disease

Strategy	Generic (Brand) Name	Dose	Side Effects
Tobacco cessation	Bupropion (Wellbutrin, Zyban) [B]	150 mg PO qd for 3 days, then 300 mg PO qd for 7–12 weeks	Diarrhea, loss of libido, nausea, tachycardia
	Nicotine supplements (gum and patch) Transdermal patch (Habitrol, Nicoderm, Nicotrol, ProStep) [D]	2 mg gum for each cigarette previously used per day 21 mg (equivalent to 1 pack of cigarettes/day) given over an 8–10 week decremental regimen	Diarrhea, nausea, tachycardia, atrial fibrillation, hypersensitivity reactions **Caution:** Using a patch with smoking increases risk of side effects.
Bronchodilators			
Short-acting beta-agonists	Albuterol (Ventolin) [C]	100–400 µg inhaled q4–6hr regular dose or prn	Tachycardia, anxiety
Atropinic agents	Ipratropium (Atrovent) [B]	40–80 µg inhaled q6hr	Dry mouth, bronchitis, URTI, palpitations, dyspnea, increased sputum, bronchospasm, hypersensitivity reactions
	Theophylline (Aerolate, Quibron, Theolair, Phyllo-contin, Pulmophylline—*Can.*) [C]	200–600 mg PO qd (single or divided doses)	Tachycardia, nausea, diarrhea, nervousness, seizure
Bronchial anti-inflammatory drugs			
Inhaled corticosteroids	Beclomethasone (Beclovent) [C]	250–1,000 µg bid	Thrush, dysphonia

URTI, upper respiratory tract infection.

DS1 1 mg/kg/day

SE1 See HYPERSENSITIVITY PNEUMONITIS.

with

RX2 **Azathioprine** (Imuran) [D]: An immunosuppressive agent that inhibits purine metabolism and the synthesis of DNA, RNA, and proteins.

DS2 Start at 1 mg/kg/day PO for 6–8 weeks, then increase by 0.5 mg/kg PO q4wk until there is a positive response, or up to a maximum dose of 2.5 mg/kg/day PO.

SE2 Fever, diarrhea, thrombocytopenia, leukopenia, anemia, secondary infection, and hepatotoxicity. Rarely, hypotension, alopecia, aphthous stomatitis, arthralgias, retinopathy, dyspnea, and hypersensitivity reactions.

or

RX3 **Cyclophosphamide** (Cytoxan, Neosar; Procytox—*Can.*) [D]: A potent immunosuppressive agent that also prevents cell division by crosslinking DNA strands and decreasing DNA synthesis.

DS3 50–100 mg/m^2/day PO as continuous therapy

SE3 **Alopecia,** but hair will usually regrow. May cause **sterility, potentially fatal acute hemorrhagic cystitis or urinary fibrosis**, **leukemia,** and, less common, **thrombocytopenia** and **anemia. Rarely,** syndrome of inappropriate secretion of antidiuretic hormone, renal tubular necrosis (usually resolves with discontinuation of the drug), congestive heart failure, pulmonary fibrosis, hemorrhagic myocarditis, and allergic reactions. Cyclophosphamide **may also potentiate the cardiac toxicity of anthracyclines.** Dosage adjustment needed for renal or hepatic failure.

or

RX4 **Cyclosporine** (Neoral, Sandimmune) [C]: Inhibits the production and release of interleukin II and interleukin II–induced activation of resting T lymphocytes.

DS4 **Note:** Neoral and Sandimmune are not bioequivalent and cannot be used interchangeably. Usual dose is 1–3 mg/kg/day PO for both drugs. Plasma concentration should be monitored every 4–7 days and dose adjusted accordingly.

SE4 Nephrotoxicity, hepatotoxicity, hypertension, psoriasis, headache, hirsutism, hypertrichosis, increased triglycerides, female reproductive disorder, diarrhea, gum hyperplasia, dyspepsia, tremor, and infection.

or

RX5 **Colchicine** [C]: Decreases leukocyte motility and inflammatory response.

DS5 Dosage can range from 0.6–2 mg/day PO in 2–3 divided doses.

SE5 Diarrhea, abdominal pain, and alopecia. Rarely, azoospermia, agranulocytosis, aplastic anemia, bone marrow suppression, hepatotoxicity, myopathy, and peripheral neuritis. Contraindicated in serious renal, gastrointestinal, hepatic, or cardiac disorders and blood dyscrasias.

PRIMARY PULMONARY HYPERTENSION

KY Primary pulmonary hypertension is defined as a mean pulmonary artery pressure > 25 mm HG in resting conditions or > 30 mm HG on exertion, without a secondary cause (e.g., congestive heart failure, mitral valve disease, recurrent pulmonary embolism, veno-occlusive disease). A contributive factor to the disease is the occurrence of small vessel thrombosis in the evolution of this disease. Prognosis of this disease is poor, with 2.8-year median survival. Approximately 20%–30% of patients will respond to vasodilator therapy, which, in turn, can slow down the evolution to cor pulmonale and death. Anticoagulation is believed to limit the thrombotic component of the disease and, therefore, is indicated. Ultimately, single lung, double lung, and heart-lung transplantation are the only treatments that can alter the longevity of a primary pulmonary hypertension patient.

TX The treatment design is based on disease severity and vasodilator challenge in a monitored setting. If under direct pulmonary artery pressure monitoring, vasodilator administration (nitric oxide, adenosine, or epoprostenol) causes a 20% drop in pulmonary vascular resistance, chronic vasodilator therapy with calcium channel blockers or continuous epoprostenol (Flolan) infusion through a portable pump can be added to anticoagulation therapy. Newer options include oral agents such as bosentan (Tracleer) and sidenafil (Viagra). **Unresponsive patients with poor functional status are directed to transplant teams for assessment.**

RX Table 20–4

DS Table 20–4

SE Table 20–4

VENOUS THROMBOEMBOLIC DISEASE

KY Venous thromboembolic diseases include deep **venous thrombosis** and **pulmonary embolism** (PE) as two components of the same disease process. **Three pathophysiologic components that lead to venous thrombosis are stasis, endothelial injury, and hypercoagulability.** Stasis explains the tendency for clots to form around valvular areas; however, it is not in itself sufficient. This type of clot is formed mainly of fibrin and red blood cells. Endothelial injury is a second component, and it can be macroscopic (e.g., surgery) or microscopic. The third component is an abnormality of the coagulation system. Antithrombin III, protein C, and protein S are the most important circulating anticoagulant proteins, and they can all be deficient. Failure of thrombolysis may also occur. A high level of homocysteine is recognized as a risk factor for thrombosis. Once a clot has formed on a venous wall, it expands toward the center of the lumen and can eventually cause occlusion. At first, it is only loosely adherent and, with its expansion, its proximal end can float freely in the lumen. At this point, it can break at the base and lead to PE; become adherent and organized, leading to a new lumen and endothelium (the valves are lost in

Table 20-4. Pharmacologic Treatments for Primary Pulmonary Hypertension

Class	Generic (Brand) Name	Dose	Side Effects
Vitamin K anticoagulant (see Ch 9 Hematology)	Warfarin (Coumadin) [D]	INR ≥ 2	Abdominal discomfort, edema, fever, hemorrhage, hyper-sensitivity reactions, lethargy, microembolization (occurs rarely and usually is shown after several weeks of therapy), priapism, purple toes syndrome caused by cholesterol, stroke, vasculitis
Calcium channel blockers (see Ch 3 Cardiology)	Nifedipine (Adalat, Procardia) [C]	30–180 mg PO qd	Fluid retention, postural hypotension, reflex tachycardia, swelling of lower extremities
	Diltiazem (Cardizem) [C]	120–360 mg PO qd	Postural hypotension, swelling of lower extremities, transient atrioventricular block
Prostaglandin	Epoprostenol (Flolan) [B]	2 ng/kg/minute	Hypotension, pulmonary edema, thrombocytopenia
Endothelin antagonist	Bosentan* (Tracleer) [X]	125–250 mg PO bid	High incidence of significant transaminase elevations, indicating potential for hepatic injury. Avoid use in patients with hepatic impairment. Avoid concurrent use with cyclosporine or glyburide.

INR = International Normalized Ratio.

*Only available through a limited distribution program directly from the manufacturer.

Table 20–5. Treatment of Venous Thromboembolic Disease*

Generic (Brand) Name	Dose	Mechanism of Action	Side Effects and Cautions
Heparin (Hep-Lock, Calcilean, Hepalean—*Can.*) [C]	See Ch 9 Hematology	Potentiates antithrombin III activity and inhibits factors IIa and Xa.	Hemorrhage, heparin-induced thrombocytopenia† **Contraindications** are listed in Ch 9 Hematology.
Low molecular weight heparin: Enoxaparin (Lovenox) [B]	1 mg/kg SC q12hr	Potentiates antithrombin III activity and inhibits factor Xa.	Hemorrhage **Contraindications** are similar to those listed for heparin in Ch 9 Hematology.
Dalteparin (Fragmin) [B]	200 U/kg SC qd		
Tinzaparin (Innohep) [B]	175 U/kg SC qd		
Warfarin derivatives (Coumadin, Simtron)[D]	Starting dose of 5 mg PO qd, titrated to an INR of 2 (also see Ch 9 Hematology)	Interferes with the formation of the reduced form of vitamin K, which is needed to act as a cofactor in the posttranslational carboxylation of glutamate residues on factors II, VII, IX, and X; protein C; and protein S	Hemorrhage **Contraindications** are the same as those described for heparin (Ch 9 Hematology), plus first trimester and last month of pregnancy.

Drug	Dosage	Mechanism of Action	Adverse Effects
Danaparoid (Orgaran) [B]	Loading dose of 2,250 U IV bolus, followed by 400 U/hr for 4 hours, then 300 U/hr for 4 hours Maintenance dose: 150–200 U/hr Prophylactic dose: 750 U SC q12hr	Mixture of heparin, dermatan, and chondroitin sulfate—inhibits factor Xa in a way similar to heparin. Cross-reactivity with heparin is approximately 10%.	Abdominal discomfort, allergic reactions, anemia, edema, hemorrhage, urinary tract infection
Argatroban [B]	2 μg/kg/minute IV	A highly selective thrombin inhibitor—reversibly binds to the active (both free and clot-associated) thrombin. Inhibits fibrin formation and the activation of factors V, VIII, XIII; protein C; and platelet aggregation.	Abdominal discomfort, arrhythmias, fever, hemorrhage, hypotension, infection, myocardial infarction
Hirudin‡	Initial bolus of 0.1–0.4 mg/kg IV, then an infusion rate of 0.06–0.15 mg/kg/hr IV	Binds tightly to the active site of thrombin, even when it is attached to fibrin. Specifically blocks the different actions of thrombin.	Disseminated intravascular coagulation, hemorrhage

INR = international normalized ratio.

*Also see Ch 9 Hematology.

†In patients who have developed heparin-induced thrombocytopenia, warfarin should be withheld until the platelet count is normal. In the meantime, an alternative anticoagulant agent such as danaparoid can be used to treat these patients.

‡Not available in the United States.

the process producing the postphlebitic syndrome); or dissolve with no side effects.

TX **Prompt therapy of PE, when present, reduces mortality from 30% to 2%. Anticoagulants are used to treat venous thromboembolic disorders.** Table 20–5 lists the anticoagulants used; see Ch 9 Hematology for more detailed information on each of the anticoagulant agents.

RX Table 20–5 and Ch 9 Hematology

DS Table 20–5 and Ch 9 Hematology

SE Table 20–5 and Ch 9 Hematology

21

Rheumatology

SAMUEL WONG,
BERNARD F. BISSONNETTE

The study of rheumatology is indeed complex. Many rheumatologic entities are not restricted to the musculoskeletal system and the supporting soft tissue but have multi-organ involvement. The treatment of other organ systems affected by the primary rheumatologic condition is discussed only briefly. Only the most common rheumatologic conditions are discussed here, along with their appropriate treatments.

ANKYLOSING SPONDYLITIS

KY Its etiology is unknown, but it has a strong relationship with HLA B27 histocompatibility antigen. It typically affects young males. Sacroiliac joint and spinal joints are mainly affected, but hip and shoulder joints and, to a lesser extent, peripheral joints are also affected. Enthesopathies are common. Extra-articular manifestations include acute iritis, apical lung fibrosis, aortic arch involvement leading to aortic insufficiency, decreased chest wall compliance, cauda equina syndrome, and amyloidosis.

TX **The cornerstone of treatment is patient education** to maintain correct spine posture. **No cure is available. Nonsteroidal anti-inflammatory drugs (NSAIDs) are first-line treatment.** Some disease-modifying antirheumatic drugs (DMARDs) are used to control symptoms, but they do not alter the course of the disease. New biologic agents are potential therapeutic options (Table 21-3).

RX1 **NSAIDs**

DS1 Table 21–1

SE1 Table 21–2

with or without

RX2 **Intra-articular glucocorticoid injection**

DS2 10–80 mg in affected joint depending on size of joint. Injection into the sacroiliac joint requires fluoroscopic guidance.

SE2 Table 21–1

with or without

RX3 **Sulfasalazine** (Azulfidine—*U.S.*; Salazopyrin—*Can.*) [B/D at term]: Mode of action still remains unclear. This DMARD is suggested to act as an anti-inflammatory, immunosuppressive, and bacteriostatic drug.

DS3 2,000 mg PO daily

SE3 Table 21–3

Table 21-1. Nonsteroidal Anti-inflammatory Drugs (NSAIDs)

Generic (Brand) Name	Dose PO	Indications	Side Effects and Cautions
Acetylsalicylic acid (Aspirin, Novasen—*Can.*) [C/D in third trimester]	325–650 mg q4hr	All inflammatory arthropathies; dose: 650 mg q4hr Second line for degenerative arthropathies without signs of inflammation; dose: 325–650 mg q4hr Musculoskeletal pain	GI perforation, GI obstruction, bleeding, renal hypertension, decreased creatinine clearance Contraindications: recent GI bleeding, asthma with nasal polyps, coagulopathy Use with caution in IBD
Diclofenac (Voltaren) [B/D in third trimester]	50–150 mg qd divided bid–tid	Same as above	Same as above
Diclofenac with misoprostil (Arthrotec) [X]	50–150 mg qd divided bid–tid	Same as above	Same as above Diarrhea from misoprostil
Etodolac (Lodine—*U.S.*; Ultradol—*Can.*) [C/D in third trimester]	200–300 mg bid	Same as above	Same as above Slightly better GI safety profile than other NSAIDs
Ibuprofen (Advil, Motrin) [B/D in third trimester]	300–600 mg q4hr	Same as above	Same as above
Indomethacin (Indocin—*U.S.*; Indotec—*Can.*) [B/D in third trimester]	150–200 mg qd divided bid–tid (*PEDS:* — 2–5 mg/kg/day divided tid–qid)	Same as above	Same as above

Ketoprofen (Orudis—*U.S.*; Rhodis—*Can.*) [B/D in third trimester]	150–200 mg qd divided tid-qid	Same as above	Same as above
Ketorolac tromethamine (Toradol) [C/D in third trimester]	10 mg qid	Same as above	Same as above
Nabumetone (Relafen) [C/D in third trimester]	1,000–2,000 mg qd divided bid	Same as above	Same as above Slightly better GI safety profile compared with other NSAIDs
Naproxen (Aleve, Anaprox, Naprelan, Naprosyn—*U.S.*; Naxen, Synflex—*Can.*) [B/D in third trimester]	250–500 mg bid (*PEDS*—*15–20 mg/kg/day divided bid*)	Same as above	Same as above
Piroxicam (Feldene) [B/D in third trimester]	10 mg bid or 20 mg qd	Same as above	Same as above
Tiaprofenic acid (Surgam)	600 mg divided bid or tid	Same as above	Same as above
Tolmetin sodium (Tolectin) [C/D in third trimester]	400 mg tid (*PEDS*—*25–30 mg/kg/day divided tid*)	Same as above	Same as above

*GI = gastrointestinal; IBD = inflammatory bowel disease.

Table 21–2. Glucocorticoid Delivery and Characteristics

Route of Delivery	Dose	Indications	Side Effects	Note
Oral	Dose depends on severity of symptoms: lowest possible dose should be used (i.e., prednisone 5–60 mg PO qd).	Acute rheumatoid arthritis Myositis and dermatomyositis Polymyalgia rheumatica Systemic lupus erythematosus Vasculitis	Avascular necrosis, cataract, cushingoid features, gastric ulcer, glaucoma, glucose intolerance, hypertension, increased susceptibility to infections, mood changes, myopathy, osteoporosis, osteonecrosis, skin fragility	Used to control inflammatory conditions. Used as a bridge when starting other DMARD therapy. When prednisone is used in conjunction with other DMARDs, it should be titrated to the lowest possible dose that controls symptoms. Use with caution with active infection. Avoid if possible in children; even 5 mg qd can **suppress bone growth.** Alternate-day therapy may prevent this but is not as effective.
Intravenous	Depends on severity of symptoms: as high as 1,000 mg bolus methylprednisolone.	Severe inflammatory conditions (i.e., vasculitis, cerebritis, nephritis)	Same as above	Short-term use only.
Intra-articular Depomedrol (intermediate acting) Triamcinolone acetonide (long acting)	Depends on joint size: 10–80 mg	Acutely inflamed joint Osteoarthritis (occasionally an indication)	Same as above	Maximum of three injections into same joint per year. Allow 3 months between injections to the same joint. Do not inject through psoriatic plaques due to risk of infection.

DMARD = disease-modifying antirheumatic drug.

with or without

RX4 **Methotrexate** (Rheumatrex) [D]: See SYSTEMIC LUPUS ERY-THEMATOSUS (SLE).

DS4 10–25 mg PO/IM weekly. Use folic or folinic acid to minimize side effects.

SE4 Table 21–3

ARTHRITIS

See ARTHRITIS ASSOCIATED WITH INFLAMMATORY BOWEL DIS-EASE, JUVENILE RHEUMATOID ARTHRITIS (JRA), OSTEOARTHRI-TIS (OA), PSORIATIC ARTHRITIS, REITER'S SYNDROME AND REACTIVE ARTHRITIS, RHEUMATOID ARTHRITIS (RA), and SEP-TIC ARTHRITIS.

ARTHRITIS ASSOCIATED WITH INFLAMMATORY BOWEL DISEASE

KY Approximately 10%–20% of persons with Crohn's or ulcerative colitis will develop arthritis. Lower-extremity joints are more commonly affected. Common extra-articular manifestations include erythema nodosum, pyo-derma gangrenosa, and painful oral ulcers. Control of the inflammatory bowel disease is important; resection of diseased bowel is associated with regression of arthritic symptoms.

TX **Therapy is supportive.**

RX1 **NSAIDs**

DS1 Table 21–1

SE1 Table 21–1

with or without

RX2 **Intra-articular glucocorticoid injection.**

DS2 10–80 mg in affected joint depending on size of joint. Injection to the sacroiliac joint requires fluoroscopic guidance.

SE2 Table 21–2

CRYSTAL-INDUCED ARTHRITIS

Gout

KY Sufferers are typically undersecretors of uric acid as opposed to over-producers. Conditions that cause overproduction of uric acid include hypoxanthine guanine phosphoribosyltransferase deficiency, glucose-6-phosphatase deficiency, myeloproliferative and lymphoproliferative disor-ders, multiple myeloma, thalassanemias, and hemolytic anemia.

TX1 **Asymptomatic hyperuricemia should not be treated. Once started, medication for prophylaxis against gout is lifelong.**

(Text continues on page 384)

Table 21–3. Disease-Modifying Antirheumatic Drugs (DMARDs)

Generic (Brand) Name	Dose	Indications
Azathioprine (Imuran) [D]	Starting dose: 1 mg/kg/day (maximum 2.5 mg/kg/day) in single or divided doses for 8 weeks, then increase by 0.5 mg/kg/day q4wk as required	Psoriatic arthritis RA (second-line treatment) SLE Scleroderma
Cyclophosphamide (Cytoxan, Neosar—*U.S.*; Procytox—*Can.*) [D]	0.5–1.0 g/m^2 IV bolus monthly for 6 months, then every 3 months for 10 doses	Major SLE organ involvement, including cerebritis/nephritis/vasculitis Scleroderma Vasculitis
Cyclosporine (Neoral, Sandimmune) [C]	2 mg/kg/day PO in divided doses for the first 6 weeks (maximum 5 mg/kg/day)	Major SLE organ involvement, including cerebritis/nephritis/vasculitis Psoriatic arthritis Scleroderma Vasculitis
Gold, oral: Auranofin (Ridaura) [C]	6 mg/day PO or 3 mg PO bid (maximum 9 mg/day) (**PEDS:**—0.1 mg/kg/day PO)	Psoriatic arthritis RA (second-line treatment)
Gold, parenteral: Auranofin (Ridaura) [C]	IM water based, aurothiomalate: Test dose of 10–25 mg, then 25–50 mg weekly. Maintenance dose: 25–50 mg IM q2wk after 20 weeks (q2–4wk). Oil based, aurothioglucose 50 mg IM weekly	Psoriatic arthritis RA (second-line treatment)
Hydroxychloroquine (Plaquenil) [C]	Initial dose: 400–600 mg PO qd Maintenance dose: (4–12 weeks) 200–400 mg PO qd (In SLE: 400 mg PO qd—bid initially, then 200–400 mg PO qd) (**PEDS:**—5–7 mg/kg/day PO)	Psoriatic arthritis RA (first-line treatment)
Methotrexate (Rheumatrex) [D]	Starting dose: 7.5 mg PO weekly. Usual steady dose: 15–25 mg PO weekly	Psoriatic arthritis RA (first-line treatment) SLE Scleroderma
Penicillamine (Cuprimine, Depen) [D]	Starting dose: 125–250 PO qd (maximum 1,000 mg/day, then increase by 125–250 mg q1–3mo as required.) (**PEDS:**—5–10 mg/kg/day)	RA (second-line treatment) Scleroderma

Side Effects	Note
Elevated LFT, GI intolerance, increased risk of infections, infections, myelo-suppression, nausea, vomiting	Effective, but has higher toxicity than other DMARDs. Use other DMARDs first, especially in persons with kidney or liver disease.
Alopecia, HSV and other infections, hemorrhagic cystitis, leucopenia malignancies, nausea, thrombo-cytopenia, vomiting	High toxicity limits use. IV pulse has fewer side effects. IV pulse must be proceeded with substantial IV hydration to avoid hemorrhagic cystitis. Drug of choice for RA vasculitis unresponsive to steroids.
Renal (routine monitoring for creatinine), hypertrichosis, numerous CNS (including central and peripheral), pancreatitis, hepatotoxicity, hypertension, myelo-suppression, bleeding, tender gums	Neoral and Sandimmune are not inter-changeable because of narrow thera-peutic window. **Use with caution in active infection.**
Dermatitis, diarrhea, glomerulonephritis, drug-induced ITP, stomatitis	Not as effective as other DMARDs in first-line treatment of RA.
Dermatitis, glomerulonephritis, stomatitis, drug-induced ITP, myelosuppression	
Hemolytic anemia in G-6-PD deficiency, neuromyopathy, retinopathy (patient should visit ophthalmologist q6mo)	Avoid if person has retinal abnormality, G-6-PD deficiency.
GI toxicity, liver toxicity, interstitial lung fibrosis, pneumonitis	Use folic acid (> 1 mg/day) or folinic acid after methotrexate administration to lessen side effects. Avoid alcohol.
GI intolerance, myelosuppression, rash, renal and hematologic abnormalities, stomatitis, immune thrombocytopenia, and proteinuria	Effective but higher toxicity than other DMARDs. Take on an empty stomach. Avoid if person has penicillin allergy.

(continued)

Table 21–3. Disease-Modifying Antirheumatic Drugs (DMARDs) *(Continued)*

Generic (Brand) Name	Dose	Indications
Sulfasalazine (Azulfidine— U.S.; Salazopyrin— Can.) [B/D at term]	2–3 g/day PO in divided doses (maximum 50 mg/week) (**PEDS:**—*10 mg/m²/week*)	Psoriatic arthritis RA (first-line treatment)

BIOLOGICAL AGENTS

Etanercept (Enbrel) [B]	25 mg SC twice/week (**PEDS:**—*0.4 mg/kg SC twice/week*)	RA (second-line treatment when other DMARDs have failed) Potential treatment for AS and psoriatic arthritis
Infliximab (Remicade) [B]	3 mg/kg IV infusion at weeks 0, 2, and 6, and q8wk thereafter. Drug is given in combination with methotrexate.	RA (second-line treatment when other DMARDs have failed) Potential treatment for AS and psoriatic arthritis
Leflunomide (Arava) [X]	Loading dose: 100 mg PO for 3 days, then 20 mg/day PO	RA (first-line treatment) Inhibitor of dihydroorotate dehydrogenase (a key enzyme in the de novo synthesis of uridine mono-phosphate) Activated lymphocytes depend on the pyrimidine de novo synthesis to achieve metabolic needs for clonal expansion and terminal differentiation into effector cells Also inhibits chemotaxis of neutrophils to joints

CHF = congestive heart failure; CNS = central nervous system; DMARD = disease-modifying antirheumatic drug; G-6-PD = glucose-6-phosphate dehydrogenase; GI = gastrointestinal; HSV = herpes simplex virus; ITP = idiopathic thrombocytopenia; LFT = liver function test (levels); RA = rheumatoid arthritis; SLE = systemic lupus erythematosus; URTI = upper respiratory tract infection.

Side Effects	Note
Agranulocytosis, GI intolerance, hemolytic anemia in G-6-PD deficiency, liver toxicity	Take with food to avoid side effects. Avoid in persons with sulfa allergy, kidney or liver disease.
Injection site reaction, infections (especially URTI), development of autoantibodies (may develop drug-induced SLE); possible aggravation of multiple sclerosis, immune thrombocytopenia, and proteinuria	Entanercept inhibits tumor necrosis factor.
Development of antibodies to infliximab (unknown relevance), development of autoantibodies (may develop drug-induced SLE) Infection: increased risk of opportunistic infection Infusion-related reactions URTI Caution in CHF: Infliximab increases the incidence of mortality and hospitalization in CHF patients.	Infliximab inhibits tumor necrosis factor.
Alopecia, diarrhea, increased risk of infections, liver toxicity, rash	

RX1a **NSAIDs:** Typically **indomethacin, naproxen,** and **diclofenac** are used.

DS1a Table 21–1

SE1a Table 21–1

with

RX1b **Colchicine [C, oral/D, parenteral]:** The exact mechanism is not known. It is not an analgesic or a uricosuric. Colchicine is known to decrease the inflammatory response to urate crystal deposition by inhibiting the migration of leukocytes, to interfere with urate deposition by decreasing lactic acid production by leukocytes, to interfere with kinin formation, and to diminish phagocytosis.

DS1b 1–1.2 mg PO loading dose followed by 0.5–0.6 mg q2hr until clinical improvement or toxicity occurs (gastrointestinal [GI] symptoms). **Maximum dose:** 8 mg/day. **Avoid IV administration** because interstitial infiltration of IV can cause severe soft-tissue trauma.

SE1b Table 21–4

with or without

RX1c **Corticosteroid**

DS1c **Intra-articular dose** depends on the size of the joint. Small joints, that is, metatarsal phalangeal joints, require only 10 mg. Large joints, that is, knees (rarely affected by gout), require 40 mg per injection. **Oral dose** consists of prednisone 40–60 mg/day PO for 1–4 days. **Intramuscular dose** of methylprednisone (DepoMedrol) or triamcinolone acetonide (Kenalog) are both 40–60 mg for 1–4 days.

SE1c See Table 21–2

TX2 **Prophylactic treatment:** prophylaxis is considered if the following are present: multiple attacks annually, tophaceous gout, gouty erosions, uric acid renal calculi, or urate nephropathy.

RX2a **Allopurinol** (Aloprim, Zyloprim—*U.S.*; Lopurin, Purinol—*Can.*) [C]. **Drug of choice and treatment is lifelong.** Allopurinol is an inhibitor of xanthine oxidase, the enzyme required in the synthesis of uric acid, thereby decreasing serum uric acid levels. It further lowers serum uric acid levels by increasing the reutilization of xanthine and hypoxanthine for the synthesis of nucleotide and nucleic acid synthesis by acting on the enzyme hypoxanthine-guanine phosphoribosyltransferase. By increasing the level of nucleotides, the drug produces a negative feedback signal to inhibit the synthesis of purines, which results in decreased uric acid levels.

DS2a 100–800 mg/day in divided doses

SE2a Table 21–4

with or without

RX2b **Probenecid** (Benemid, Benemid) [B]: **This uricosuric drug should not be started during an attack of gout.** Probenecid inhibits tubular reab-

Table 21–4. Anticrystalline Therapy

Generic (Brand) Name	Dose (PO)	Indications	Side Effects and Cautions
Allopurinol (Aloprim, Zyloprim—*U.S.*; Lopurin, Purinol—*Can.*) [C]	100–800 mg qd in divided doses	Gout prophylaxis*	Hives, itching, LFT abnormalities Caution: Allopurinol should not be used for acute gouty attacks.
Colchicine [C, oral/D]	Prophylactic dose: 0.5–1.8 mg PO 1–4 times/week Treatment dose in acute attack: 1–1.2 mg PO loading dose, followed by 0.5–0.6 mg PO q2hr until clinical improvement is achieved or toxicity occurs (GI) (maximum 8 mg/day)	Prophylaxis for gout and pseudo-gout (CPPD *crystal disease*) Treatment for acute gout and pseudogout (CPPD *crystal disease*)	GI upset, alopecia, agranulocytosis, aplastic anemia, myelosuppression, hepatotoxicity, myopathy Caution: Avoid IV route if possible because extravasation of colchicine is extremely irritating to underlying tissue.
Probenecid (Benemid) [B]	500 mg PO qd for 1 week; then increase to a maximum of 1 g PO bid thereafter	Gout prophylaxis	Headache, joint pain and swelling, rash Caution: Do not use for acute gouty attacks or if suspect uric acid renal calculi:
Sulfinpyrazone (Anturane—*U.S.*; Antazone, Anturan—*Can.*) [C/D near term]	200–400 mg od (maximum 800 mg od)	Gout prophylaxis*	Bone marrow suppression, rash, headache, polyuria, increased bleeding time, hepatic necrosis, nephrotic syndrome, uric acid renal calculi

CPPD = calcium pyrophosphate dihydrate; GI = gastrointestinal; LFT = liver function test (levels).
*Asymptomatic hyperuricemia should not be treated because once started, medication for prophylaxis against gout is lifelong.

sorption of urate, thereby increasing the urinary excretion of uric acid and decreasing serum urate levels.

DS2b See Table 21–4

SE2b See Table 21–4

with or without

RX2c **Sulfinpyrazone** (Anturane—*U.S.*; Antazone, Anturan—*Can.*) [C/D near term]: See ANKYLOSING SPONDYLITIS.

DS2c See Table 21–4

SE2c See Table 21–4

Pseudogout or Calcium Pyrophosphate Dihydrate (CPPD) Crystal Disease

KY CPPD crystal disease is a condition in which CPPD accumulates in the synovial membranes and cartilage (chondrocalcinosis) of joints, causing inflammation. Possible causes include excessive inorganic pyrophosphate concentration in the synovial fluid, inorganic pyrophosphate arising from hydrolysis of chondrocyte nucleoside triphosphates in the joint, inordinate pyrophosphate levels from increased production or decreased catabolism, and idiopathic processes (joint trauma, surgical meniscal removal, hyperparathyroidism, hypothyroidism, hemochromatosis, Wilson's disease, and ochronosis).

TX **Underlying causes should be treated** (e.g., hemochromatosis, hyperparathyroidism). **Acute treatment** is the same as that for acute gout. **Prophylactic treatment** consists of colchicine.

RX1 Acute treatment: Same as that for acute gout.

DS1 See Gout.

SE1 See Gout.

RX2 **Prophylactic treatment:** Colchicine.

DS2 0.6–1.2 mg PO qd

SE2 Table 21–4

JUVENILE RHEUMATOID ARTHRITIS (JRA)

KY The clinical course and outcome are quite different from the adult form. Various forms of JRA include systemic-onset JRA, polyarticular-onset JRA, and pauciarticular JRA.

TX The treatment approach is similar to that used in adult RA. The main difference is that in JRA the use of **acetylsalicylic acid is avoided,** because of its association with Reye's syndrome (with concomitant varicella and influenza viral infections). **With pauciarticular JRA, prompt screening for the early development of iridocyclitis by slit-lamp examination can prevent permanent visual loss or blindness.**

RX1 **Narcotic analgesics**

DS1 Table 21–5

SE1 Table 21–5 with or without

RX3 **Glucocorticoids, oral**

DS3 1–40 mg PO daily depending on severity of symptoms

SE3 There is a **risk of bone growth suppression** even with doses as low as 5 mg. See Table 21–2.

or

RX2 **NSAIDs:** Ibuprofen (Advil, Motrin), naproxen (Aleve, Naprosyn) and tolmetin (Tolectin) are approved for use in children.

DS2 Table 21–1

SE2 Table 21–1

with or without

RX4 **Glucocorticoids, intra-articular**

DS4 10–40 mg in each affected joint depending on the size of the joint

SE4 See Table 21–2

with or without

RX5 **DMARDs:** Methotrexate and intramuscular gold injections are most commonly used. Etanercept, hydroxychloroquine, penicillamine, and sulfasalazine are also used.

DS5 Table 21–3

SE5 Table 21–3

OSTEOARTHRITIS (OA)

KY The most common of the arthropathies. Incidence increases with aging. All joints of the body can be affected.

TX **Medical treatment is focused on controlling pain.** Type of analgesia used depends on the severity of the degeneration: mild, moderate, or severe. Increasingly used are nutritional supplements purported to reduce pain and regenerate damaged cartilage (glucosamine and chondroitin). Chondroitin and glucosamine can be taken concurrently with other treatments for OA. Viscosupplementation could be considered for mild to moderate OA of the knee.

RX1 **Acetaminophen** (Tylenol) [B]: Blocks pain impulse generation peripherally.

DS1 325–650 mg PO q4hr prn; should not exceed maximum dose of 4 g/day

SE1 **Risk of hepatic impairment.** In situations of **overdose (> 150 μg/mL at 4 hours)**, acetaminophen causes **hepatotoxicity.**

Table 21-5. Narcotics* Used as Analgesics in Rheumatic Diseases

Generic (Brand) Name	Dose (PO)	Side Effects	Note
Codeine [C/D depending on dose and duration of use]	8–80 mg q4hr prn	Cognitive impairment, constipation, dry mouth, nausea, pruritus, respiratory depression, sedation, urinary retention	Psychological and physical dependence may occur. Drug has no anti-inflammatory properties.
Codeine, sustained-release (Codeine Contin—*Can.*)	100–300 mg bid (may be increased if there is insufficient pain control)	Same as above	Same as above
Codeine with acetaminophen	1–2 tablets† q4hr prn	Same as above Caution: Dosing should not exceed acetaminophen 4 g/day.	Same as above
Fentanyl patch (Duragesic) [B/D depending on duration of use or high doses at term]	25–100 ug q3 days	Decreased severity of side effects described above	Less likelihood of developing psychological and physical dependence.
Meperidine (oral) (Demerol, Meperitab) [B/D depending on dose and duration of use]	50–150 mg q4hr (may be increased if there is insufficient pain control)	Same as above	Same as above
Morphine [B/D depending on dose and duration of use]	5–20 mg q4hr	Same as above	Same as above
Morphine, sustained-release (MS Contin)	10–40 mg bid (may be increased if there is insufficient pain control)	Same as above	Same as above

Oxycodone (Endocodone, Oxycontin, Percolone, Roxicodone, Intensol—*U.S.*; Supendol—*Can.*) [B/D depending on dose and duration of use]	5–10 mg q4hr (may be increased if there is insufficient pain control)	Same as above	Same as above
Oxycodone, sustained-release (OxyContin)	10–40 mg bid (may be increased if there is insufficient pain control)	Same as above	Same as above
Oxycodone with acetaminophen (Endocet, Percocet, Roxicet, Roxilox, Tylox—*U.S.*; Oxycet—*Can.*)[C]	1–2 tablets‡ q4hr prn	Same as above Caution: Dosing should not exceed acetaminophen 4 g/day.	Same as above
Oxycodone with aspirin (Endodan, Percodan—*U.S.*; Oxycodan—*Can.*) [D]	1–2 tablets§ q4hr prn	Same as above See Table 21–1 for aspirin side effects and cautions.	Psychological and physical dependence may occur. Drug has anti-inflammatory properties owing to aspirin component.

*In cases of overdose, administer naloxone (Narcan) 0.2–0.4 mg IV 15 minutes prn and place patient under close supervision for possibility of respiratory depression (because half-life of opioid is longer than that of naloxone), which will require repeated naloxone administration.

†Codeine with acetaminophen: 1 tablet contains 7.5–60 mg of codeine phosphate and 325 mg of acetaminophen.

‡Oxycodone with acetaminophen: one tablet/capsule contains 5 mg of oxycodone hydrochloride and 325 mg of acetaminophen.

§Oxycodone with aspirin: one tablet contains 4.5 mg of oxycodone hydrochloride, 0.38 mg of oxycodone terephthalate, and 325 mg of aspirin.

> **ANTIDOTE**
>
> The **antidote for acetaminophen poisoning is acetylcysteine (Mucomyst—*U.S.*; Parvolex—*Can.*).** 140 mg/kg PO; followed by 17 doses of 70 mg/kg PO q4hr. Repeat dose if vomiting occurs within 1 hour of any administered dose.

or

RX2 **Ibuprofen** (Advil, Motrin) [B/D in third trimester: Provides pain relief in patients with mild OA.]

DS2 Table 21–1

SE2 Table 21–1

or

RX3 **Selective COX 2 inhibitors:** Used as first-line treatment for pain relief in moderate or severe OA and as second-line treatment for patients with mild OA for whom acetaminophen and ibuprofen are not successful.

DS3 Table 21–6

SE3 Table 21–6

or

RX4 **NSAIDS:** Used as second-line treatment for pain relief in patients with moderate or severe OA for whom selective COX 2 inhibitors are not successful.

DS4 Table 21–1

Tables 21–6. COX 2 Selective NSAIDs

Generic (Brand) Name	Dose (PO)	Indications	Side Effects and Cautions
Celecoxib (Celebrex) [C/D in third trimester]	200 mg qd for OA 200 mg bid for RA	OA RA	Associated with increased cardiovascular events. Headache, GI upset, URTI, sinusitis, pharyngitis, peripheral edema, insomnia, hypertension, cardiac arrhythmias, GI hemorrhage
Mobicoxib (Mobicox)	7.5 mg qd–bid	OA	
Rofecoxib (Vioxx) [C/D in third trimester]	25 mg qd	OA, acute pain	Hypersensitivity reactions: avoid in patients with known allergic reactions to aspirin and NSAIDs. Use celecoxib with caution in patients with sulfonamide allergy.

GI = gastrointestinal; MI = myocardial infarction; NSAIDs = nonsteroidal anti-inflammatory drugs; OA = osteoarthritis; RA = rheumatoid arthritis; URTI = upper respiratory tract infection.

SE4 Table 21–1

with or without

RX5 **Opioids:** Used in cases of severe OA to relieve pain.

DS5 Table 21–5

SE5 Table 21–5

with or without

RX6 **Intra-articular steroid injection**

DS6 Table 21–2 and Table 21–7

SE6 Table 21–2

with or without

RX7 **Dietary supplementation** with chondroitin and glucosamine

DS7 Chondroitin: 800–1,000 mg PO qd in divided doses for 3 months. Glucosamine: 500 mg PO tid for 3 months.

SE7 Amount of active ingredient is dependent on the manufacturer. No significant side effects.

with or without

RX8 Hyaluronic acid (Synvisc): Viscosupplementation may be considered in mild to moderate OA of the knee.

DS8 Weekly intra-articular injections in the knee for 3–5 weeks.

SE8 Local irritation and infection.

POLYMYALGIA RHEUMATICA

KY Etiology is unknown, but the condition has a close association with giant cell arteritis. It is more common in elderly females. Patients present with fever, weight loss, malaise, and symptoms in the neck, shoulder, and hip girdle, as well as morning stiffness.

TX Mainstay of treatment is the use of **oral prednisone.** Duration of treat-

Table 21–7. Dose Equivalency of Various Glucocorticoids

Half-life	Generic Name	Relative Anti-inflammatory Effect
Short acting	Cortisone	0.8
	Hydrocortisone	1.0
Intermediate acting	Prednisone	3.5
	Prednisolone	4.0
	Methylprednisolone	5.0
	Triamcinolone	5.0
Long acting	Dexamethasone	30
	Betamethasone	30

ment may be months. Tapering of medication should begin after several months of therapy to the lowest dose that will control symptoms. The dose may have to be increased if the patient has a flare-up while on a tapering schedule. If the patient is symptom free for 1 year, then therapy can be discontinued.

RX **Prednisone**

DS 10–30 mg PO qd

SE See Table 21–2

PSORIATIC ARTHRITIS

KY Psoriatic arthritis affects 10%–15% of persons with psoriasis. The arthritis can precede or follow the development of the skin lesions. Etiology of psoriasis and psoriatic arthritis is unknown. Psoriatic arthritis can present in several ways: mono/oligoarthritis (the most common initial presentation), polyarthritis (the most common form, very similar distribution of affected joints as RA), arthritis mutilans, axial disease, and enthesitis.

TX Treatment of psoriatic joint disease is similar to treatment of RA. New biologic agents are potential therapeutic options (Table 21-3).

RX1 **NSAIDs**

DS1 Table 21–1

SE1 Table 21–1

or

RX2 **DMARDs:** Methotrexate (for both skin and joint disease), sulfasalazine (only for joint manifestations), hydroxychloroquine, gold, azathioprine, or cyclosporine.

DS2 Table 21–3

SE2 Table 21–3

with or without

RX3 **Intra-articular glucocorticoid injection**

DS3 10–80 mg in affected joint depending on size of joint

SE3 Table 21–2

REITER'S SYNDROME / REACTIVE ARTHRITIS

KY Follows GI (*Shigella, Salmonella, Campylobacter,* and *Yersinia*), genitourinary (*Chlamydia trachomatis, Ureaplasma urealyticum*), or upper respiratory tract (*Chlamydia pneumoniae*) infections. Arthritis typically occurs 2–4 weeks after infection. **Reiter's syndrome is composed of the triad of arthritis, urethritis, and conjunctivitis.** Arthritis is typically asymmetrical and affects fewer than four joints (oligoarthritis). Lower-extremity, sacroiliac, and spinal joints are commonly affected. Enthesopathies are also common. **Extra-articular manifestations** include kera-toderma blennorrhagicum, circinate balanitis, oral ulcers, nail changes, anterior uveitis, and aortitis.

TX Disease is typically self-limiting, lasting 3–12 months. However, antibiotics to eradicate the organism may be beneficial.

RX1 NSAIDs

DS1 Table 21–1

SE1 Table 21–1

with or without

RX2 **Intra-articular glucocorticoid injection**

DS2 10–80 mg in the affected joint depending on the size of the joint. Injection to the sacroiliac joint requires fluoroscopic guidance.

SE2 Table 21–2

with or without

RX3 **DMARDs:** azathioprine, methotrexate, and sulfasalazine

DS3 Table 21–3

SE3 Table 21–3

RHEUMATOID ARTHRITIS (RA)

KY RA is an autoimmune, seropositive (i.e., rheumatoid factor), multisys-tem disease of unknown etiology. It has been postulated that there is pro-liferation of synovial cells and an inflammatory response, which leads to the local migration of lymphocytes, plasma cells, and mast cells. Com-pounded by the edema and neovascularization, there is subsequent hyper-trophy and hyperplasia of the synovial cells. The expanding synovium imposes on the joint space and eventually erodes into the subchondral bone and covers the cartilage as a pannus. Articular cartilage is ultimately destroyed through direct resorption and a lack of nutrient synovial fluid, leading to definitive joint destruction and fusion. Extra-articular manifesta-tions include rheumatoid nodules, vasculitis, sicca complex, Felty's syn-drome, keratoconjunctivitis, scleritis and episcleritis, pulmonary involve-ment, cardiac involvement (i.e., pericarditis), central nervous system (CNS) involvement (from nerve entrapment and vasculitis resulting in a mononeu-ritis multiplex), and anemia.

TX The treatment paradigm for seropositive arthropathies such as RA has recently been changed. **In RA, erosions to the articular surface occur early in the course of the disease** (within 2 years of disease onset in pol-yarticular seropositive RA). **The early use of DMARDs has been shown to slow progression of these articular changes.** Later-onset use of DMARDs may allow this window of opportunity to pass. Another change in the paradigm is the recognition that **occasionally a single drug is not effective in the control of the arthritis;** increasingly, combination DMARDs are being used. However, the optimal DMARD combination to use or even which DMARD is the most appropriate first-line drug still needs to be determined.

RX1 **DMARD:** When starting DMARD therapy, low- or high-dose **glu-cocorticoid** (10–40 mg qd) is started at the same time, as a bridge therapy before the start of any therapeutic effect from the DMARD. Possible DMARD treatment strategies include (1) the step-up approach—using DMARD early at the highest doses necessary, followed by the addition of another DMARD if therapeutic result is not achieved; (2) the step-down bridge—starting with combination DMARD therapy and weaning off the number of drugs to the minimum, using disease activity as a strict guide (the most toxic drug is withdrawn first); and (3) the overlap-and-switch—when switching from one DMARD to another, the first is continued for a limited time with the next one before being discontinued.

DS1 Table 21–3

SE1 Table 21–3

with or without

RX2 **Prednisone**

DS2 10–40 mg PO qd

SE2 Table 21–2

with or without

RX3 **NSAID**

DS3 Table 21–1

SE3 Table 21–1

with or without

RX4 **Celecoxib** (Celebrex) [C/D in third trimester]

DS4 200 mg PO bid

SE4 Table 21–6

with or without

RX5 **Intra-articular steroid injection:** This may be beneficial if only a few joints are affected.

DS5 Table 21–2 and Table 21–7

SE5 Table 21–2

  with or without

RX6 **Acetaminophen** (Tylenol): See OSTEOARTHRITIS (OA).

DS6 325–650 mg q4hr prn

SE6 See OSTEOARTHRITIS (OA).

or

RX7 **Narcotic analgesics** depending on the severity of the symptoms.

DS7 Table 21–5

SE7 Table 21–5

SCLERODERMA

See SYSTEMIC SCLEROSIS AND SCLERODERMA.

SEPTIC ARTHRITIS

Bacteria, viruses, fungus, *Mycobacterium,* and protozoa may cause septic arthritis. Predisposing conditions include intravenous substance abuse, age (> 60 years), joint surgery, diabetes, dialysis, human immunodeficiency virus, neoplasia, and RA.

Bacterial Infection

KY **Must be treated quickly and aggressively to prevent destruction of the joint.** Typically presents as an acute monoarthritis (80%) or oligoarthritis (< 20%). Most common pathogens include Gram-positive bacteria in children (*Staphylococcus aureus, Streptococcus* species, and *Haemophilus influenzae* type B) and intravenous drug users (*S. aureus Streptococcus* species) and Gram-positive (*S. aureus*) and Gram-negative bacteria in the elderly. Note that the incidence of gonococcal-related septic arthritis has been decreasing.

TX **Aspirate joint for Gram stain and culture before initiating empiric treatment.** Joint may require repeated aspiration or surgical drainage. Initiate empirical antibiotic treatment before Gram stain and culture results are known. **Note: fluoroquinolones should not be used empirically because of the high incidence of resistance. Start with IV antibiotics.** Use appropriate organism-specific antibiotic for 3–6 weeks once the organism has been identified by culture. **Oral medication may be used after 2 weeks of IV therapy.** Continue treatment for longer duration in immunocompromised patients. For patients with an infected prosthetic joint that cannot be removed, treatment may be lifelong.

RX1 **Penicillins: Bactericidal agents** (Table 21–8) that inhibit bacterial cell wall synthesis. **Used in the treatment of suspected Gram-positive bacteria.**

DS1 Table 21–8

SE1 **Hypersensitivity** occurs in approximately 1%–4% and **anaphylaxis** in approximately 0.01% of treatment courses. **Hematologic reactions,** such as anemia and thrombocytopenia have also been reported. There is a **risk of seizures in the presence of renal insufficiency.**

or

RX2 **First-generation cephalosporins:** These agents are used in **suspected cases of Gram-positive bacterial infection.** These bactericidal antimicrobial agents act by inhibiting bacterial cell wall synthesis.

DS2 Table 21–9

Table 21–8. Penicillins

Generic (Brand) Name	Dose
Ampicillin (Marcillin, Polycillin, Principen—U.S.; Ampicin, Penbritin —Can.) [B]	20–30 mg/kg/day PO divided into 4 equal doses 50–200 mg/kg/day IV divided into 4–6 equal doses
Cloxacillin (Cloxapen—U.S.; Orbenin—Can.) [B]	20–30 mg/kg/day PO divided into 4 equal doses 50–200 mg/kg/day IV divided into 4–6 equal doses
Methicillin (Staphcillin— Can.) [B]*	50–200 mg/kg/day IV divided into 4–6 equal doses
Nafcillin (Nallpen—U.S.; Unipen—Can.) [B]	50–200 mg/kg/day IV divided into 4–6 equal doses
Oxacillin (Bactocill) [B]	20–30 mg/kg/day PO divided into 4 equal doses 50–200 mg/kg/day IV divided into 4–6 equal doses
Penicillin G benzathine (Bicillin, Permapen—U.S.; Megacillin—Can.) [B]	Aqueous benzyl 100,000–200,000 IU/kg/day IV divided into 4–6 equal doses Procaine 800 mg IM Benzathine 800 mg IM
Penicillin V potassium (Suspen, Truxcillin, Veetids—U.S.; Pen-Vee —Can.) [B]	20–30 mg/kg/day PO divided into 4 equal doses
Piperacillin (Pipracil) [B]	8,000 mg IM divided into 2,000 mg per injection site or 4,000 mg IV q4–6hr
Ticarcillin (Ticar) [B]	300 mg/kg/day IV divided into 4–6 equal doses

*Methicillin is not available in the United States.

SE2 The risk of an **allergic reaction** to a cephalosporin is increased in known penicillin-allergic patients.

or

RX3 Second- and third-generation cephalosporins: Used in **suspected enteric or Gram-negative bacterial infections.**

DS3 Table 21–9

SE3 The risk of an **allergic reaction** to a cephalosporin is increased in known penicillin-allergic patients. Third-generation cephalosporins are associated with transient elevation of aspartate aminotransferase levels, reversible blood urea nitrogen elevation, and disturbance of the vitamin K–dependent clotting pathway. Ceftriaxone is associated with a transient formation of gallbladder sludge.

Table 21-9. Cephalosporins

Generic (Brand) Name	Dose	Sensitive Organisms
First Generation		
Cephalexin (Keflex) [B]	250 mg PO q6hr	Staphylococci (not MRSA)
Cefazolin (Ancef, Kefzol) [B]	500–1,000 mg IM/IV q6–8hr	Streptococci
		Klebsiella pneumoniae
		Proteus mirabilis
Second Generation		
Cefaclor (Ceclor) [B]	250 mg PO q8–12hr (maximum 2g/day)	Staphylococci (not MRSA)
Cefotetan (Cefotan) [B]	1,000–2,000 mg IM/IV q12hr	Streptococci
Cefoxitin (Mefoxin) [B]	1,000–2,000 mg IM/IV q6–8h	Haemophilus influenzae
Cefuroxime (Ceftin, Kefurox, Zinacef) [B]	250 mg PO bid	Moraxella catarrhalis
		Enterobacteriaceae
		Anaerobic activity (not enterococci or Listeria monocytogenes)
Third Generation		
Cefixime (Suprax) [B]	400 mg PO qd	Aerobic Gram-negative bacilli (not Pseudomonas aeruginosa)
Cefotaxime (Claforan) [B]	1000–2,000 mg IM/IV q8hr	H. influenzae
Ceftriaxone (Rocephin) [B]	500–1,000 mg IM/IV q12hr	M. catarrhalis
		Neisseria meningitidis
		Streptococci
Ceftazidime (Ceptaz, Fortaz, Tazicef, Tazidime) [B]	250–2,000 mg IM/IV q8–12hr	Aerobic Gram-negative bacilli including P. aeruginosa
		H. influenzae
		M. catarrhalis
		N. meningitidis

MRSA = methicillin-resistant Staphylococcus aureus.

or

RX4 **Aminoglycosides** (Gram-negative): Gentamicin (Cidomycin, Garamycin), tobramycin (Nebcin, Tabrex), amikacin (Amikan), netilmicin (Netromycin). These bactericidal agents inhibit protein synthesis by binding the 30S subunit of the bacterial ribosome. Because these agents cannot be absorbed after oral administration, IV or IM injection is required. Excretion of these agents is mostly by the kidneys.

DS4 These agents can be administered as a single daily dose or in divided doses. The recommended total daily dose is 5–7 mg/kg.

SE4 **Nephrotoxicity** and **ototoxicity.** In renal insufficiency, aminoglycosides should be avoided or the dosing interval should be extended.
or

RX5 **Vancomycin** (Vancocin) [C]: This glycopeptide antibiotic acts against many Gram-positive bacteria by inhibiting cell wall synthesis and selectively inhibiting RNA synthesis. This agent is used in suspected cases of methicillin-resistant *S. aureus* bacterial infection.

DS5 Drug is poorly absorbed by mouth but can be given intravenously. The usual IV dose for an adult is 500 mg q6hr or 1,000 mg q12hr. **Each dose should be administered at no more than 10 mg/min or over at least 60 minutes, whichever is longer.** In patients with impaired renal function, the dose must be adjusted and the serum levels must be checked for toxic accumulation, which can occur over several weeks of treatment.

SE5 Anaphylaxis, nephrotoxicity, ototoxicity, and reversible neutropenia. **Rapid infusion over several minutes can lead to hypotension, shock, and even cardiac arrest.**

Lyme Disease

KY Lyme disease (*Borrelia burgdorferi*) is caused by tick bites and early localized disease features, including erythema migrans. Early disseminated disease (days to months after tick bite) can present with cardiac and neurologic manifestations. Late disease (months to years after tick bite) features include migratory episodes of polyarthritis, so-called tertiary neuroborreliosis.

TX **Antibiotic treatment** is curative. **Important: Immediate treatment will prevent progression to stages with serious sequelae.**

RX Table 21–10 and Table 21–11

DS Table 21–10 and Table 21–11

SE Table 21–10 and Table 21–11

Mycobacterium Infection

KY *Mycobacterium* includes tuberculosis (TB), atypical mycobacterium, and leprae. The classic articular presentation of *Mycobacterium tuberculosis* is spinal TB or Pott's disease. TB infection of peripheral joints is uncommon. Pott's disease may cause destruction of the vertebral endplates, abscess formation within the spinal canal and psoas muscle, and arachnoiditis.

Table 21–10. Oral Therapy of Early Lyme Disease*

Generic (Brand) Name	Dose (PO)
Adults	
Amoxicillin (Amoxil) [B]	250–500 mg qid
Doxycycline (Vibramycin—*U.S.*; Doxycin—*Can.*) [D]	100 mg bid
Tetracycline (Brodspec—*U.S.*; Tetracyn—*Can.*) [D]	250–500 mg qid
Children	
Amoxicillin	40 mg/kg/day divided dose
Erythromycin	30 mg/kg/day divided dose
Penicillin V potassium	25–50 mg/kg/day divided dose

*Duration of therapy for all drugs is 3–4 weeks.

TX Treat *Mycobacterium* to treat the arthritis. Isoniazid (INH), rifampin, and pyrazinamide for regions of low INH resistance. If the incidence of INH resistance is unknown, add streptomycin or ethambutol. For multidrug-resistant TB, use INH, rifampin, and pyrazinamide with streptomycin or ethambutol and add second-line antibiotics, such as amikacin and quinolones (ciprofloxacin, sparfloxacin, or levofloxacin). Combined rifampin/INH (Rifamate) as well as a rifampin/INH/pyrazinamide (Rifater) drugs are available for better compliance. See Ch 10 Infectious Diseases for further information on TB.

RX1 **Isoniazid** (INH) (Nydrazid—*U.S.*; Isotamine—*Can.*) [C]: This specific bactericidal agent is active against organisms of the genus *Mycobacterium,* specifically *M. tuberculosis, Mycobacterium bovis,* and *Mycobacterium kansasii.*

DS1 300 mg PO qd for 6 months

SE1 GI intolerance, hepatitis, hypersensitivity reactions, and rash. Peripheral neuropathy has been reported predominantly in malnourished patients and can be prevented by the concomitant use of pyridoxine (vitamin B_6). Can cause drug-induced SLE.

Table 21–11. Intravenous Therapy of Early Disseminated and Late Lyme Disease*

Generic Name	Dose
Adults	
Ceftriaxone	2 g/day in single or divided doses
Cefotaxime	3 g bid
Chloramphenicol	50 mg/kg/day, 4 divided doses
Penicillin G benzathine	20 million U, 6 divided doses
Children	
Cefotaxime	90–180 mg/kg/day
Ceftriaxone	75–100 mg/kg/day
Penicillin G benzathine	300,000 U/kg/day, 6 divided doses

*Duration of therapy for all drugs is 2–4 weeks.

with

RX2 **Rifampin** (Rifadin, Rimactane.) [C]: Inhibits DNA-dependent RNA polymerase, causing suppression of RNA synthesis in susceptible bacteria. Active against microorganisms of the genus *Mycobacterium,* including *M. tuberculosis, M. kansasii, Mycobacterium marinum, Mycobacterium avium*-intracellulare (*M. avium* complex), and *Mycobacterium leprae.* It also acts against some Gram-negative bacteria, including *Neisseria meningitidis* and *H. influenzae* type b, and some Gram-positive bacteria, including *S. aureus* and *S. epidermidis.*

DS2 600 mg PO qd for 6 months

SE2 Hepatitis, fever, and rash. The combination of rifampin and ethambutol in high doses can lead to thrombocytopenia. Overdose causes lethargy, liver involvement and jaundice, and an orange discoloration of the skin, urine, sweat, saliva, tears, and feces.

with

RX3 **Pyrazinamide** (Tebrazid.) [C]: This synthetic analog of nicotinamide acts against metabolically active tubercle bacilli. Its exact mode of action is unclear.

DS3 25 mg/kg PO qd for 2 months

SE3 Hepatotoxicity and hyperuricemia.

with or without

RX4 **Streptomycin** [D]: An aminoglycoside primarily active against Gram-negative aerobes with limited action against some Gram-positive aerobes (i.e., staphylococci).

DS4 15 mg/kg/day (maximum 1 g) IM qd or 25–30 mg/kg (maximum 1.5 g) IM twice weekly or 25–30 mg/kg (maximum 1 g) IM 3 times/week.

SE4 Ototoxicity and nephrotoxicity.

or

RX5 **Ethambutol** (Myambutol—*U.S.*; Etibi—*Can.*) [B]: Bacteriostatic agent against *M. tuberculosis.* Also disrupts the cell membrane, facilitating entry into the cell by other drugs.

DS5 15–25 mg/kg/day (maximum 2.5 g/day) PO

SE5 Reversible **retrobulbar neuropathy** resulting in **defective red-green vision with subsequent field constriction or blindness.** Baseline visual acuity test **and regular monitoring every 4–6 weeks is recommended.**

with or without

RX6 **Amikacin** (Amikin) [C]: Aminoglycoside.

DS6 5–7.5 mg/kg/dose IM q8hr

SE6 Ototoxicity, nephrotoxicity, neurotoxicity, and hypersensitivity.

or

RX7 **Ciprofloxacin** (Cipro, Ciloxan) [C]: Fluoroquinolone.

DS7 500 mg PO bid or 400 mg IV q8–12hr

SE7 Not recommended for children because of possible damage to developing cartilage. Headache, GI upset, seizure, and hypersensitivity reactions.

Viral Infection

KY Common viruses associated with arthritis include parvovirus B19, hepatitis B and C, rubella, human immunodeficiency virus, and alphavirus. Rare viral causes of arthritis/arthralgias include adenovirus, coxsackie viruses, Epstein-Barr virus, and cytomegalovirus.

TX **Treat infectious agent,** if possible. Otherwise, treatment is supportive with NSAIDs.

RX **NSAIDs**

DS Table 21–1

SE Table 21–1

SJOGREN'S SYNDROME

KY **Primary form** most commonly presents as dry eyes (keratoconjunctivitis sicca) and dry mouth (xerostomia). **Secondary form** comprises the previously mentioned associated symptoms with other autoimmune diseases, that is, RA, SLE, and systemic sclerosis.

TX **For keratoconjunctivitis:** Consider the use of artificial tears and/or Cevimeline (Evoxac) [C] 30 mg PO tid.

For xerostomia: Consider the use of sugarless candy and chewing gum to stimulate salivary gland function; and/or Pilocarpine [C] with an initial dose of 20 mg/day PO, titration up to 30 mg/day. **For secondary form symptoms:** The use of DMARDs is similar to SLE.

RX DMARDs: Azathioprine, methotrexate, cyclophosphamide, cyclosporine.

DS See Table 21–3

SE See Table 21–3

SYSTEMIC LUPUS ERYTHEMATOSUS (SLE)

KY Etiology of primary form is unknown. Great female preponderance (9:1 female-male ratio). **Multisystem involvement,** including joints, skin, mucosal linings, serous membranes, vascular vessels, kidney, lungs, heart, CNS, GI system, muscles, and hematopoietic (including increased risk of thrombosis with antiphospholipid antibody syndrome). Arthralgias and arthritis are the most common manifestations of SLE. **Drug-induced lupus** exists, and those with a definite association include chlorpromazine, methyldopa, hydralazine, procainamide, and INH. **Drugs with a possible association** include phenytoin, penicillamine, and quinidine.

TX Therapy is organ specific. Therapy listed here is for the treatment of acute inflammatory manifestations, that is, arthritis, vasculitis, and cerebritis.

RX1 **Acetaminophen:** See OSTEOARTHRITIS (OA).

DS1 See OSTEOARTHRITIS (OA).

SE1 See OSTEOARTHRITIS (OA).

with or without

RX2 **Narcotic analgesics**

DS2 Table 21–5

SE2 Table 21–5

or

RX3 **NSAIDs**

DS3 Table 21–1

SE3 Patients with lupus nephritis may be especially susceptible to the renal side effects of NSAIDs (Table 21–1).

with or without

RX4 **Hydroxychloroquine** (Plaquenil) [C]: Beneficial in the **treatment of cutaneous manifestations of SLE.**

DS4 See Table 21–3

SE4 See Table 21–3

or

RX5 **Azathioprine** (Imuran) [D]: Beneficial in the treatment of **nephritis caused by SLE.**

DS5 See Table 21–3

SE5 See Table 21–3

with or without

RX6 **Methotrexate** (Rheumatrex) [D]: Mechanism of action is through the competitive inhibition of folic acid reductase and, thus, interferes with tissue-cell reproduction.

DS6 See Table 21–3

SE6 See Table 21–3

with or without

RX7 **Cyclophosphamide** (Cytoxan, Neosar—*U.S.*; Procytox—*Can.*) [D]: Antineoplastic agent used in cases of **severe SLE organ involvement including cerebritis and vasculitis.**

DS7 See Table 21–3

SE7 See Table 21–3

with or without

RX8 **Cyclosporine** (Neoral, Sandimmune) [C]

DS8 See Table 21–3

SE8 See Table 21–3

with or without

RX9 **Glucocorticoids:** Topical or intralesional for **rashes.** Intra-articular for **arthritis.** Oral or intravenous for **diffuse activity** (Table 21–2 and Table 21–7).

DS9 **Minor disease activity** (serositis, arthritis): Prednisone < 0.5 mg/kg PO qd.

Major disease activity (nephritis, CNS involvement): Prednisone (or equivalent) 1 mg/kg PO qd in single or divided doses. **Maximum: 4 weeks' duration and then taper dose.** Intravenous methylprednisolone bolus up to 1,000 mg IV over 30 minutes for 3 days.

SE9 See Table 21–2

SYSTEMIC SCLEROSIS AND SCLERODERMA

KY Etiology is unknown. Characterized by widespread fibrosis and vasculopathy (proliferative and obliterative) NOT vasculitis. Subtypes include diffuse cutaneous scleroderma (significant visceral involvement including lung, kidneys, GI tract, and heart), limited cutaneous scleroderma (CREST syndrome = calcinosis, Raynaud's phenomenon, esophageal involvement of scleroderma, sclerodactyly and telangiectasia), overlap syndrome (with features of RA, SLE, polymyositis, and scleroderma), localized scleroderma, and undefined connective tissue disease.

TX The use of DMARDs is similar to that for RA; however, treatment with DMARDs is not as effective. Medications include penicillamine, cyclophosphamide, cyclosporine, azathioprine, and methotrexate (Table 21–3). As with SLE, **treatment is organ specific.** Moisturizing creams and emulsifying ointments should be used for skin care.

Scleroderma-related fibrosis (includes intimal hyperplasia of small arteries, i.e., Raynaud's phenomenon, renal crisis, and pulmonary hypertension, and extravascular tissue fibrosis, i.e., skin, interstitial lung disease, and tendon involvement), consider Recombinant Human Relaxin: 25 μg/kg total daily dose given by continuous IV infusion, colchicine, photophoresis, and cyclophosphamide (for lung fibrosis). There is no adequate treatment for **cardiopulmonary involvement.** For **renal crisis, angiotensin-converting enzyme inhibitors are the drugs of choice.** Calcium channel blockers and prostacyclin analogs (Iloprost) are second-line treatment options.

Treatment of **Raynaud's phenomenon** consists of vasodilators. First line is calcium channel blockers. Prazosin and topical nitroglycerin has also been used. Prostacyclin analogs (Iloprost) are a consideration.

For **GI manifestations,** consider broad-spectrum antibiotics for bacterial overgrowth and proton pump inhibitors due to dysmotility and prokinetic agents to improve GI motility.

Following are general treatments for **musculoskeletal manifestations** for scleroderma.

RX1 **Acetaminophen:** See OSTEOARTHRITIS (OA).
DS1 See OSTEOARTHRITIS (OA).
SE1 See OSTEOARTHRITIS (OA).

with or without

RX2 **Narcotic analgesics**

DS2 See Table 21–5

SE2 See Table 21–5

or

RX3 **NSAIDs**

DS3 See Table 21–1

SE3 See Table 21–1

with or without

RX4 **Prednisone:** Used in the treatment of **myositis.**

DS4 See Table 21–2

SE4 See Table 21–2

with or without

RX5 **DMARDs:** For the treatment **of musculoskeletal manifestations and scleroderma-related fibrosis.**

DS5 See Table 21–3

SE5 See Table 21–3

VASCULITIDES

KY Includes polyarteritis nodosa, allergic granulomatosis and angiitis, Wegener's granulomatosis, Kawasaki disease, Takayasu arteritis, hypersensitivity vasculitis, Henoch-Schönlein purpura, Behçet syndrome, giant cell arteritis (or temporal arteritis), vasculitis associated with rheumatic diseases (RA, SLE), and thromboangiitis obliterans. Etiology is unknown.

TX The **cornerstone of treatment is the use of glucocorticoids.** The use of **other cytotoxic agents,** that is, cyclophosphamide, depends on the status of the patient. **Salicylates and high-dose IV immunoglobulins** are indicated in the treatment of Kawasaki's arteritis.

RX1 **Prednisone**

DS1 1–2 mg/kg PO qd

SE1 See Table 21–2

with or without

RX2 **Cyclophosphamide**

DS2 0.5–1.0 g/m^2 IV bolus followed by 1–4 mg/kg/day PO

SE2 See Table 21–3

22

Urology

SIDNEY B. RADOMSKI, SERGIO B. GIANCOLA

ERECTILE DYSFUNCTION

Impotence

KY Impotence is defined as the inability to acquire or sustain an erection of sufficient rigidity for sexual intercourse $> 75\%$ of the time. Drugs (sympathetic blockers), endocrine abnormalities, psychogenic causes, diabetes, neurologic problems, and urologic disease are predisposing factors.

TX Therapy for men with erectile dysfunction is aimed to restore the capacity to acquire and sustain penile erections and to reactivate libido. **Optimal treatment varies with the cause of impotence.** Table 22–1 lists commonly and less commonly used treatment options. The more commonly used pharmacologic treatments are discussed herein.

RX1 **Testosterone:** Its replacement is indicated in men with evidence of hypogonadism and low free serum testosterone and decreased libido. **Its routine use in all cases of erectile dysfunction is not warranted.**

DS1 See Ch 5 Endocrinology.

SE1 See Ch 5 Endocrinology.

or

RX2 **Sildenafil** (Viagra): A selective inhibitor of phosphodiesterases (PDE) type 5. With sexual stimulation, nitric oxide is released in the penis. This stimulates the production of cyclic guanosine monophosphate (cGMP), which in turn relaxes penile smooth muscle to allow increased blood flow into the penis. PDE type 5 breaks down cGMP; sildenafil prevents the breakdown of cGMP to allow increased blood flow into the penis. The success of this drug is variable from 50%–80% depending on the etiology of the erectile dysfunction.

DS2 Dosage ranges from 25–100 mg PO 1–1.5 hours before sexual activity. Stimulation is required for an erection. The medication should be taken on an empty stomach.

SE2 Side effects are associated with the vasodilatory properties of sildenafil, including headache, lightheadedness, dizziness, flushing, distorted vision, and syncope. A transient effect on color vision and myocardial infarction have also has been reported. Dosage should be decreased in liver or kidney disease and in patients taking potent cytochrome P450 inhibitors such as erythromycin, cimetidine, ketoconazole, and protease inhibitors. **It is contradicted in patients using any form of nitrates either occasionally or on a regular basis. The combination of nitrates and sildenafil causes dramatic hypotension**

Table 22–1. Treatments Available for Impotence

Generic (Brand) Name	Dose
Oral medications Sildenafil (Viagra)	25–100 mg PO 1–1.5 hours before sexual activity. Stimulation is required for an erection. Effective for approximately 4 hours.
Trazodone (Trazon)	50–100 mg PO qd
Yohimbine	5.4–6 mg PO tid
Intracavernous injection Alprostadil (Caverject, Edex)	5–20 μg injected into the base of the penis 10–20 minutes before sexual activity. Erection can be attained for about 1 hour.
VIP, phentolamine (Invicorp)	Inject 10–20 minutes before sexual activity. Stimulation is required for erection.
Intraurethral application Alprostadil (MUSE)	Alprostadil in gel or tablet form: 100–1,000 μg inserted into the meatus of the penis by applicator 5–10 minutes before sexual activity. Erection can be attained for approximately 1 hour. Can be used twice daily.

(decrease of 50 mm Hg). If a patient taking sildenafil has an acute ischemic syndrome, nitrates should not be given within 24 hours, and even longer in patients with renal or hepatic dysfunction or intracavernous agents.

RX3 Alprostadil [formerly prostaglandin E_1] (Caverject, Edex): Relaxes trabecular smooth muscle by dilation of cavernosal arteries by a corporeal veno-occlusive mechanism when injected along the penile shaft.

DS3 Dosage ranges from 5–20 μg intracavernous injection.

SE3 Penile pain is dose related and probably caused by the low pH of the mixture. Priapism can occur. **Contraindicated in hyaline membrane disease, persistent fetal circulation, dominant left-to-right shunt, respiratory distress syndrome, conditions predisposing to priapism, penile anatomical deformities, and those with penile implants or intraurethral agents.**

Mechanism of Action	Side Effects and Cautions
Inhibits phosphodiesterase type 5, which causes cyclic guanosine monophosphate to accumulate in the penis.	**Contraindicated** with concomitant nitrate use (see text).
An antidepressant with selective inhibition of central serotonin uptake and some alpha-adrenergic blocking activity. Relaxes smooth muscle to allow increased penile blood flow.	Dizziness, lethargy, priapism
Blocks presynaptic alpha-2-receptors, increases libido, and possibly increases flow and decreases outflow.	Anxiety, gastrointestinal upset, possible increased hypertension, insomnia
Causes smooth-muscle relaxation in corpus cavernosa.	May be painful and is not recommended for daily use. Priapism can occur. **Contraindication** listed in text.
Causes relaxation of penile vascular smooth muscle.	Priapism
Directly affects vascular and ductus arteriosus smooth muscle, causing vasodilation and allowing blood flow to and entrapment in the lacunar spaces of the penis.	Not recommended with pregnant partners.

RX4 **Intraurethral alprostadil**/prostaglandin E_1 (Muse): Corporal smooth muscle relaxant.

DS4 Dose of 100–1,000 μg placed in the urethra via an applicator.

SE4 Hypotension and urethral and penile pain. Contraindications are the same as those listed for intracavernous injectable alprostadil (Caverject).

Priapism

KY Priapism is defined as an unwanted, painful erection lasting > 4 hours. Predisposing factors include sickle cell anemia, multiple myeloma, and leukemia. Priapism is a considerable side effect described with the use of alprostadil and papaverine.

TX **Priapism is a medical emergency** often requiring urgent urologic intervention to evacuate blood clogged within the corpora cavernosa. First

Table 22–2. Alpha-Adrenergic Agonists Used in the Treatment of Priapism

Generic (Brand) Name	Dose (Intracavernous Injection)	Side Effects and Cautions
Phenylephrine (Neo-Synephrine)*	(Dilution of 0.2 mg in 2 mL of saline) 250–500 µg q5min until detumescence is achieved	The patient must be monitored carefully after injection of these agents because of potential cardiac side effects (i.e., tachycardia and hypertension).
Epinephrine	10–20 µg	

*Clinically used most often.

line of treatment involves intracavernous injection of an alpha-adrenergic agonist. If medical therapy fails, a spongiocavernosa shunt is required.

RX **Alpha-adrenergic agonists:** Cause arterial vasoconstriction.

DS Table 22–2

SE Table 22–2

FAILURE TO EMPTY VOIDING DYSFUNCTION

Benign Prostatic Hyperplasia (BPH) (Urethral Causes)

KY BPH increases in frequency progressively with age in men older than 50 years. Common, but not specific, symptoms of BPH are increased frequency of urination, nocturia, hesitancy, urgency, and weak urinary stream. These symptoms usually occur slowly and progress gradually over years.

TX Current medical management of BPH is based on two premises. The first involves the accepted fact that prostatic growth can physically cause outflow obstruction. This growth is influenced by androgen stimulation. The second is that there is a significant amount of smooth muscle in the prostate that can cause dynamic obstruction through increased muscle tone. This muscle is influenced by adrenergic stimulation.

RX1 **5-Alpha-reductase inhibitors:** These drugs block the conversion of testosterone to dihydrotestosterone (DHT) within prostate cells. DHT is the major intracellular androgen and stimulates prostatic growth. It is through this form of stimulation that prostatic hypertrophy may develop. Patients who are on 5-alpha-reductase inhibitors will have decreased serum and prostatic DHT and therefore decreased stimulation for prostatic growth. Prostatic size, therefore, decreases and urinary flow increases through reduction in the obstructing effect of a large prostate gland. Note that it may take several months for a clinically significant reduction in prostate volume to occur. **It is important to note that a decrease in prostate-specific antigen may occur; an important consideration if prostate-specific antigen is being used to screen for prostate cancer as the levels may be artificially low because of the medication.**

DS1 Table 22–3

Table 22–3. Treatment Options for Benign Prostatic Hyperplasia

Class	Generic (Brand) Name	Dose	Side Effects
5-alpha-reductase inhibitors	Finasteride (Proscar)	5 mg PO qd	Impotence, decreased libido, decreased volume of ejaculate, breast tenderness/enlargement
Alpha-adrenergic blockers	Doxazosin (Cardura)	Start at 1 mg PO qd and increase as tolerated up to 10 mg PO qd	Peripheral vasodilation, hypotension, dizziness, headache, asthenia, somnolence, nasal congestion, palpitations
	Terazosin (Hytrin)	Start at 1 mg PO qhs and then increase as tolerated by patient (e.g., 1 mg/week) to 5–10 mg PO qhs	
Alpha-1A-adrenergic blockers	Tamsulosin (Flomax)	0.4 mg PO qd	Abnormal ejaculation, decreased volume of ejaculation, dizziness, postural hypotension, syncope, asthenia

SE1 Table 22–3

or

RX2 **Alpha-adrenergic blockers:** Smooth muscle within the prostate and bladder neck has been found to have alpha$_1$-adrenergic receptors. Blockage of these receptors significantly improves urinary flow, presumably through relaxation of smooth muscle both in the prostate as well as in the bladder neck. Relaxation of the muscle around the prostatic urethra and the bladder neck results in decreased outflow resistance from the bladder, thereby accounting for the improved flow seen in patients taking this medication.

DS2 Table 22–3

SE2 Table 22–3

or

RX3 **Alpha-1A-adrenergic blockers: Tamsulosin** (Flomax) belongs to this class of drugs and is a highly selective receptor antagonist for the alpha-1A-adrenoceptor subtype, which predominates in the human prostate. It has been shown that this drug is effective in the treatment of symptomatic BPH with only minor effects on blood pressure and vasodilatation.

DS3 Table 22–3

SE3 Table 22–3

Detrusor External Sphincter Dyssynergia (Urethral Causes)

KY This problem occurs in patients who have sustained a spinal cord injury between the brain stem and sacral cord. It results in a spastic external sphincter (striated muscle).

TX There is no effective treatment available at this time. Diazepam and baclofen are used but have not proven very effective.

RX1 **Diazepam** (Valium) [D]: Binds to stereospecific benzodiazepine receptors on the postsynaptic gamma-aminobutyric acid (GABA) neuron, enhancing the inhibitory effect of GABA on neuronal excitability. This causes increased neuronal membrane permeability of chloride ions, which produces hyperpolarization (a less excitable state) and stabilization.

DS1 2–10 mg PO bid–qid

SE1 Drowsiness and hypotension. **Contraindicated in patients with narrow-angle glaucoma.** Diazepam has also been associated with **an increased frequency of grand mal seizures.**

or

RX2 **Baclofen** (Lioresal) [C]: Inhibits the transmission of both monosynaptic and polysynaptic reflexes at the spinal level, resulting in the relief of muscle spasticity.

DS2 5 mg PO tid

SE2 Drowsiness and hypotension. **Use with caution in patients with renal impairment and seizure disorder.**

Weak Detrusor Muscle (Bladder Causes)

KY This problem is commonly encountered in the diabetic patient with decreased sensation and chronic overstretching of the detrusor smooth muscle. It is also common in the elderly, although it is not exactly clear why bladder contractility decreases with age.

TX Bladder contractility depends on stimulation of the muscarinic cholinergic receptor sites at the postganglionic parasympathetic neuromuscular junctions. Unfortunately, there is no medication that actually improves bladder contractility.

RX **Bethanechol** (Urecholine) [C]: This cholinergic agonist theoretically stimulates the parasympathetic-rich detrusor muscle to cause bladder contractility. Although this drug has been used to improve contractility of the detrusor, there is no evidence that it can actually cause a contraction of the bladder.

DS 10–50 mg PO bid–qid or 2.5–5 mg SC tid–qid

SE Flushing, diarrhea, nausea, vomiting, and bronchospasm. **Contraindicated** in patients with bronchial asthma, bowel obstruction, ulcer disease, benign prostatic hypertrophy, bradycardia, vasomotor instability, atrioventricular conduction defects, hypotension, or parkinsonism. **Intramuscular and intravenous use of this drug is contraindicated** because it can cause a severe cholinergic reaction.

FAILURE TO STORE VOIDING DYSFUNCTION

Bladder Instability or Hyperreflexia (Bladder Causes)

KY Uncontrollable contractions of the bladder can be either **idiopathic (instability)** or caused by a **neurologic cause (hyperreflexia).** Instability is common in elderly healthy females, males with BPH, and women with stress urinary incontinence. The exact mechanism that results in uncontrollable spasms is not clear. It may be related to supersensitivity at the cholinergic receptor sites. Neurologic conditions such as a spinal cord injury, Parkinson's disease, and stroke can cause bladder spasms. Loss of central control of the bladder is likely to be responsible for this problem.

TX The drugs used for this condition are musculotropic relaxants that directly relax smooth muscle.

RX Table 22–4

DS Table 22–4

SE Table 22–4

Table 22–4. Treatment Options for Bladder Instability or Hyperreflexia

Generic (Brand) Name	Dose (PO)
Dicyclomine (Antispas, Bentyl, Byclomine, Dibent, DiSpaz, Or-Tyl—*U.S.*; Bentylol—*Can.*) [B]*	20 mg qid and increase to 40 mg qid
Flavoxate (Urispas) [B]*	100–200 mg tid–qid
Imipramine (Tofranil) [D]†	10–25 mg qd–qid
Imipramine + oxybutynin	Imipramine: 10–25 mg qd + Oxybutynin: 5–20 mg qd
Oxybutynin (Ditropan) [B]*	2.5–5 mg qd–qid
Oxybutynin XL (Ditropan XL) [B]*	5–20 mg qd
Propantheline (Pro-Banthine—*U.S.*; Propanthel—*Can.*) [C]*	15 mg tid + 30 mg qhs
Tolterodine (Detrol) [C]*	1–2 mg bid
Tolterodine LA (Detrol LA) [C]*	4 mg qd

BPH = benign prostatic hyperplasia; CHF = congestive heart failure; CNS = central nervous system; GI = gastrointestinal; MI = myocardial infarction.

*Anticholinergic drugs.

†Tricyclic antidepressant.

Interstitial Cystitis

KY Interstitial cystitis is a complex and uncommon disease entity resulting in bladder dysfunction with severe frequency and suprapubic pain. Its diagnosis and treatment remain a challenge.

TX Effective drug therapy is still lacking; however, extensive literature exists on this treatment.

RX1 **Pentosan polysulfate sodium** (Elmiron) [B]: Corrects the proposed defect in the bladder epithelial permeability barrier, glycosaminoglycan layer, causing interstitial cystitis. The effectiveness of this drug remains unclear. It is a low-molecular-weight heparin–like compound with anticoagulant and fibrinolytic effects.

Side Effects and Cautions

Same as for oxybutynin

Tachycardia, drowsiness, headache, GI upset, hypersensitivity reactions, leukopenia, increased intraocular pressure, blurred vision
Contraindicated in patients with GI obstruction or hemorrhage and BPH.

Sedation, orthostatic hypotension, arrhythmias, tachycardia, hypertension, palpitations, MI, heart block, CHF, stroke
Contraindicated with concurrent monoamine oxidase inhibitor usage and acute recovery phase from MI.

Anticholinergic side effects may be increased with this combination.
Contraindications are the same as those listed for oxybutynin and imipramine.

Dry mouth, constipation, dry eyes, fatigue, tachycardia, palpitations
Contraindicated in patients with acute glaucoma, urinary retention, and bowel obstruction.
Additive sedation with CNS depressants and alcohol and additive anticholinergic effects with antihistamines and anticholinergic agents.

This slow-release preparation has lower peak blood levels resulting in fewer side effects than oxybutynin. **Contraindications** are the same as those listed for oxybutynin.

Same as for oxybutynin

Side effects similar to those for oxybutynin but less dry mouth. **Contraindications** are the same as those listed for oxybutynin.

DS1 Dosage of 100–200 mg PO tid. Medication needs to be continued for 6–12 months before effects are recognized in some patients.

SE1 Bleeding is possible with use of this medication, and caution is advised to predisposed patients. Alopecia occurs in < 1% and is reversible when the drug is discontinued. Thrombocytopenia is rare.

or

RX2 **Amitriptyline** (Elavil, Vanatrip—*U.S.*; Levate—*Can.*) [D]: This tricyclic antidepressant has been shown to be effective in patients with interstitial cystitis; pain and urinary frequency improve. The exact mechanism of action in interstitial cystitis is unclear, but amitriptyline is a potent blocker of H1-histaminergic receptors also effectively used in other pain syndromes (see Ch 17 Pain Management).

DS2 25–75 mg PO qd

SE2 See Ch 19 Psychiatry.

Stress Urinary Incontinence (Urethral Causes)

KY Stress urinary incontinence is the occurrence of stress leakage caused by sphincter opening, in the absence of bladder contraction, with increase in intra-abdominal pressure. This condition is the most common cause of urinary incontinence in young women. It may also occur in men after transurethral or radical prostatectomy. There are three proposed causes of stress incontinence: (1) insufficient urethral support from pelvic endofascia and muscles, (2) complete failure of urethral closure, and (3) urethral instability.

TX Medications in the treatment of this condition play a role, but other treatments, including surgery, are the mainstay.

RX Table 22–5

DS Table 22–5

SE Table 22–5

GENITOURINARY INFECTIONS

Urinary tract infections (UTIs) in pregnancy are discussed in Ch 13 Obstetrics. Pediatric UTIs are discussed in Ch 18 Pediatrics.

Complicated UTI

KY In general, the complicating cause resulting in these infections should be dealt with in addition to treating the UTI. For example, outlet obstruction caused by BPH should be treated by relieving the obstruction (i.e., medication or surgery). As with uncomplicated infections, Gram-negative organisms are most common. However, other organisms, such as enterocci, can be present owing to these complicating causes.

TX Treatment depends on the urine culture results: If there is no resistance to the antibiotics used in uncomplicated infection, then these same antibiotics can be used; if resistance is demonstrated, then fluoroquinolones (ciprofloxacin, norfloxacin and levofloxacin) are used to treat the infection; and, if urine cultures are not available in the case of complicated infections, then treat with fluoroquinolones. Treatment courses in complicated UTI should be for 7 days because of the increased incidence of resistance in these patients.

RX Table 22–6

DS Table 22–6

SE Table 22–6

Table 22–5. Treatment Options for Stress Urinary Incontinence

Class	Generic (Brand) Name	Dose	Side Effects
Alpha-adrenergic agonists	Ephedrine [C]	25–50 mg PO q6hr up to 150 mg/day	Hypertension, anxiety, insomnia, cardiac arrhythmias Serious cardiovascular effects have been reported with these agents.
	Pseudoephedrine (Sudafed) [C]	30–60 mg PO q6hr	
Estrogen	Oral	1–2 mg qd, adjusted as necessary to limit symptoms	Venous thromboembolism, pulmonary embolism, hypertension, increased size of uterine leiomyomata, migraine
	Topical	2–4 g/day intravaginally for 2 weeks; reduce to 1–2 g/day for 2 weeks; followed by maintenance of 1 g 1–3 times/week	Association with estrogen therapy and the development of endometrial and breast carcinoma.
	Intravaginal ring (Estring)		

Table 22-6. Treatment of Genitourinary Infections

Generic (Brand) Name	Dose	Indications	Side Effects and Cautions
Amoxicillin (Amoxil) [B]	500 mg PO tid	Pyelonephritis UTIs	Hypersensitivity, pseudomembranous colitis, diarrhea Concurrent administration may decrease the efficacy of oral contraceptive pills and increase the effects of warfarin. Dose must be decreased in renal impairment.
Ampicillin [B] + gentamicin [aminoglycoside] [C]	Ampicillin: 1–2 g IV q6hr + Gentamicin: 1 mg/kg IV q8 hr	Pyelonephritis	Ampicillin: hypersensitivity, seizures, hemolytic anemia, thrombocytopenia Decrease dose in renal impairment. Gentamicin: ototoxicity, nephrotoxicity **Contraindicated** in conditions that depress neuromuscular transmission.
Ceftriaxone (Rocephin) [B]	1 g IV qd	Pyelonephritis	Diarrhea, eosinophilia, thrombocytosis, hypersensitivity
Cephalexin (Keflex) [B]	250 mg PO postcoital	Recurrent UTIs	Hypersensitivity, pseudomembranous colitis, diarrhea Dose must be decreased in renal impairment.
Fluoroquinolones Ciprofloxacin (Ciloxan, Cipro) [C]	250–500 mg PO bid	Complicated UTIs	**Prolongation of Q-T interval,** GI upset, dizziness, seizures, hypersensitivity
Levofloxacin (Levaquin) [C]	250 mg PO qd	Epididymo-orchitis	
Norfloxacin (Chibroxin, Noroxin) [C]	400 mg PO bid	Pyelonephritis	

Nitrofurantoin (Furadantin, Macrobid, Macrodantin—*U.S.*; Nephronex—*Can.*) [B]	50–100 mg PO bid-qid	UTIs
	50 mg PO postcoital	Recurrent UTIs
		Hypersensitivity, pseudomembranous colitis, dizziness, insomnia, Q-T prolongation, pulmonary fibrosis in long-term use **Contraindicated** in patients with renal impairment.
Piperacillin and tazobactam sodium (Zosyn—*U.S.*; Tacozin—*Can.*) [B]	3.375 g IV q8hr	Pyelonephritis
		Diarrhea, hypertension, insomnia, headache, hypersensitivity
Tetracycline (Achromycin, Brodspec—*U.S.*; Tetracyn—*Can.*) [D]	250–500 mg PO q6hr	Epididymo-orchitis
		Hypersensitivity, photosensitivity, diarrhea, pseudomembranous colitis, discoloration of teeth, enamel hypoplasia in young children **Contraindicated** in children and pregnancy.
Trimethoprim and sulfamethoxazole (TMP-SMX) (Septra) [C/D at term]	1 DS tablet PO bid*	Epididymo-orchitis Pyelonephritis UTIs
	1 RS tablet PO postcoital†	Recurrent UTIs
		GI upset, dermatologic reactions **Life-threatening reactions** such as severe dermatologic and hepatotoxic reactions. **Contraindicated** in megaloblastic anemia caused by folate deficiency, hepatic or renal impairment, and pregnancy.

DS = double strength; RS = regular strength; GI = gastrointestinal; UTIs = urinary tract infections.

*Trimethoprim 160 mg and sulfamethoxazole 800 mg.

†Trimethoprim 80 mg and sulfamethoxazole 400 mg.

Epididymo-orchitis

KY These infections can occur in any age group. In children, they are typically caused by Gram-negative organisms. These children need to be investigated for congenital anomalies, such as ureteropelvic junction obstruction and ectopic ureters. In the young adult male, these infections are usually caused by *Chlamydia trachomatis*, and further investigations are not generally required. In older men, obstruction is usually the cause, and Gram-negative organisms are most common. These men need further investigation (i.e., ultrasound and cystoscopy).

TX Treatment options are listed in Table 22–6.

RX Table 22–6

DS Table 22–6

SE Table 22–6

Pyelonephritis

KY Acute uncomplicated pyelonephritis is suggested by pyuria, flank pain, fever, or costovertebral angle tenderness in the presence or absence of cystitis symptoms. Usually there is an acute onset, with signs and symptoms existing for < 3 days before diagnosis. White cell casts indicate a renal origin, but they are not always present. In addition to the signs and symptoms of uncomplicated pyelonephritis, complicated UTIs may also be associated with nonspecific signs and symptoms, such as malaise, fatigue, nausea, or abdominal pain. Symptoms may be insidious, occurring for weeks to months before diagnosis.

TX In uncomplicated cases of pyelonephritis with no evidence of sepsis, oral antibiotics are acceptable, including trimethoprim and sulfamethoxazole (TMP-SMX), amoxicillin, or fluoroquinolones. Length of treatment is 7–14 days. Patient follow-up is required as sepsis can develop rapidly. Septic patients with complicated pyelonephritis require hospital admission and IV antibiotics; concomitant ampicillin and aminoglycoside IV administration, piperacillin-tazobactam IV administration, or ceftriaxone IV administration. Length of treatment is 14 days.

RX Table 22–6

DS Table 22–6

SE Table 22–6

Recurrent UTIs

KY Recurrent UTIs in women often occur postcoital. Prophylactic antibiotics may be warranted if these infections are numerous over 1 year, ≥ 4 per year.

TX **Prophylactic antibiotic regimens** consist of one antibiotic tablet at bedtime, or one tablet postcoital can be very effective with little resistance occurring with time. Drugs used are TMP-SMX, nitrofurantoin, cephalexin, or ciprofloxacin. **Caution should be used when nitrofuran-toin is used long term because of the potential of pulmonary fibrosis in women older than 50 years**.

RX Table 22–6

DS Table 22–6

SE Table 22–6

Uncomplicated UTI

KY Uncomplicated means without any significant cause promoting infection, such as stones, BPH, and retention. These typically occur in women, rather than men, in the younger age groups. As men age, prostatic obstruction results in an increase in lower UTIs, although still less than in elderly women.

TX The most common organism present in these cases is *Escherichia coli*, which is present in approximately 70%–85% of all community-acquired UTIs in young women.

RX Table 22–6

DS Table 22–6

SE Table 22–6

MALE SEXUALLY TRANSMITTED DISEASES

Sexually transmitted diseases in the female patient are discussed in Ch 8 Gynecology.

Genital Ulcers

KY The diagnosis of acute genital ulcers is perplexing because the initial clinical impression by infectious disease specialists may be wrong in up to 40% of cases. The classic sexually transmitted diseases in this class include syphilis, chancroid, genital herpes, lymphogranuloma venereum, and granuloma inguinale.

TX The treatment regimens for sexually transmitted genital ulcers are described in Table 22–7.

RX Table 22–7

DS Table 22–7

SE Table 22–7

Gonococcal Urethritis

KY Urethritis, the usual manifestation of male sexually transmitted diseases, represents the response of the urethra to inflammation of any cause. Symptoms include urethral discharge accompanied by a burning or itching sensation on urination.

(Text continues on page 422)

Table 22-7. Treatment of Male Sexually Transmitted Diseases

Disease	Generic (Brand) Name and Dose	Side Effects and Cautions
Gonococcal urethritis	Oral regimens: Cefixime 400 mg PO single dose + doxycycline 100 mg PO bid for 7 days Ciprofloxacin 500 mg PO single dose + doxycycline 100 mg PO bid for 7 days Ofloxacin 400 mg PO single dose + doxycycline 100 mg PO bid for 7 days	Table 22–8
	Parenteral regimens: Ceftriaxone 250 mg IM single dose + doxycycline 100 mg PO bid for 7 days	
Nongonococcal urethritis	Doxycycline 100 mg PO bid for 7 days Erythromycin 500 mg PO qid for 7 days Ofloxacin 300 mg PO bid for 7 days Tetracycline 500 mg PO qid for 7 days	Table 22–8
Genital ulcers Chancroid	Azithromycin (Zithromax) 1 g single dose	Hypersensitivity, GI upset, ventricular arrhythmias **Contraindicated** in patients with hepatic impairment.
	Ceftriaxone 250 mg IM single dose	Table 22–6
	Erythromycin 500 mg bid for 7 days	Table 22–8

Genital herpes	Acyclovir (Zovirax) 200 mg 5 times/day for 5–10 days	GI upset, headache, acute renal failure, leukopenia, thrombocytopenia, hypersensitivity, anaphylaxis, seizures Use with caution in patients with renal impairment.
Granuloma inguinale	Tetracycline 500 mg PO qid	Table 22–8
Lymphogranuloma venereum	Doxycycline 100 mg PO bid for 21 days	Table 22–8
Syphilis	Benzathine penicillin G 2.4 MU IM single dose Doxycycline 100 mg PO bid for 14 days	Table 22–8

GI = gastrointestinal.

TX Gonococcal urethritis is caused by the organism *Neisseria gonor-rhoeae.* Treatment consists of either **oral or parenteral antibiotics** as described in Table 22–7.

RX Table 22–7

DS Table 22–7

SE Table 22–7

Nongonococcal Urethritis

KY Nongonococcal urethritis is a syndrome with several causes but without an etiologic diagnosis. The most important cause is *C. trachomatis,* which can account for 50% of all cases.

TX When diagnosed, nongonococcal urethritis should be treated with tetracycline, doxycycline, or erythromycin. Alternatively, ofloxacin can also be used. The sexual partner(s) should also be treated accordingly.

RX Table 22–7

DS Table 22–7

SE Table 22–7

PROSTATITIS

Acute Prostatitis

KY Patients present with prostatodynia, fever, elevated white blood cell count, dysuria, and difficulty voiding.

TX Treatment is initiated with concomitant administration of **IV ampicillin and an aminoglycoside** until urine culture results are available. The cause is usually Gram-negative organisms. The **total length of treatment is at least 6 weeks;** IV antibiotics for 5–7 days followed by oral antibiotics (**TMP-SMX or fluoroquinolones**).

RX Table 22–8

DS Table 22–8

SE Table 22–8

Chronic Prostatitis

KY Chronic prostatitis may be difficult to diagnose and treat, and in some instances prostatodynia occurs. Patients often present with perineal or suprapubic pain and irritative and obstructive voiding symptoms.

TX Urine cultures can be negative. **Empiric treatment with antibiotics can be attempted** and has been shown to have varying results. Treatment choices include **TMP-SMX** or **fluoroquinolones for 1–3 months.**

RX Table 22–8

DS Table 22–8

SE Table 22–8

Table 22-8. Treatment of Prostatitis

Generic (Brand) Name	Dose	Side Effects and Cautions
Acute prostatitis*		
Ampicillin (Penbritin)	Ampicillin: 1–2 g IV q6hr	Table 22-6
+	+	
Gentamicin [aminoglycoside]	Gentamicin: 1 mg/kg IV q8hr	
TMP-SMX (Septra)	1 DS† tablet PO bid for 6 weeks	Table 22-6
Fluoroquinolones		
Ciprofloxacin (Cipro)	250–500 mg PO bid for 6 weeks	
Levofloxacin (Levaquin)	250 mg PO qd for 6 weeks	
Norfloxacin (Noroxin)	400 mg PO bid for 6 weeks	
Chronic prostatitis		
TMP-SMX (Septra)	1 DS† tablet PO bid for 1–3 months	Table 22-6
Fluoroquinolones		Table 22-6
Ciprofloxacin (Cipro)	250–500 mg PO bid for 1–3 months	
Levofloxacin (Levaquin)	250 mg PO qd for 1–3 months	
Norfloxacin (Noroxin)	400 mg PO bid for 1–3 months	
Nonbacterial prostatitis		
Tetracycline (Tetracyn)	250–500 mg PO qd for 10 days	Table 22-6
Doxycycline (Vibramycin)	100 mg PO bid for 1 day	Hypersensitivity, GI upset, diarrhea, oral candidiasis
		Permanent discoloration of teeth and enamel hypoplasia when used during tooth development. **Contraindicated** in pregnancy and hepatic impairment.

(continued)

423

Table 22-8. Treatment of Prostatitis (*Continued*)

Generic (Brand) Name	Dose	Side Effects and Cautions
Erythromycin (Eryc, Erythrocin—*U.S.*; Diomycin, Erybid—*Can.*)	250–500 mg PO qid for 10 days	**Q-T prolongation and ventricular arrhythmias,** including torsade de pointes **Contraindicated** in hepatic impairment and with concomitant astemizole, pimozide, and terfenadine use.
Ibuprofen (Advil)	400 mg PO qid	Hypersensitivity, bleeding Can compromise existing renal function.
Indomethacin (Indocin—*U.S.*; Indotec—*Can.*)	25–50 mg PO tid	Hypersensitivity, bleeding. **Contraindicated** in patients with renal impairment and thrombocytopenia.
Oxybutynin (Ditropan)	2.5 mg PO qd–bid	Table 22-4
Prostatodynia		
TMP-SMX (Septra)	1 DS† tablet PO bid for 10–14 days	Table 22-6
Tetracycline (Tetracyn)	250–500 mg PO qid for 10–14 days	Table 22-6
Alpha-adrenergic blockers		
Doxazosin (Cardura)	Start at 1 mg PO qd and increase as tolerated up to 10 mg PO qd	Table 22-3
Terazosin (Hytrin)	Start at 1 mg PO qhs and increase as tolerated (e.g., 1 mg/week) to 5–10 mg PO qhs	

DS = double strength; TMP-SMX = trimethoprim and sulfamethoxazole.

*Acute prostatitis is treated with concomitant ampicillin and aminoglycoside IV for 5–7 days and then, if Gram-negative organisms, TMP-SMX or fluoroquinolones.

†Trimethoprim 160 mg and sulfamethoxazole 800 mg.

Nonbacterial Prostatitis

KY The etiology of nonbacterial prostatitis is unknown.

TX Although cultures generally exclude the usual bacterial pathogens, a trial of tetracycline, doxycycline, or erythromycin may be a reasonable option. In addition, these patients will require reassurance and encouragement to exercise and engage in normal sexual activity; need to avoid caffeine, alcohol and spicy foods; need to have warm sitz baths; and need to take anti-inflammatory drugs (ibuprofen or indomethacin) or anticholinergic agents (oxybutynin).

RX Table 22–8

DS Table 22–8

SE Table 22–8

APPENDIX

Table of Conversion from Conventional Units to Système International (SI) Units of Commonly Used Measurements

Component	Specimen	Conventional Unit	SI Unit
Acetaminophen, toxicity	Serum	> 120 µg/mL at 2–4 hours	> 794 µmol/L at 2–4 hours
Albumin	Serum	3.5–5.0 g/dL	35–50 g/L
Bicarbonate (HCO_3^-)	Plasma	21–28 mEq/L	21–28 mmol/L
Calcium	Serum	8.5–10.5 mg/dL	2.1–2.6 mmol/L
CD4	Serum	410–1,590 cells/µL 410–1,590/mm³	0.41–1.59 × 10⁹/L
Chloride	Plasma, serum	96–106 mEq/L	96–106 mmol/L
Cholesterol (total)	Serum	Desirable: < 200 mg/dL Borderline: 200–239 mg/dL High: ≥ 240 mg/dL	< 5.17 mmol/L 5.17–6.18 mmol/L ≥ 6.21 mmol/L
Cholesterol, high-density lipoprotein (HDL)	Plasma	Male: 35–65 mg/dL Female: 35–80 mg/dL	0.91–1.68 mmol/L 0.91–2.07 mmol/L
Cholesterol, low-density lipoprotein (LDL)	Plasma	60–130 mg/dL	1.55–3.37 mmol/L

Creatine kinase (CK)	Serum	50–200 U/L
Creatine kinase isoenzymes, MB fraction	Serum	0–5 ng/mL
		< 10 U/L
Creatinine	Plasma, serum	0.6–1.2 mg/dL
Creatinine clearance	Serum, urine	75–125 mL/min
D-Dimer	Plasma	< 0.5 µg/mL
Ferritin	Plasma, serum	Male: 30–300 ng/mL
		Female: 10–200 ng/mL
Folate (folic acid)	Plasma, serum	Normal: 3.1–17.5 ng/mL
		Borderline deficient:
		2.2–3.0 ng/mL
		Deficient: < 2.2 ng/mL
		Excessive: > 17.5 ng/mL
Glucose	Urine	< 0.05 g/dL
Glucose, fasting	Plasma, serum	70–110 mg/dL
Hemoglobin (adult)	Whole blood	Male: 13–18 g/dL
		Female: 12–16 g/dL

50–200 U/L
0–5 µg/L
< 10 U/L
53–106 µmol/L
1.24–2.08 mL/s
< 0.5 mg/L
30–300 µg/L
10–200 µg/L
7.0–39.7 nmol/L
5.0–6.8 nmol/L
< 5.0 nmol/L
> 39.7 nmol/L
< 0.003 mmol/L
3.9–6.1 mmol/L
8.1–11.2 mmol/L
7.4–9.9 mmol/L

(continued)

Table of Conversion from Conventional Units to Système International (SI) Units of Commonly Used Measurements *(Continued)*

Component	Specimen	Conventional Unit	SI Unit
Hemoglobin A_{1C}	Whole blood	4%–7% total hemoglobin	0.04–0.07 proportion of total hemoglobin
Hemoglobin A_2	Whole blood	2%–3%	< 0.02–0.03
Insulin	Plasma	11–240 μU/mL	79–1,722 pmol/L
Iron (total)	Serum	60–150 μg/dL	10.7–26.9 μmol/L
Leukocyte (white blood cell) count (WBC)	Whole blood	4.5–$11 \times 10^3/mm^3$ 45–11,000/μL	4.5–$11 \times 10^9/L$
Lipase	Serum	14–280 mIU/mL	14–280 U/L
Platelet count (thrombocytes)	Whole blood	150–$450 \times 10^3/mm^3$ 150–$450 \times 10^3/μL$	150–$450 \times 10^9/L$

	Specimen	Conventional units	SI units
Potassium	Plasma, serum	3.5–4.5 mEq/L	3.5–5.0 mmol/L
Salicylate intoxication	Plasma, serum	> 50 mg/dL	> 3.62 mmol/L
Sodium	Plasma	135–145 mEq/L	135–145 mmol/L
Thyroid-stimulating hormone (TSH)	Serum	0.5–5 µIU/mL	0.5–5 µIU/L
Thyroxine	Serum	Free (FT_4): 0.9–2.3 ng/dL; Total (T_4): 5.5–12.5 µg/dL	12–30 pmol/L; 71–160 nmol/L
Troponin I (cardiac)	Serum	< 0.6 ng/mL (> 1.5 ng/mL consistent with acute myocardial infarction)	< 0.6 µg/L (> 1.5 µg/L consistent with acute myocardial infarction)
Vitamin B_{12}	Serum	1–10 µg/mL	3.2–32.4 µmol/L

INDEX

Page numbers in *italics* denote figures; those followed by a t denote tables